Praise for Men's Health For Dummies

"No matter how take-charge they think they are, most men don't take much charge of their health. Now, thanks to Charles Inlander's *Men's Health For Dummies,* every man can take charge of his body, mind and health. A must-read if you care at all about feeling well and staying well."

> — Ted David, CNBC network anchor

"A smart read! Translating the newest medical discoveries into plain and fun-to-read English, Inlander tells men how to *get* healthy and how to *stay* healthy. If you want to reach your maximum potential physically and mentally, this is the resource you need."

> — Sydney Walker III, M.D.
> Director, Southern California
> Neuropsychiatric Institute

"We men worry a lot about 'fitness' but far less about what it takes for real health. Charles Inlander has boiled down tons of information to give us simple, easy-to-read rules that can make us fitter and healthier."

> — Victor Cohn, former Science Editor of *The Washington Post,* author of *News & Numbers: A Guide to Reporting Scientific Claims and Controversies in Health and Other Fields*

"Charlie cuts right to the chase. You will get the essential health information you need clearly and concisely."

> — Joe Graedon, pharmacologist, author of the bestselling *People's Pharmacy* books

"With baby boomers aging and health costs rising, one of the most important tasks we face as a society is to persuade people to live healthier lives. This book gives men straightforward, basic advice on how to do that. I recommend it to men of all ages who want to be active and healthy well into their senior years."
— Steven Findlay, Health Policy Analyst,
National Coalition on Health Care

"This book is an excellent and direct approach to achieving and maintaining positive health status and possibly an excellent way to improving one's quality of life."
— J. Lyle Bootman, Ph.D.
Dean and Professor, University of Arizona
Health Sciences Center; Executive Director,
Health Outcomes & Pharmacoeconomics
Center (HOPE)

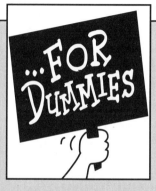

TM

References for the Rest of Us!™

BESTSELLING BOOK SERIES

Do you find that traditional reference books are overloaded with technical details and advice you'll never use? Do you postpone important life decisions because you just don't want to deal with them? Then our ...*For Dummies*® business and general reference book series is for you.

...*For Dummies* business and general reference books are written for those frustrated and hard-working souls who know they aren't dumb, but find that the myriad of personal and business issues and the accompanying horror stories make them feel helpless. ...*For Dummies* books use a lighthearted approach, a down-to-earth style, and even cartoons and humorous icons to dispel fears and build confidence. Lighthearted but not lightweight, these books are perfect survival guides to solve your everyday personal and business problems.

> "More than a publishing phenomenon, 'Dummies' is a sign of the times."
>
> — The New York Times

> "...you won't go wrong buying them."
>
> — Walter Mossberg, Wall Street Journal, on IDG Books' ...For Dummies books

> "A world of detailed and authoritative information is packed into them..."
>
> — U.S. News and World Report

Already, millions of satisfied readers agree. They have made ...*For Dummies* the #1 introductory level computer book series and a best-selling business book series. They have written asking for more. So, if you're looking for the best and easiest way to learn about business and other general reference topics, look to ...*For Dummies* to give you a helping hand.

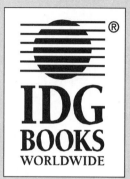

IDG
BOOKS
WORLDWIDE
®

1/99

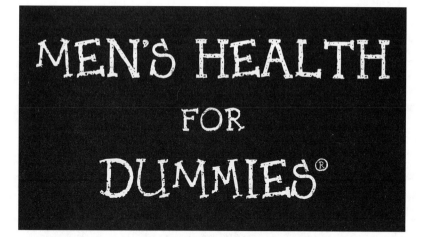

MEN'S HEALTH FOR DUMMIES®

by Charles Inlander
and the People's Medical Society

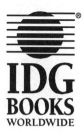

IDG Books Worldwide, Inc.
An International Data Group Company

Foster City, CA ♦ Chicago, IL ♦ Indianapolis, IN ♦ New York, NY

Men's Health For Dummies®

Published by
IDG Books Worldwide, Inc.
An International Data Group Company
919 E. Hillsdale Blvd.
Suite 400
Foster City, CA 94404
www.idgbooks.com (IDG Books Worldwide Web site)
www.dummies.com (Dummies Press Web site)

Library of Congress Catalog Card No.: 99-61113

ISBN: 0-7645-5120-5

Printed in the United States of America

10 9 8 7 6 5 4 3 2 1

1B/QU/QT/ZZ/IN

Distributed in the United States by IDG Books Worldwide, Inc.

Distributed by CDG Books Canada Inc. for Canada; by Transworld Publishers Limited in the United Kingdom; by IDG Norge Books for Norway; by IDG Sweden Books for Sweden; by Woodslane Pty. Ltd. for Australia; by Woodslane (NZ) Ltd. for New Zealand; by TransQuest Publishers Pte Ltd. for Singapore, Malaysia, Thailand, Indonesia, and Hong Kong; by ICG Muse, Inc. for Japan; by Norma Comunicaciones S.A. for Colombia; by Intersoft for South Africa; by Le Monde en Tique for France; by International Thomson Publishing for Germany, Austria and Switzerland; by Distribuidora Cuspide for Argentina; by Livraria Cultura for Brazil; by Ediciones ZETA S.C.R. Ltda. for Peru; by WS Computer Publishing Corporation, Inc., for the Philippines; by Contemporanea de Ediciones for Venezuela; by Express Computer Distributors for the Caribbean and West Indies; by Micronesia Media Distributor, Inc. for Micronesia; by Grupo Editorial Norma S.A. for Guatemala; by Chips Computadoras S.A. de C.V. for Mexico; by Editorial Norma de Panama S.A. for Panama; by American Bookshops for Finland. Authorized Sales Agent: Anthony Rudkin Associates for the Middle East and North Africa.

For general information on IDG Books Worldwide's books in the U.S., please call our Consumer Customer Service department at 800-762-2974. For reseller information, including discounts and premium sales, please call our Reseller Customer Service department at 800-434-3422.

For information on where to purchase IDG Books Worldwide's books outside the U.S., please contact our International Sales department at 317-596-5530 or fax 317-596-5692.

For consumer information on foreign language translations, please contact our Customer Service department at 1-800-434-3422, fax 317-596-5692, or e-mail rights@idgbooks.com.

For information on licensing foreign or domestic rights, please phone +1-650-655-3109.

For sales inquiries and special prices for bulk quantities, please contact our Sales department at 650-655-3200 or write to the address above.

For information on using IDG Books Worldwide's books in the classroom or for ordering examination copies, please contact our Educational Sales department at 800-434-2086 or fax 317-596-5499.

For press review copies, author interviews, or other publicity information, please contact our Public Relations department at 650-655-3000 or fax 650-655-3299.

For authorization to photocopy items for corporate, personal, or educational use, please contact Copyright Clearance Center, 222 Rosewood Drive, Danvers, MA 01923, or fax 978-750-4470.

is a registered trademark under exclusive license to IDG Books Worldwide, Inc., from International Data Group, Inc.

About the Author

Charles B. Inlander, President of the People's Medical Society, is a highly acclaimed health commentator on National Public Radio's *Marketplace*. He is a faculty lecturer at the Yale University School of Medicine and writes regularly for *Nursing Economics, The New York Times, Glamour,* and *Boardroom*.

ABOUT IDG BOOKS WORLDWIDE

Welcome to the world of IDG Books Worldwide.

IDG Books Worldwide, Inc., is a subsidiary of International Data Group, the world's largest publisher of computer-related information and the leading global provider of information services on information technology. IDG was founded more than 30 years ago by Patrick J. McGovern and now employs more than 9,000 people worldwide. IDG publishes more than 290 computer publications in over 75 countries. More than 90 million people read one or more IDG publications each month.

Launched in 1990, IDG Books Worldwide is today the #1 publisher of best-selling computer books in the United States. We are proud to have received eight awards from the Computer Press Association in recognition of editorial excellence and three from Computer Currents' First Annual Readers' Choice Awards. Our best-selling ...*For Dummies*® series has more than 50 million copies in print with translations in 31 languages. IDG Books Worldwide, through a joint venture with IDG's Hi-Tech Beijing, became the first U.S. publisher to publish a computer book in the People's Republic of China. In record time, IDG Books Worldwide has become the first choice for millions of readers around the world who want to learn how to better manage their businesses.

Our mission is simple: Every one of our books is designed to bring extra value and skill-building instructions to the reader. Our books are written by experts who understand and care about our readers. The knowledge base of our editorial staff comes from years of experience in publishing, education, and journalism — experience we use to produce books to carry us into the new millennium. In short, we care about books, so we attract the best people. We devote special attention to details such as audience, interior design, use of icons, and illustrations. And because we use an efficient process of authoring, editing, and desktop publishing our books electronically, we can spend more time ensuring superior content and less time on the technicalities of making books.

You can count on our commitment to deliver high-quality books at competitive prices on topics you want to read about. At IDG Books Worldwide, we continue in the IDG tradition of delivering quality for more than 30 years. You'll find no better book on a subject than one from IDG Books Worldwide.

John Kilcullen
Chairman and CEO
IDG Books Worldwide, Inc.

Steven Berkowitz
President and Publisher
IDG Books Worldwide, Inc.

Eighth Annual
Computer Press
Awards ≥1992

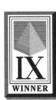

Ninth Annual
Computer Press
Awards ≥1993

Tenth Annual
Computer Press
Awards ≥1994

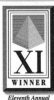

Eleventh Annual
Computer Press
Awards ≥1995

IDG is the world's leading IT media, research and exposition company. Founded in 1964, IDG had 1997 revenues of $2.05 billion and has more than 9,000 employees worldwide. IDG offers the widest range of media options that reach IT buyers in 75 countries representing 95% of worldwide IT spending. IDG's diverse product and services portfolio spans six key areas including print publishing, online publishing, expositions and conferences, market research, education and training, and global marketing services. More than 90 million people read one or more of IDG's 290 magazines and newspapers, including IDG's leading global brands — Computerworld, PC World, Network World, Macworld and the Channel World family of publications. IDG Books Worldwide is one of the fastest-growing computer book publishers in the world, with more than 700 titles in 36 languages. The "...For Dummies®" series alone has more than 50 million copies in print. IDG offers online users the largest network of technology-specific Web sites around the world through IDG.net (http://www.idg.net), which comprises more than 225 targeted Web sites in 55 countries worldwide. International Data Corporation (IDC) is the world's largest provider of information technology data, analysis and consulting, with research centers in over 41 countries and more than 400 research analysts worldwide. IDG World Expo is a leading producer of more than 168 globally branded conferences and expositions in 35 countries including E3 (Electronic Entertainment Expo), Macworld Expo, ComNet, Windows World Expo, ICE (Internet Commerce Expo), Agenda, DEMO, and Spotlight. IDG's training subsidiary, ExecuTrain, is the world's largest computer training company, with more than 230 locations worldwide and 785 training courses. IDG Marketing Services helps industry-leading IT companies build international brand recognition by developing global integrated marketing programs via IDG's print, online and exposition products worldwide. Further information about the company can be found at www.idg.com. 1/24/99

Author's Acknowledgments

Creating a reference book is a collaborative effort. No one person can take all the credit (or the blame!). And *Men's Health For Dummies* is no exception. This book is the product of many people, each of whom has earned my sincere respect and total appreciation.

Special thanks to my associates at the People's Medical Society. An entire crew of my talented colleagues are the primary reason this book is a reality. Annette Doran, who served as the editorial project manager, deserves the most credit. This was her first major People's Medical Society project, and she oversaw the entire development of the book. Working with researchers, writers, editors, and me, she made sure everything was done at the level of excellence we expect.

Nor was she alone: Other People's Medical Society staff contributed mightily, including Michael Donio, Jennifer Hay, and Janet Worsley Norwood. Karla Morales, our vice president for editorial services, oversaw the entire project with her usual diligence and powerful talent. She deserves a medal.

Thanks to Gail Ross, our literary agent, board member, and friend, for engineering the relationship between our organization and IDG Books.

Many wonderfully talented writers and researchers contributed to this book. My special appreciation to each of them: Lee Beadling, Marcy S. Caplin, MSN, RN, CS, Jack Curtin, Mary Erpel, Anthony J. Garbowski, Rob Goldberg, Lisa M. Hanson, Tom Harper, John R. Hillman, Jr., Gerald Irving, Kristin Kraft, Patricia Mary McAdams, David M. Pushic, Maria G. Richard, John Riddle, Enid Rosenblatt, Mindy Weinstein-Toran, Kimberly Tucci, Paul Wirth, and Barbara C. Worthington.

Working with IDG Books has been a unique pleasure. Tami Booth, executive editor, conceived of the idea and wanted to work with us. It's been a wonderful working relationship. Tim Gallan, an IDG senior project editor, guided us and assisted us in making this a more readable and informative work. Tammy Castleman served as the copy editor, Kathryn Born as illustrator, and David Rudnick and Mark Stolar as technical editors. Obviously, without their considerable talents, this book would still be just an idea.

Publisher's Acknowledgments

We're proud of this book; please register your comments through our IDG Books Worldwide Online Registration Form located at http://my2cents.dummies.com.

Some of the people who helped bring this book to market include the following:

Acquisitions and Editorial

Senior Project Editor: Tim Gallan

Executive Editor: Tammerly Booth

Senior Copy Editor: Tamara Castleman

Technical Editors: David Rudnick, Instructor in Urology, Massachusetts General Hospital; Mark Stolar, Associate Professor of Clinical Medicine at Northwestern University Medical School

Editorial Manager: Leah Cameron

Acquisitions Coordinator: Karen S. Young

Editorial Coordinator: Maureen Kelly

Editorial Assistant: Donna Love

Production

Project Coordinator: Regina Snyder

Layout and Graphics: J. Tyler Connor, Maridee V. Ennis, Angela F. Hunckler, Jane E. Martin, Brent Savage, Kate Snell, Michael A. Sullivan, Brian Torwelle

Illustrator: Kathryn Born

Proofreaders: Christine Berman, Kelli Botta, Henry Lazarek, Jennifer Mahern, Rebecca Senninger, Ethel M. Winslow, Janet M. Withers

Indexer: Liz Cunningham

General and Administrative

IDG Books Worldwide, Inc.: John Kilcullen, CEO; Steven Berkowitz, President and Publisher

IDG Books Technology Publishing: Brenda McLaughlin, Senior Vice President and Group Publisher

Dummies Technology Press and Dummies Editorial: Diane Graves Steele, Vice President and Associate Publisher; Mary Bednarek, Director of Acquisitions and Product Development; Kristin A. Cocks, Editorial Director

Dummies Trade Press: Kathleen A. Welton, Vice President and Publisher; Kevin Thornton, Acquisitions Manager

IDG Books Production for Dummies Press: Michael R. Britton, Vice President of Production and Creative Services; Cindy L. Phipps, Manager of Project Coordination, Production Proofreading, and Indexing; Kathie S. Schutte, Supervisor of Page Layout; Shelley Lea, Supervisor of Graphics and Design; Debbie J. Gates, Production Systems Specialist; Robert Springer, Supervisor of Proofreading; Debbie Stailey, Special Projects Coordinator; Tony Augsburger, Supervisor of Reprints and Bluelines

Dummies Packaging and Book Design: Patty Page, Manager, Promotions Marketing

♦

The publisher would like to give special thanks to Patrick J. McGovern, without whom this book would not have been possible.

♦

Contents at a Glance

Cartoons at a Glance

By Rich Tennant

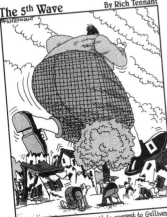

"So whose bright idea was it to suggest to Gulliver that he get more exercise?"

page 5

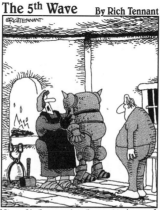

"Okay, Sir Loungealot, I was able to pound out another inch in the waist, but you're gonna have to start taking care of yourself or buy a new suit of armor."

page 51

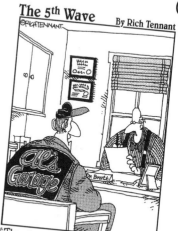

"There's a 'thbump, thbump' when I walk up stairs and then I hear a low 'ka-chink, ka-chink' going around corners, and I'm having trouble getting my horn to work."

page 91

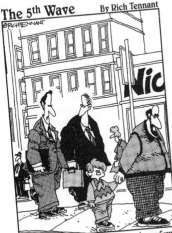

"I got a little confused about how to perform an NPT test. I thought you could use a postage meter." *See Chapter 7

page 299

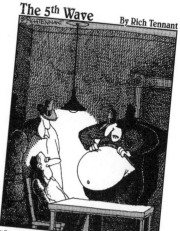

"Look—just tell us what we want to know. Don't make me use this on you!"

page 355

Fax: 978-546-7747 • E-mail: the5wave@tiac.net

Table of Contents

Introduction

Yeah, yeah, you've heard it said hundreds of times: Men simply don't care about their health.

Well, we're here to tell you that simply isn't true. Oh sure, you may not run to the doctor every time you have an ache or pain. Yep, you've been programmed to grit your teeth and suffer through sports and emotional injuries. And there's no doubt about it — you often do throw caution to the wind and order that big 16-ounce porterhouse steak, showing you're as macho as the next guy.

But deep down, most men do care about staying healthy. Remember, it was men who started the jogging craze, went to the gym at lunchtime, and asked their employers to create on-site wellness programs. Today you see men throwing their fear of gender self-degradation to the wind and enrolling in coed aerobics programs and even water ballet classes! Who said men worry about being labeled health pansies? And because it was always assumed that men don't care about their health, there have been few books or materials written to help guide a man to a long and healthy life. Most men have had to figure it out for themselves — a little information here, a little information there. It's confusing and frustrating. And too often they've gotten it wrong.

What This Book Is About

Men's Health For Dummies was written for you, the average busy Joe who doesn't want to spend hours in the classroom taking notes you'd rather toss out. But whether or not you consider yourself average (or Joe for that matter), this book is for any man who wants to know what's what about male health.

So the People's Medical Society wants to help you get it right. Our goal is to give you the one book you'll need to understand your body, maintain your health, and deal with the health care system. That's a big goal, but we feel we've done it in the pages that follow.

And that leads to why this book is so special. The information you find in these pages is not opinion. The People's Medical Society has scoured medical texts, journals, and studies for the most up-to-date and credible information we could find on each of the subjects we discuss. We didn't rely on just one doctor or one study. We wanted to make sure that what you read is valid information.

Obviously, you're now convinced you own the perfect book. Just about everything you need to know to maintain your health and get through the health care system is found in the following pages. But remember, this book cannot do certain things. For example, an accurate diagnosis cannot be made from a book. Nor can the correct dosage of a medication be prescribed. This book is a reference guide, to be used in conjunction with a medical professional. Don't make the foolish assumption that you can do it all alone. In fact, that's why we help guide you in picking a medical professional. So here's the official disclaimer. While it certainly protects us, it really is meant to protect you.

> **Official Disclaimer For Dummies:** The information in this reference is not intended to substitute for expert medical advice or treatment; it is designed to help you make informed choices. Because each individual is unique, a physician must diagnose conditions and supervise treatments for each individual health problem. If an individual is under a doctor's care and receives advice contrary to information provided in this reference, the doctor's advice should be followed, as it is based on the unique characteristics of that individual.

How This Book Is Organized

Enough of the preliminaries — time get down to the main event! How do you use this book? Well, the first thing to know is how we've organized it. Actually, it's pretty logical. What we've done is make this book easy to use and easy to read. We've divided the book into five sections. Each section stands alone — meaning that you can just about open it to any page (without having to read the previous ten pages) and still find what you need. So here are the different sections and an overview of what you'll find in each:

Part I: Calling the Shots: Taking Charge of Your Health

This part tells you how to maintain good health through healthy habits, wise medical decisions, and good health care coverage. Chapter 1 has the recipe you need for a healthy body and mind that is achieved through good nutrition and exercise. Vitamins and minerals from A to zinc are also in this chapter. Chapter 2 is loaded with information that you need to maintain good health such as choosing a doctor and dentist and understanding preventive care and screening tests. Chapter 3 tells you what you need to know about health insurance, managed care, Medicare, and Medicaid, plus death and dying issues.

Part II: Righting the Wrongs

This part is about regaining good health. Chapter 4 tells you how to calculate your healthy weight and, if needed, how to lose weight and keep it off. Chapter 5 gives you the facts about addictions to alcohol, nicotine, and drugs and where to get help for yourself or loved ones. Chapter 6 is about stress and how to manage it in your daily life. Chapter 7 is packed with self-care techniques ranging from home tests to emergency care and first aid.

Part III: All That Ails You

This is the fattest (uh, most pumped-up) section of the book. Chapter 8 is about those aches and pains — such as colds and flu — that enter in and quickly exit out of your life (admittedly, sometimes not so quickly) and what you can do about them. Chapter 9 is loaded with information about your muscles, joints, and bones and what to do if they're not their healthiest best. Chapter 10 gives you the facts about hair loss and what options you have for keeping a hairy scalp or replacing hair on your head. Chapter 11 takes a close look at the structure of your skin and common skin problems from athlete's foot and jock itch to acne and moles. Chapter 12 wakes you up to the facts of sleep disorders and also tells you footloose guys how to prevent jet lag. Chapter 13 answers your questions about depression.

Chapter 14 shows you how to cool the burning of ulcers and treat other problems that make your digestive tract feel like a wild boa constrictor. Chapter 15 is about problems with the male plumbing such as urinary tract infections and testicular problems. Of course, this chapter explains your options for treating such conditions. Chapter 16 gives you the facts about prostate disease, including how to prevent it and treat it if it occurs. Chapter 17 tells you what to do to keep your ol' ticker in top shape, prevent and control high blood pressure, recognize the signs of a stroke, and lower your cholesterol level. Chapter 18 answers your questions about cancer, takes some of the fear out of the disease, and offers the hope of current and future treatments. Chapter 19 is about allergies, asthma, and diabetes — those health conditions and diseases that remain with you for life — and how to live fully with them.

Part IV: Your Sexual Health

Now you didn't purchase this book just for the sexual health part, did you? But just in case you did, you won't be disappointed — this section makes it clear that there's more to a man's sexual health than simply a prescription for Viagra. Chapter 20 tells you about sexual development, male menopause, and peak sexual functioning. Chapter 21 is devoted to contraception, both reversible and permanent forms of birth control. Chapter 22 gives the facts about sexually transmitted diseases and safer sex options. Chapter 23 is about infertility and various treatments to help you become that family man you always wanted to be. Chapter 24 is loaded with information on sexual difficulties ranging from erection problems and premature ejaculation to sexual desire disorder and painful intercourse.

Part V: The Part of Tens

No *...For Dummies* book would be complete without "The Part of Tens." This section provides ten valuable Internet health resources for you to investigate and explains ten common surgical and diagnostic procedures.

Icons Used in This Book

To help you find important information in this book a little more efficiently, we've included little pictures in the margins, called icons. Here are the icons and what they mean:

This icon point out tips, tricks, and hints that will help you take better care of yourself.

This icon indicates that you need to exercise caution.

We use this icon to flag information that you shouldn't forget.

This icon tells you that we're presenting optional facts and figures — trivia, more or less — that you may find interesting but can skip if you want.

Part I

Calling the Shots: Taking Charge of Your Health

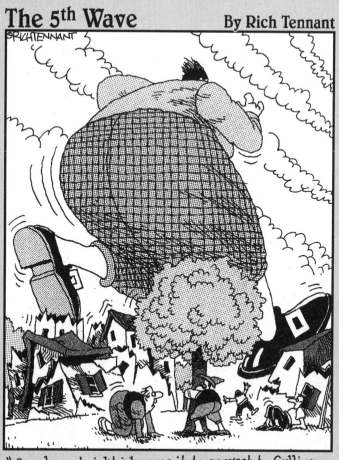

"So whose bright idea was it to suggest to Gulliver that he get more exercise?"

In this part . . .

We provide advice on developing good health habits, which not only includes a balanced diet and a decent amount of exercise but also involves choosing a doctor, getting routine physical exams, and knowing what to expect from your health insurance.

Chapter 1

Recipe for a Healthy Body and Mind

*Y*our health is in your hands, but that needn't scare you. In fact, research shows that you can definitely influence the state of both your physical and mental health. You can learn to eat right, get enough exercise, and relieve stress. Not doing these things can jeopardize your health. So if you're ready to take charge of your health, start by reading this chapter.

Diet

Diet counts. Food keeps your body going, and to keep it going well, you have to put the right foods in it. Here are some facts you should know:

- ✔ Four of the ten leading causes of death in men are directly linked to diet.

- ✔ A proper diet reduces the risk of premature death from the "Big Ones": heart disease, cancer, stroke, and diabetes.

- ✔ Eating the right foods can lower a person's risk of high blood pressure, obesity, and high cholesterol. (Men develop these conditions more often than women do, by the way.)

The good news is that you can change your diet without torturing yourself. You just have to know what to eat and how much of it to eat.

Your body takes nutrients from food. Fats, proteins, carbohydrates, vitamins, and minerals are all nutrients. In addition, your body gets water from food. About 60 percent of a man's body weight is water. So a 155-pound guy is made up of almost 88 pints of water! Water maintains the correct chemical balance in your body and contributes to your blood volume. The following sections describe what each of these nutrients is all about.

Fats

From everything you've heard and read, you may consider fat the food villain. But you need a certain amount of fat for proper nutrition. Fat comes from animal or vegetable sources and provides energy for your body. If you require the energy right away, your body breaks down the fat into glucose, which gives you the needed energy. Carbohydrates and proteins have less energy (calories) per gram than fat, but your body can get its energy source from carbohydrates and proteins more easily than from fatty foods.

When you don't need energy right away, your body stores fat within your cells. Stored fat can cause problems. Aside from making your jeans fit tightly, too much fat can increase your risk of heart disease and certain cancers.

Fat can be divided into four types, and some fats are better for you than others.

Saturated fats

These fats are the ones you should most strenuously avoid. Solid at room temperature, saturated fats are found in the white marbling and the visible fat around meats, and in butter, cheese, whole milk, and ice cream. Saturated fats are also in coconut, palm-kernel, and palm oils. (The fat is liquid in these oils.) Even if you don't use these oils consciously, they may still be part of your diet because these three plant oils are widely used in commercial baked goods such as cookies and crackers. Saturated fats also raise the blood levels of the "bad" cholesterol — low-density lipoproteins (LDLs) — which contributes to the development of the fatty deposits that block arteries, causing heart disease (see Chapter 17).

Trans fatty acids

No more than 10 percent of your calories should come from saturated fats *and* trans fatty acids combined — about 18 to 26 grams daily, for most men. Trans fatty acids are in products that have *hydrogenated vegetable oils* (oils that have been processed with hydrogen to make them hard), such as some types of margarine and vegetable shortening. Trans fatty acids raise "bad" cholesterol levels and lower "good" cholesterol levels — high-density lipoproteins (HDLs). HDLs help escort fats from the body, lowering cholesterol levels.

REMEMBER

Fat in your diet

The maximum amount of fat you should have in your diet is 30 percent. That means that no more than 30 percent of all the calories you consume in one day should come from fat. So if you consume 2,500 calories per day, 800 calories or fewer should come from fat.

Polyunsaturated fats

Polyunsaturated fats are liquid at room temperature and are the predominant fat in common vegetable oils such as corn, safflower, sunflower, cottonseed, and soybean. Research suggests that although they don't raise bad cholesterol levels, they do lower good cholesterol levels.

Monounsaturated fats

These are the ones you want! The main portion of your fat intake should come from monounsaturated fats. Monounsaturated fats seem to lower the bad cholesterol levels without dropping the good cholesterol levels. You can find these fats in olive and canola oils.

Proteins

Proteins are your special buddies. Without protein, your body cannot grow or maintain itself. Your tissues and organs all contain protein. Proteins also bring in the amino acids that are essential to your body, but that your body doesn't produce itself. Proteins can be a source of heat and energy for your body, too. Proteins come from animal and plant sources such as fish, beef, poultry, eggs, dairy products, nuts, and beans.

But as important as protein is, don't overdo it. As things stand, the average American man's diet is too high in protein. The recommended daily allowance for protein actually depends on your weight — about .37 grams of protein per pound. So a 150-pound guy needs 56 grams of protein per day or about 12 ounces of meat per day. For a vegetarian or meatless choice, consider about $2^1/_4$ cups of soybeans per day. Men who exercise regularly, though, may need more protein than men of the same weight who don't exercise regularly (and no, 18 holes of Gameboy golf doesn't count as regular exercise).

How to calculate fat content

Calculate the number of calories from fat by multiplying the number of grams of fat in the food by 9 (the number of calories in 1 gram of fat). To figure the percentage of calories by fat, divide the number of calories from fat by the total number of calories.

Carbohydrates

Carbohydrates are your body's main source of energy. They're essential sources of vitamins and minerals. At least half of your daily calories should come from carbohydrates. Without carbohydrates, your body relies on other sources of energy, such as proteins and fats. This can result in a condition known as "starvation ketosis." Muscle tissue breaks down making the blood too acid, which can leave you feeling rundown and queasy.

Carbohydrates can be simple (sugars such as glucose, fructose, and galactose) or complex (starches and fibers). Fiber can either be *soluble* (it dissolves in water) or *insoluble* (doesn't dissolve). Insoluble fiber is thought to scrap away *carcinogens* (cancer-causing agents) from the walls of the organs in your digestive system. Fiber also helps to relieve constipation and can lower your risk of colon and rectal cancers.

Federal Nutrition Guidelines

The latest *Dietary Guidelines for Americans*, published by the Department of Agriculture and Health and Human Services in 1995, suggests that you keep a balanced, varied diet, rich in grain products, fruits, and vegetables, and low in sugar, sodium, and total fat. The guidelines also recommend that if you drink alcohol, you should limit yourself to no more than 2 drinks per day (a drink is defined as 12 ounces of beer, 4 ounces of wine or champagne, or 1¹/₂ ounces of liquor).

Men, in particular, should keep their weight within a healthy range instead of gaining weight with age. But if you need to lose weight, you should aim for a one-half to one pound loss per week. Lose the weight through exercise and healthful food choices with lower total calories, rather than rapid or "crash" weight-loss programs (see Chapter 4).

Who says that the government never did anything for you? Here's a handy little guide on the current dietary recommendations called the U.S. Government Food Guide. Figure 1-1 translates the recommendations into servings and shows a pyramid of the six food categories. The category with the most servings is at the bottom, and the one with the fewest number of servings is at the top. Here are the six food groups and their serving sizes:

- Use items in the fat, oil, and sweet group sparingly.

- For the milk, yogurt, and cheese group, one serving equals 1 cup of milk or yogurt, 2 ounces of natural cheese, or 2 ounces of processed cheese.

- For the meat, poultry, fish, dry beans, eggs, and nuts group, one serving equals 2 to 3 ounces of cooked lean meat, fish, or poultry; 1 to 1$^1/_2$ cups cooked of dry beans; 2 to 3 eggs; or 4 to 6 tablespoons of peanut butter.

- For the fruit group, one serving equals 1 medium apple, banana, or orange; $^1/_2$ cup of chopped, cooked, or canned fruit; or $^1/_2$ cup of fruit juice.

- For the vegetable group, one serving equals 1 cup of raw, leafy vegetables; $^1/_2$ cup of other vegetables (cooked or chopped raw); or $^1/_2$ cup of vegetable juice.

- For the bread, cereal, rice, and pasta group, one serving equals 1 slice of bread, 1 ounce of ready-to-eat cereal, or $^1/_2$ cup of cooked cereal, rice, or pasta.

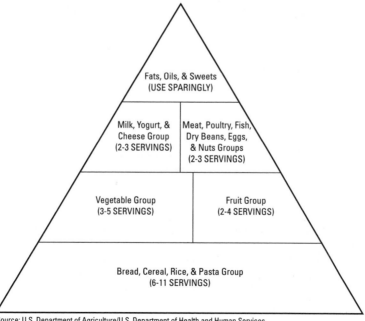

Figure 1-1:
The U.S.
Government
Food
Pyramid.

Fats, Oils, & Sweets
(USE SPARINGLY)

Milk, Yogurt, &
Cheese Group
(2-3 SERVINGS)

Meat, Poultry, Fish,
Dry Beans, Eggs,
& Nuts Groups
(2-3 SERVINGS)

Vegetable Group
(3-5 SERVINGS)

Fruit Group
(2-4 SERVINGS)

Bread, Cereal, Rice, & Pasta Group
(6-11 SERVINGS)

Source: U.S. Department of Agriculture/U.S. Department of Health and Human Services

Vitamins and Minerals

Vitamins and minerals are essential to life. Vitamins and minerals, found in foods and available in supplements, support your reproductive health, strengthen your immune system, contribute to growth, and keep your body's systems functioning.

Vitamins

Vitamins are organic substances that your body uses to make *coenzymes.* Coenzymes help your body to use energy from food and produce immune cells. There are 13 known vitamins, 4 of which are fat soluble (they dissolve in fat): A, D, E, and K. Nine are water soluble (they dissolve in water): vitamin C and the eight B vitamins — B1 (thiamin), B2 (riboflavin), niacin, B6, B12 (cobalamin), folic acid, pantothenic acid, and biotin. The body quickly excretes water soluble vitamins; they must be replenished regularly. Fat-soluble vitamins hang around in your body for a long period of time and require some fat in the diet for absorption.

Vitamin A

Vitamin A is a clear, yellow oil. Some yellow and orange vegetables contain *carotenoids,* which your body uses to convert to vitamin A. Vitamin A helps maintain the *epithelial cells,* found in your eyes, skin, blood vessel lining, and other internal and external surfaces of the body. Some signs that you're not getting enough vitamin A include night blindness, dry eyes and mouth, and poor tooth development. Sources of vitamin A include green and yellow fruits and vegetables, fish liver oils, and animal liver.

Watch your intake because vitamin A can build up in your body. Daily levels of more than 50,000 I.U. (International Units) on a long-term basis may be toxic.

The B vitamins

The B vitamins work together in several metabolic functions and many are found together in the same foods. However, each has individual characteristics and functions, and some, such as folic acid and niacin, have been found to be especially effective under certain conditions.

Thiamin, niacin, riboflavin, biotin, pantothenic acid, and B6 all work together to convert food into energy, making them essential to growth and development. They are also necessary to the process that creates red blood cells, hormones, and neurotransmitters (though B6, B12, and folic acid appear to play a bigger role in the nervous system than do the other Bs).

Two B vitamins — niacin and B6 — can cause problems if taken in large doses via supplements. Doctors sometimes prescribe niacin for people with high cholesterol; depending on the type of niacin, it can cause uncomfortable flushing and itching.

Niacin can cause liver damage in doses over 3 grams daily.

Folic acid may play a role in preventing heart disease by holding down blood levels of a damaging substance known as *homocysteine,* which has been linked to heart disease. Folic acid used to be one of the most common vitamin deficiencies in the United States until manufacturers began fortifying bread and other grain-based foods with it.

You can find B vitamins in a wide range of foods; however, not every food contains them all. But generally, whole grains, meats, and beans are good sources. Some foods are especially good sources of individual Bs. For example, milk and dairy foods are the most important source of riboflavin, providing half our intake. *Vegans* — vegetarians who don't eat any animal products — have to take supplements of B12 to balance their diets.

Vitamin C (ascorbic acid)

Vitamin C is a white powder that dissolves easily in water. This vitamin is thought to prevent cancer, cataracts, and damage from pollutants, and may reduce the effects of the common cold. Vitamin C helps produce connective tissue throughout your body (in skin, muscles, gums, blood vessels, and bone). If you bruise easily or have bleeding gums, you're probably not getting enough of this vitamin. Other signs of deficiency include muscular weakness, nosebleeds, frequent infections, slow wound healing, and scurvy, a disease marked by anemia, weakness, spongy gums, and bleeding under the skin. Good sources of vitamin C include citrus fruits, red bell peppers, strawberries, broccoli, Brussels sprouts, and papaya. If you're prone to gout or kidney stones, avoid *megadoses* (a dose greatly in excess of a prescribed or recommended amount) of vitamin C.

Vitamin D

Vitamin D is an amber-colored oil in its supplement form. This vitamin regulates how much calcium and phosphorous your body needs to help your bones grow and develop. Some signs that you're not getting enough of this vitamin are soft, thin bones, bone pain, and muscle weakness. Vitamin D is limited to a few foods such as fatty fish, liver, egg yolks, and fortified milk and cereals. Your body also manufactures its own vitamin D when exposed to sunlight. More than 1,000 I.U. of vitamin D on a daily basis can be toxic.

Vitamin E

Vitamin E is another fat-soluble vitamin. Unlike other vitamins, which control metabolic reactions or functions of hormones, vitamin E has one primary role — to act as an antioxidant (see the sidebar "Antioxidants"). Vitamin E can reduce your risk of heart disease by preventing the *oxidation* (formation of molecules that can damage cells) of artery-clogging cholesterol (LDL). Vitamin E is also useful in preventing scars from forming on damaged skin. Some signs that you need vitamin E are lethargy, inability to concentrate, loss of balance, and anemia. Look to these sources for your supply of vitamin E: hazelnut, wheat-germ, and sunflower oils, mayonnaise, eggs, and fortified cereals.

Vitamin K

Vitamin K, a fat-soluble vitamin, is a yellowish oil. This vitamin helps your blood to clot, an important factor when you've cut your skin. Most likely, you get enough of this vitamin in your daily diet, but some signs of deficiency are easy bleeding and bruising and frequent nosebleeds. Pork, lettuce, carrots, avocados, olive oil, and dark-green, leafy vegetables — such as kale, spinach, and parsley — are good sources of vitamin K. The only precaution connected to this vitamin is that large amounts can interfere with blood-thinning drugs.

Minerals

Minerals are substances found in nonliving things such as metals and rocks. There are 15 essential minerals: manganese, copper, calcium, phosphorus, sodium, potassium, sulfur, zinc, chlorine, iron, iodine, molybdenum, selenium, magnesium, and chromium. Minerals care for your body's functions such as blood clotting, blood pressure regulation, and the beating of your heart. Minerals also maintain your thyroid gland, body temperature, and brain function. What follows are a few common minerals.

Calcium

Calcium is a silvery-white metallic element that just loves your bones and teeth! This mineral keeps your body healthy by aiding in *nerve conduction* (sending messages along your central nervous system), maintaining your immune system, helping in blood clotting, metabolism, and muscle contraction, and keeping your heart strong. Calcium also helps prevent osteoporosis (see Chapter 9) and muscle cramps, and it may even help prevent colon cancer. You're not getting enough calcium if you have the following signs: abnormal heartbeat, muscle pain, cramps, numbness, dementia, or stiffness in your hands and feet. Most likely, your major source of calcium is milk and dairy products, but you can also find it in foods such as kale, turnip greens, kelp, tofu, salmon, sardines (with bones), and soybeans. Doses up to 2,500 mg per day are considered safe for those without a history of kidney stones.

Antioxidants

Antioxidants are like a little police force that helps limit certain chemical reactions in your body. These chemical reactions — the same ones that cause butter to turn rancid and iron to rust — involve oxygen (they're known as *oxidative reactions*).They result in the formation of what are called *free radicals,* that is, molecules that can damage cells within your body. In some cases, this damage can lead to diseases such as heart disease and cancer.

Antioxidants, which include vitamins C and E, beta-carotene (a substance that becomes vitamin A), and selenium (the only mineral in the group), "terminate" the free radicals, making them harmless. Studies show that antioxidants may help lower the risk of cancer, prevent cataracts, and reduce damage to the lungs caused by pollution.

Chromium

Chromium is an essential trace mineral, which means it's only needed in small amounts. This mineral helps your body burn glucose (blood sugar) for energy. Signs that you're not getting enough include weight loss, diabetes-like symptoms (see Chapter 19), and nerve degeneration. Chromium is in liver, Brewer's yeast, black pepper, thyme, beef, poultry, whole grains, beer, and oysters. Little is known about the possible toxic effects of chromium.

Copper

More than just a pretty metal, this essential mineral helps your body form new red blood cells, stores and carries iron through your blood system, and may help prevent heart disease and cancer. You're probably not getting enough if you become pale, your blood pressure increases, your body can't handle glucose, you have connective tissue or bone disorders, and your body's "thermostat" isn't working properly. Copper is found in beef and chicken livers, crab, chocolate, sunflower seeds, peanut butter, oysters, and beans.

Iodine

Iodine is a nonmetallic, blackish-gray element. This mineral helps your thyroid gland regulate your body's metabolism. You're probably getting enough iodine unless you don't eat shellfish, fish, or iodized salt. But some sure signs of iodine deficiency are chronic fatigue, dry skin, sudden weight gain, or a *goiter* (an enlarged thyroid). Daily doses as small as 2,000 mg can be toxic.

Iron

A major element on earth, iron is part of *hemoglobin,* a protein that carries oxygen in your red blood cells throughout your body. Many people don't get enough iron in their diets; they're usually cranky and can't seem to concentrate. Most likely they have anemia, too. But iron is in many food sources such as liver, meats, poultry, fish, beans, whole grains, and most dark-green, leafy vegetables. Many experts advise against taking iron supplements without a doctor's okay because too much iron can cause constipation and increase the risk of heart disease. The risks of long-term use of moderate-to-high doses (25 to 75 mg per day) are unknown.

Magnesium

Magnesium is a silvery-white metallic element related to calcium and zinc and is very important because it's responsible for every major biological process in your body. It helps keep your heartbeat steady, keeps your blood vessels toned, and helps your muscles to contract. You're probably not getting enough magnesium if you have high blood pressure, heart disease, weakness, nausea, muscle cramps, dizziness, depression, and an irregular heartbeat. Supplementing your diet is okay, provided you don't have kidney problems. Magnesium is found in whole grains, nuts, avocados, beans, and dark-green, leafy vegetables. People with kidney problems should take no more than 600 mg per day, and only with their doctor's permission.

Sodium, potassium, and chloride

These three minerals act as *electrolytes* (elements that carry electric currents) in body fluids, and they work together to maintain fluid balance and pressure in your cells. They regulate blood pressure, heart rate, muscle contraction, nerve transmission, and acidity. Sodium and chloride are virtually never too low in American diets because they're the prime ingredient in table salt. In fact, most people eat too much of them, which can cause high blood pressure. However, many people don't eat enough potassium, which is mostly found in fruits, potato skins, whole grains, and milk. People with kidney problems, people taking a diuretic called spironolactone, and people taking angiotensin converting enzyme (blood pressure medication) should take potassium supplements only with their doctor's permission.

Selenium

Selenium, a trace mineral, is an antioxidant and works similarly to vitamins C and E and beta-carotene. It also helps to boost your body's immune system. Some signs that you're not getting enough include muscle loss, muscle pain, and heart problems. You can get selenium from these foods: broccoli, mushrooms, Brewer's yeast, cabbage, celery, whole grains, fish, and organ meats (such as the heart and kidneys). Taking more than 5 mg can cause "garlic breath," nausea, damaged fingernails, vomiting, and nervous system problems.

Zinc

Zinc is a silvery-blue metal. It helps in the structure and function of your cell's membranes; assists in the production of more than 200 enzymes; helps heal wounds; makes your skin healthy; helps you to taste, smell, and see things; and maintains your testosterone levels. Zinc is also thought to help prevent prostate cancer. Some clear signs that you're not getting enough zinc are slow growth; poor appetite; sex glands that are not functioning properly; abnormalities in taste, smell, and vision; skin changes; and an increase in infections. Zinc is found in beef, lamb, oysters, and crab, but if meat isn't your thing, you can get zinc from wheat germ. If you do supplement your diet with zinc, you should use very low doses because as little as 25 mg have been found to decrease the immune system function.

How Much Do I Need?

The RDAs (Recommended Dietary Allowances), developed by the Food and Nutrition Board of the National Academy of Sciences, is a guide that tells you the amount of nutrients you need to stay healthy. But the RDAs are not necessarily the ideal amounts for optimal health. Rather, they are the amounts that will prevent deficiency and related health problems in most people. Keep in mind that the RDAs are only suggested minimum amounts. Talk with your doctor or nutritionist about what doses are appropriate for you before changing your vitamin and mineral intake.

Because the RDA amounts show only what prevents deficiency rather than what keeps you healthy, the U.S. government and the nutrition community are working to set new standards of healthy intake for nutrients. The standards are called Dietary Reference Intakes, or DRIs. The DRIs include

- ✔ **Estimated Average Requirement (EAR):** The level estimated to be adequate for half the healthy people in an age or gender group.

- ✔ **Recommended Dietary Allowance (RDA):** The level estimated to meet the needs of as many as 97 percent of healthy people in an age or gender group.

- ✔ **Adequate Intake (AI):** The level estimated to reduce the risk of certain diseases rather than merely prevent deficiency. The AI is used when there isn't enough scientific evidence to determine an EAR.

- ✔ **Tolerable Upper Intake Limits (ULs):** The highest level of daily intake that is unlikely to cause problems.

These standards are undergoing quite an upheaval right now. It could be as long as five to seven years before DRIs are established for all the nutrients covered in the RDAs.

Physical Fitness

You may not be Arnold Schwarzenegger, but even his body needs the right foods and exercise to keep it healthy. Your body is like a car. Give it fuel (food) and maintain it (exercise), and it gets you where you need to go. Neglect it, and it rusts (in the case of your body, gets sick).

Exercise can be what you want it to be: a planned workout or a change in your daily routine that makes your body move more. For example, take the stairs instead of the elevator or park your car farther away and walk. Any movement that you make to improve your physical fitness is exercise.

Benefits of physical fitness

Exercise keeps your heart, lungs, and muscles in working order, and it lowers your risk of coronary heart disease by strengthening the heart muscles and ridding the body of excess fat and calories. Exercise helps to prevent or eliminate other things you can do without: obesity, stress, high blood pressure, and high cholesterol. Exercise can also do the following:

- Fight non-insulin-dependent diabetes by increasing insulin sensitivity (that is, helps insulin to work better), which improves blood-glucose levels and helps in the long-term control of the disease.
- Protect against back pain. Exercise keeps the muscles and joints of your back strong and flexible.
- Help you to sleep more soundly.
- Relieve stress and boost self-esteem.
- Help you to sleep more soundly.
- Reduce sexual tension.

Aerobic exercise

Aerobic exercise makes your heart pump, your muscles move, and your body break into a sweat. "Aerobic" means "with oxygen." When you exercise aerobically (for example, swimming, walking, running), your muscles demand oxygen that's being carried by the blood. As a result, aerobic exercise trains your heart, lungs, and entire cardiovascular system to process and deliver oxygen more quickly and efficiently to every muscle in your body. As your heart becomes stronger and more efficient, a larger amount of blood can be pumped with each heartbeat, thus supplying a larger amount of oxygen to your muscles. The more oxygen your muscles get, the harder they can work to keep you a lean, mean fighting machine.

Handling stress through diet and exercise

According to the American Medical Association, stress is anything that disturbs a person's mental and physical well-being. Stress is commonly defined as a response to conditions or events, both routine and out of the ordinary. Stress can be caused by factors as diverse as physical violence, a loss of a job, birth or death, or even getting stuck in a traffic jam.

Your body reacts to stress as if it's physically threatened. It gets ready for "fight or flight." (This is known as the stress response.) Adrenaline is released, your heart beats faster, the passageways of your lungs expand, and the blood vessels of your skin and digestive system narrow to increase the blood supply to the muscles. Once you have either fought or flown, the body returns to normal.

But you can't fight or flee from every stressful situation, a dilemma that can make you susceptible to health problems such as migraines, indigestion, high blood pressure, backaches, and insomnia. However, you can cope with stress in many ways (which we cover in more depth in Chapter 6), but an easier way is through diet and exercise.

Stick to nutritious foods. Cut out sugary sweets (they boost your stress level by stimulating adrenaline). Go easy on caffeine and nicotine because they wreak havoc with your nerves and stimulate your mind (see Chapter 5). Exercise regularly to work away tension. After 10 to 20 minutes of intense exercise, the brain releases *epinephrine* and *endorphins,* tension-lowering chemicals. Epinephrine is the stress hormone that gives you a surge of energy to help sustain activity while improving blood circulation. However, it doesn't increase stress because it's balanced by endorphins, stress-fighting chemicals that make you feel good.

Anaerobic exercise

The word "anaerobic" means "without oxygen." So when you exercise anaerobically, your muscles are working at such an intense level (weight lifting, for example) that your blood can't supply them with enough oxygen to keep them working. This point of intensity is called the *anaerobic threshold* (coined by Karl Wasserman, a California physiologist, in 1972). When you reach this threshold, your body can't continue at the same intensity, at least not for long. As you may guess, each time you reach an anaerobic threshold, you have to train longer and more intensely to reach the next level.

Anaerobic exercise strengthens muscles, but it does little to improve your cardiovascular system. Because of this, you should make aerobic conditioning a priority or you could harm yourself seriously if you participate in anaerobic activities without your heart being in condition or if you have high blood pressure.

Elements of an exercise program

If you're healthy and following your doctor's advice, the benefits of exercise far outweigh any risks. But if you're over 35 and have been a couch potato for a long time, consult a doctor before starting an exercise program.

To get the most out of your workout, incorporate five basic elements into your exercise program:

- ✔ **The warm-up.** This is 5 to 10 minutes of slow exercise that uses your large muscle groups (legs, arms, and back, for example) and gets you ready for your main workout. You may want to walk at a moderate pace or use a stationary bike or a stair climber to warm up. Calisthenics such as arm circles, knee lifts, and trunk rotations are helpful. Warming up helps to prevent soreness and injury. Warm up longer on cold days. If you're older, you need to add an extra 5 to 10 minutes to warm up. Warm up until you start to sweat.

- ✔ **Aerobic exercises.** Running, swimming, walking, tennis — anything that is prolonged activity and makes your lungs and heart work.

- ✔ **Anaerobic exercises.** Strength training such as weight lifting and elastic resistance using exercise bands.

- ✔ **Flexibility.** Change your exercise program to keep it challenging and enjoyable.

- ✔ **The cool-down.** It's time to chill. You need to cool down after a workout, so do at least five minutes of slow, easy exercise such as slow walking, combined with stretching. Cooling down brings your heart rate down and lessens muscle soreness.

Chapter 2

Maintaining the Machine

• •

• •

*Y*ou clean out the gutters on your house every spring to keep the water flowing and your roof in good shape. You back up the files on your computer regularly in case a meltdown occurs. You ask friends where to find the best pizza in town. But do you take the same precautions with your body? Do you keep backup medical records? Do you choose your doctor or medication like you would choose your food? In this chapter, we give you the information you need to boost your health, obtain your medical records, choose a doctor, and make other important health-related decisions.

Men and Physicals: The Odd Couple

Maybe you're the type of guy who maintains his car better than his own body. If you remember your car's last oil change but not your last physical, it's probably been too long since you've had one.

The fact is that men schedule 150 million fewer doctor appointments than women do. If you're like most men, you avoid seeing a doctor. Why is that so? One reason offered by Andrew Kimbrell, cofounder of the Men's Health Network, is that "in their 20s, men are too strong to see a doctor. In their 30s, they're too busy, and in their 40s, they're too scared."

Experts also say that men aren't as comfortable talking about their health problems, especially if the problems are sexual in nature. Men tend to wait until a problem gets worse before they seek medical attention. Men are also less likely than women to follow through with their doctors' recommendations. Get the hint? You need to call your doctor and make an appointment.

Questions your doctor may ask you

When you come in for your physical, your doctor may ask about your medical history, your lifestyle, work, any health problems you've experienced, and family history. He will also want to know the name and dosage of any drugs you take. To help prepare yourself for these questions, make a list of all your prescription and nonprescription drugs. Or bring the medications in their original containers to the doctor visit. Your pharmacist can be a big help in preparing a medication record for you to bring along, especially if you have all your prescriptions filled at the same pharmacy.

If you are seeing this doctor for the first time, collect your medical records from your previous doctor before you go. You have to submit a written request for copies of your records or to have them transferred, so make sure that you allow several weeks.

What to expect during your appointment

Based on your age and medical and family history, your doctor may want you to have certain tests. For example, if diabetes runs in your family, the doctor may want to run a blood test to check your glucose level.

The medical tests that your doctor may order fall into four categories:

- ✔ **Screening tests:** These tests look for a potential problem in an otherwise healthy man. Some of the common screening tests you can expect — depending on your age — include blood pressure check, blood and urine tests, tuberculosis test, electrocardiogram (ECG), digital rectal exam (DRE), blood in stool test, prostate-specific antigen (PSA) blood test, skin exam, and a sigmoidoscopy.

- ✔ **Diagnostic tests:** If your screening test is abnormal, your doctor may order a diagnostic test. For example, if your PSA levels are elevated or your doctor feels an enlarged prostate during the DRE, he may recommend a biopsy to determine whether you have prostate cancer, or he may request another test to determine whether you have a noncancerous condition known as benign prostatic hyperplasia (BPH).

- ✔ **Prognostic tests:** These tests provide the doctor with additional information after he makes a diagnosis. For example, if a doctor makes a diagnosis of lung cancer, he may order a type of imaging test called an MRI (magnetic resonance imaging) scan to see whether the cancer has spread from the lungs to other areas of the body. Through additional testing, the doctor can better assess a patient's condition and probable treatment or therapy.

- ✔ **Monitoring tests:** These tests determine the effects of medical treatment on a disease or other condition.

Testing, testing, testing . . .

Medical tests may be invasive or noninvasive. A test that pierces or invades the body is invasive and carries a risk of infection or other conditions. A noninvasive test doesn't enter the body. If your doctor recommends an invasive test, always ask whether a noninvasive test is available that can provide similar information.

Physicals and preventive screening

What follows are general guidelines for medical testing and screening based on various sources, including studies, groups of medical experts, and the U.S. Preventive Services Task Force. Keep in mind that the medical community does not always agree on what tests should be performed, how often, or if at all. Also, your own health and family history may suggest a different timetable. You and your doctor should discuss what is best for you.

Basic physical exam

A physical exam should include your medical and family history and a head-to-toe examination. The exam may include checking your eyes, ears, and skin; listening to your heart; checking the inside of your mouth and throat (say ah!); measuring your height and weight; and tapping your knees to check reflexes. Keep in mind that your doctor won't check everything. If you have a problem — for example, your hearing isn't what it used to be — mention this to your doctor. He may then refer you to a hearing specialist. How often should you have a physical exam? Every three years for healthy men until age 40, and every two years after that. Yearly after age 50.

Your doctor may order some of the following tests at the same time as your physical exam:

✔ **Blood pressure check:** Your doctor uses a *sphygmomanometer* to screen you for hypertension. He wraps a cuff around your upper arm and inflates it. As air is let out of the cuff, the doctor listens to the blood pressure with a stethoscope and watches the numbers on the sphygmomanometer.

> **When:** Every one to two years for all adults 18 years and older, according to the American Academy of Family Physicians. Some experts recommend a check every time you visit your doctor because blood pressure can fluctuate rapidly due to stress, disease, or other conditions. (See Chapter 17 for more information on blood pressure.)

✔ **Blood tests:** A lab technician draws blood from a vein in your arm to screen for diabetes, high cholesterol levels, and liver and kidney function. Your doctor may also order a complete blood cell (CBC) count to determine the number counts of red blood cells, white blood cells, and platelets, and the levels of hemoglobin and hematocrit. With these tests your doctor may be able to detect certain cancers, anemia, infection, bleeding, and other blood disorders. You will have to fast for 8 to 12 hours before the test to obtain more accurate blood cholesterol and blood glucose levels.

> **When:** Every three years for healthy men until age 40, and every two years until age 50. Yearly after age 50.

✔ **Digital rectal exam:** This simple, painless exam takes less than a minute to perform. The doctor inserts a lubricated gloved finger into your rectum and feels for the prostate gland and any lesions — wounds, sores, lumps — of the rectum. (See Figure 2-1.) The anticipation of this exam is often worse than the exam itself, and if you can relax, the exam is pretty painless. Don't be alarmed if your doctor tells you that your prostate is enlarged. More than half of men over the age of 50 have an enlarged prostate caused by a noncancerous condition known as BPH. (See Chapters 15 and 16 for more information about the prostate.)

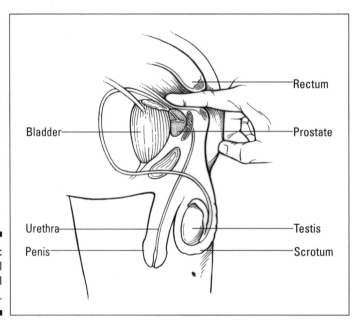

Figure 2-1:
A digital
rectal
exam.

When: Yearly after age 40, according to the American Cancer Society.

✔ **Electrocardiogram (ECG or EKG):** A technician places electrodes on your chest, arms, and legs to pick up and record electrical impulses from your heart. An EKG can detect abnormalities such as heart damage after a heart attack, an irregular heart rhythm, and an enlarged heart.

When: Every three years after age 30 if you're at risk for heart disease; every three to four years after age 50 if you're not at risk. Some experts recommend getting a baseline EKG at the age of 40 to use as a comparison with future EKGs.

✔ **Fecal occult blood test:** This test can detect minute amounts of blood not visible to the naked eye in the stool. Your doctor may obtain a stool sample during your DRE, or he may ask you to provide one. The sample is placed on a specimen card and observed for a color change after adding drops of a special solution or tablet. A color change may indicate an ulcer or a more serious disease such as cancer.

When: Every year after age 50, according to the American Cancer Society, though many experts recommend annual testing beginning at age 40.

✔ **Human immunodeficiency virus (HIV):** This blood test detects the virus that causes acquired immune deficiency syndrome (AIDS). *Remember:* A positive test means you have been exposed to the AIDS virus and that the virus is present in your body. It doesn't mean that you have AIDS. If this test is positive, your doctor will give you special counseling.

When: This test is recommended if you have multiple sex partners. If you have had unprotected sex with someone at risk for the disease or have used intravenous drugs, you should definitely have this test done. (See Chapter 22 for more information about HIV and other sexually transmitted diseases.)

✔ **Prostate-specific antigen (PSA):** PSA levels are measured by a blood test. PSA is found in all men, but its level rises with prostate cancer. Levels may also be slightly elevated with BPH and prostatitis.

When: Yearly after age 40 if you are at high risk (being African-American or having a family history of prostate cancer); yearly after age 50 if you're not at risk, according to the American Cancer Society. (See the sidebar "Making the PSA test decision.")

✔ **Skin cancer examination:** The doctor exams your skin for any changes, especially a change in the color or size of a mole or other darkly colored growth. He also looks for scaliness, bleeding, oozing, or any other changes in nodules or bumps.

When: Every three years between the ages of 20 and 39 and yearly after age 40; monthly skin self-exam (see Chapter 18 for instructions) for all adults, according to the American Cancer Society.

✔ **Testicular examination:** The doctor exams your testicles for swelling or any sign of a hernia (the famous "turn-your-head-and-cough" test).

When: Every three years after age 20, and yearly after age 40. The American Academy of Pediatrics recommends a monthly self-exam beginning at age 18 (see Chapter 7 for instructions).

✔ **Tuberculin test:** This test determines whether you have a tuberculosis (TB) infection, but it can't tell whether it's a past or present infection. A nurse introduces a protein into your skin by scratch, puncture, or injection. If you're infected with TB, a raised, hard red lump will form at the site where the protein was introduced.

When: Yearly if you're at high risk (low socioeconomic status, high TB prevalence area, exposure to TB, or immigrant), according to the Bright Futures guidelines.

✔ **Sigmoidoscopy:** Your doctor inspects your rectum and sigmoid colon (the part immediately above the rectum) by using a special tube called a *sigmoidoscope*. It has a light at the end to allow your doctor to view the colon and look for problems such as tumors and polyps. Before the test, you may need to follow a special diet for a few days and take an enema.

When: Every three to four years after age 50, according to the American Cancer Society.

✔ **Urinalysis:** You collect a urine sample in a container, and a lab technician tests for conditions such as infection, diabetes, and kidney problem.

When: Every three years for healthy men to age 40, and every two years to age 50. Yearly after age 50.

Making the PSA test decision

Some groups, such as the U.S. Preventive Services Task Force, recommend against routine testing. PSA testing is highly controversial because prostate cancer is slow-growing and is fatal in only a small fraction of those affected, and treatment by radiation and surgery can seriously hamper quality of life and may not offer any long-term benefits. Thus, you and your doctor should decide together whether to screen for prostate cancer.

Vision and glaucoma screening

Eye examinations consist of several tests that check your vision and look for any buildup of pressure in the eyes. The following are possible tests:

- ✔ **Visual acuity screening:** This test consists of reading a standard wall chart at a distance of 20 feet. Your doctor checks each eye separately. If you have glasses or contacts, be sure to wear them during the test.

- ✔ **Refraction screening:** This test, which is done in an optometrist's or ophthalmologist's office, consists of reading an eye chart with one eye covered and using different lenses.

- ✔ **Visual field measurement:** This test determines how well you see objects from below, from above, and from the sides.

- ✔ **Slit-lamp examination:** This test consists of special eyedrops that cause your pupils to dilate so that the examiner can see as far back as your retina.

- ✔ **Tonometry:** This test checks the internal pressure of your eye by using a *tonometer,* a device that uses pressurized air to record how your cornea reacts to a painless, quick puff of air. An abnormal pressure reading may indicate glaucoma.

- ✔ **Retinal examination:** This test uses an *ophthalmoscope* (a tool that looks like a fat flashlight with a disk at its end) to check your retina. You do run the possible risk, albeit it small, of a corneal infection should your cornea get scratched during this test.

A comprehensive eye and vision examination is recommended every one to two years for adults up to 64; yearly age 65 and over, according to the American Optometric Association. Anyone at increased risk for eye disease (African-Americans, or people with diabetes, high blood pressure, or any eye disease) should have exams as recommended by their eye care professionals.

Questions to ask about medical tests

If your doctor orders a test, ask the name of the test and its purpose. If you think you may have had this test done recently, tell your doctor. You may not have to repeat the test. Ask your doctor these questions:

- ✔ Why do I need this test?

- ✔ Why this particular test? Does the test provide general or specific information? If it provides general information, ask what the next step will be.

- ✔ How accurate and reliable is the test?

✔ What happens if the test is positive? Or negative?

✔ Is the test invasive or noninvasive? If the test is invasive, what are the risks involved? Can a noninvasive test provide similar information?

✔ Does the test require any special preparation?

✔ How much does it cost?

✔ Are any alternatives available if I refuse this test?

Your Medical Records

You can best recognize your medical chart as the clipboard or notebook your doctor carries in the crook of his arm when he enters your hospital or examining room. He silently flips through the pages, possibly issues a few "harrumphs" under his breath, writes some illegible notes, and then quickly shuts the cover. Your anxiety level rises a bit as you try to peek at what he's writing.

Will you live or die?

Your *medical record* is the collection of all your charts kept in a central location at the hospital or your doctor's office. This record includes information such as

✔ Biographical data

✔ Medical and family history

✔ Physical exam results

✔ Medical diagnosis

✔ Results of diagnostic and laboratory studies such as X rays, blood work, and biopsies

✔ Procedures

✔ Medication records

✔ Doctors' orders (what is prescribed for the patient)

✔ Progress notes written by doctors, nurses, consultants, and other health-care workers

✔ Informed consent forms (a doctrine that informs you about your condition and about the benefits and risks of any procedures the doctor wants to perform on you)

✔ Care plans (specifies how often nurses check vital signs, medications, incisions, and dressings; when patient goes for physical therapy; approximate discharge; and any aftercare following discharge)

Your medical record can provide you with information about your condition and diagnosis, as well as its prognosis — for better or worse. Some doctors don't want to share your record with you because you may not be able to understand their notes or they believe that the information may scare you away from having a procedure performed. If you feel that your doctor isn't explaining your condition to your satisfaction or isn't being honest with you, you may want to take a look at your medical record.

To find out whether you can access your medical records, call your state department of health (look in the blue pages or government section of the phone book). They can tell you if there is a statue, law, or health department regulation that "guarantees" access. Your health department can clarify legal issues, which you can then use to build a case for obtaining copies.

Choosing a Doctor

With the multitude of physicians available, how do you choose? The decision used to be easy, one that you probably didn't give much thought to at all. You simply went to the family doctor that your parents went to. Chances are, this doctor cared for you as a child, an adolescent, and as an adult. And then you brought your children to see him. But now you can make a decision, and you're wise to look for a doctor before you need one — not when you're feeling ill or have an emergency.

Before choosing a doctor, decide on the type of *primary care physician* (a personal physician who can provide routine care for a wide range of medical problems for you and your family) you want. You have three basic choices:

✔ **General practitioners, or G.P.s:** These doctors are not as numerous as they once were. They tend to be older men who started practice right after their internship was over. They treat a wide variety of medical problems.

Keep your own medical records

Medical records are sometimes incomplete or altered. Keeping a record of your medical care may sound hard to do, but it's not. Get some loose-leaf paper, a ruler, a pencil with an eraser, and a three-ring binder to store your records. Fill in the following information:

✔ Record your individual visits and major hospitalizations.

✔ Record laboratory tests and results.

✔ Record prescription and nonprescription medications. Be sure to include expiration dates (when the medication is no longer effective).

✔ **Family practitioners:** These doctors must go through a three-year residency to gain further knowledge in internal medicine, minor surgery, orthopedics, and preventive care. If you're looking for a doctor for the whole family, family practitioners provide gynecologic, obstetric, and pediatric care. To become qualified as a family practitioner, a doctor must also pass a comprehensive examination.

✔ **Internist:** These doctors also complete a three-year residency and pass a comprehensive exam. They have advanced training in the diagnosis and treatment of disorders of the gastrointestinal system, heart, kidney, liver, endocrine system, and other internal organs. Although an internist may practice as a family physician, he often subspecializes in another area, such as the pulmonary system.

The search is on!

Choosing the right doctor is an important decision — one that can literally mean the difference between life and death. Make sure that you put as much time and energy into your search as you would shopping for a new car! Where do you start?

Ask around

Ask your family, friends, and coworkers for recommendations. If you know someone in the health-care field, ask him or her. But keep in mind that what someone else wants or likes in a doctor may not necessarily be your choice. The fatherly, silver-haired Marcus Welby look-alike may be perfect for Aunt Josie but not for you.

If your doctor is retiring or moving on, ask him for a referral. Also ask other doctors that you have contact with, such as your kid's pediatrician or your chiropractor.

Let your fingers do the walking

Of course, you can always use the phone book. Doctors are listed alphabetically and by specialty.

Beware of doctors advertising in newspapers. Question why he is advertising. For example, did he just finish his internship? Or does he have an established practice and is trying to attract new patients because his previous patients were dissatisfied and left?

Other resources

Check a physician referral service run by the local medical society or hospital. Keep in mind that these resources limit their recommendations just to doctors who are associated with them. You may, however, be able to get information about board certifications from these services.

Managed care and your primary care physician

If you belong to a managed-care plan, expect some limitations on your choice of doctors.

If you belong to a managed-care plan, you've probably come across the term *gatekeeper*. A gatekeeper is your primary care physician who oversees your routine health care and controls your access to other health-care providers who work with the plan. Indeed, an integral part of managed care is its emphasis on primary care physicians.

In his or her role as gatekeeper, your doctor controls the access — or the gate — through which you are referred to see specialists in the plan, undergo tests and other diagnostic services, or get admitted to the hospital. Some managed-care plans require that you get a referral for some routine care, such as an eye exam. In most plans, you and your primary care doctor can choose a specialist from a list of physicians who work with the plan. Managed-care plans generally sign contracts with only a few specialists in a medical field (such as cardiology) in each locality. If you go to a specialist without a referral from your doctor, your plan may not cover or pay for that service. The same thing applies if you see a specialist who isn't under contract with the plan you belong to.

Narrowing the choices: A get-acquainted visit

Call the doctors on your list to schedule an appointment to meet face-to-face. Many doctors will meet you for a brief chat — free of charge. To be sure, ask ahead so that there'll be no surprises. If a doctor won't meet with you for a get-acquainted visit, cross him or her off your list.

Pay attention to the office environment. Are the receptionist and office staff patient and friendly? Did they offer you a friendly greeting, or did they chat behind their glass partition, ignoring you until they were ready? When you made the appointment, were they flexible in scheduling?

Ask the doctor the following questions:

- ✔ **What are your credentials?** Ask him to include his medical degree, any board certifications, specialties, and postgraduate education.

- ✔ **What hospital are you affiliated with?** Your health insurance plan may require that you go to a specific hospital.

- ✔ **Do you set aside a special "telephone hour" during the week to accept patient calls?**

✔ **Who covers for you when you're not available?**

✔ **What are the fees for an office visit?** How much is a physical exam?

✔ **Are you in practice by yourself or with a group?** Can I choose my practitioner (the answer may depend on your insurance plan)?

✔ **Do you consider me to be a partner in my health care?**

✔ **Will you tell me test results?** Or will the nurse or receptionist call me?

✔ **Will you explain tests, procedures, and medications that you recommend, including their benefits, risks, and alternative treatments?**

If you are seeing several doctors for a get-acquainted visit, jot down each doctor's answers to your questions and your thoughts about the visit after you leave the office while they are fresh in your mind.

Choosing a doctor in managed care

Choosing a doctor in managed care requires that you know your needs, ask questions, get information from many sources, and be persistent. In general, managed-care plans have more influence over doctors' interactions with and treatment of their patients than with traditional insurance plans. An added complication is the fact that in some cases, a doctor may be a full-time employee of a managed-care plan and, thus, must follow its rules and regulations.

True, your doctor is legally and ethically obligated to act in your best interest, but today — a time when managed care is growing rapidly — the burden is more on you to make sure that you get the highest level of care. Here are questions you should ask your doctor:

✔ **How does my managed-care plan pay you?** Managed-care plans may pay your doctor in different ways: capitation, fee-for-service, discounted fee-for-service, and fee schedule. *Capitation* is when your doctor receives a fixed monthly payment from your managed-care plan to provide care for you. If you use a lot of services (such as many tests and procedures), he stands to lose because he must pay for this care. *Fee-for-service* is when your managed-care plan pays your doctor after he provides care to you. How much the plan pays depends on your doctor's fees, as well as on what the plan believes is appropriate. *Discounted fee-for-service* is similar to fee-for-service, except that your doctor agrees to take less money than he would in the fee-for-service arrangement. *Fee schedule* is when your doctor is paid a fixed, predetermined sum of money, depending on the services he provides. He gets paid after he provides you with care.

✔ **If my managed-care plan pays you by capitation, do you pay the costs of referrals to specialists, lab tests, or X rays out of your own pocket?** By your doctor sharing in the cost, your managed-care plan makes certain that your doctor refers you to a specialist or orders tests or X rays only when necessary. However, an unethical doctor may short-change your health by not referring you to a specialist or by not ordering a necessary test or X ray so that he can save money.

✔ **If my plan denies a treatment or referral that you recommend, how will you work with me to resolve the issue?** You and your doctor should show the plan that the services recommended are medically appropriate and that no other reasonable alternatives are acceptable.

✔ **Do you get an annual bonus or share of profits from my managed-care plan?** Paying doctors an annual bonus is a common practice in managed care. Typically, a doctor or the group of doctors he belongs to gets a bonus based on how his practice compares with other practices in the plan. Doctors who order too many or too few tests and procedures are penalized with lower bonuses.

✔ **How does your office maintain my medical records?** Your medical records are private documents that no one should be sneaking a peek at without your permission. Some doctors and managed-care plans put medical records on computers that are accessible to other doctors and personnel. If your doctor uses a computer to store medical records or shares records with other doctors across the Internet, ask what security measures his office takes to prevent illegal access and whether he is legally required to get your permission before doing so.

Choosing a dentist

The procedure for choosing a dentist isn't all that different from choosing a doctor. Focus your questions on essentially the same areas that you asked the doctor and his staff. You probably also want to ask the dentist the following:

✔ What is your philosophy and methods of anesthesia?

✔ What is your policy towards X rays?

✔ Can you explain your infection control procedures? Pay particular attention to the use of gloves, masks, and protective clothing.

✔ Do you routinely sterilize and disinfect the instruments and work area?

✔ Do you provide prevention-oriented teaching at each visit?

✔ What is your procedure for emergency treatment?

Choosing Specialists

A specialist is a doctor who focuses on a specific body system, age group, or disorder. After obtaining an M.D. (Doctor of Medicine) or D.O. (Doctor of Osteopathy) degree, a doctor then undergoes two to three years of residency. Many specialists also take one or more years of additional training (called a fellowship) in a specific area of their specialty (called a subspecialty).

Look for a specialist who's board certified, but note that board certification doesn't mean the same thing as clinical competence.

Be aware that a doctor may also call himself a specialist in a certain field even if he's not board certified. To verify whether a doctor is certified in a specialty or subspecialty, call the American Board of Medical Specialties toll-free at 800-776-2378.

If your doctor recommends that you see a specialist for a second opinion or to verify a diagnosis, don't reach for the phone just yet. You may need to ask your doctor a few things first:

- ✔ **What is the problem?** Insist that your doctor explain your problem clearly in words that you can understand. If your doctor is put off by your questions, we suggest you reread the section "Choosing a Doctor" and find yourself another doctor.

- ✔ **If you send me to a specialist for further testing, what do you expect the tests to show?** Don't settle for anything less than specific reasons for having the test done. A response like the line from the nursery rhyme "to see what he could see, see, see . . ." is not good enough!

- ✔ **What type of specialist do you feel I need, and why that particular one?** Is your doctor choosing this specialist because he is a competent and excellent practitioner, or is he a friend of your doctor?

- ✔ **May I have the names of several specialists to investigate?** Ask whether they're board certified in their specialties. Then follow the procedure we describe earlier for choosing a doctor and see who you feel is competent.

Don't forget to call your health insurance plan and ask whether you have to choose from a list of participating specialists. You also want to ask whether you need to get approval before you see a specialist.

Osteopathy

Osteopathy is the sometimes forgotten branch of mainstream medical care. If traditional medicine (allopathic medicine) can be neatly categorized into two basic approaches — focuses on the disease versus the patient — osteopathy focuses on the latter.

Osteopaths hold that the body is an interrelated structure. Particularly important is the musculoskeletal system (bones, muscles, and joints). Consequently, hands-on diagnosis and manipulation (such as adjusting the spine or a joint or a pinched nerve) are the mainstays of osteopathy and, in short, separate osteopaths from medical doctors.

Surgery: Is It Really Necessary?

Uh, oh! Your doctor just recommended that you have surgery. What do you do? Don't rush home to pack your bags just yet because you may not need the surgery.

As many as 10 to 20 percent of all surgeries may be unnecessary. A Canadian study published in the *New England Journal of Medicine* estimated that in the United States, almost half of the more than 100,000 carotid endarterectomies done (a procedure that cleans out the arteries that supply blood to your brain) were performed on patients without symptoms of carotid disease.

If your doctor says you need surgery, ask the following questions:

- ✔ Is this surgery really necessary?
- ✔ Can we treat my problem with alternatives such as medication, diet, bed rest, or physical therapy?
- ✔ What will happen if I don't have the surgery?
- ✔ Will the problem recur even after surgery is done?
- ✔ What are the risks and potential complications of the surgery? Ask yourself whether you feel the risks outweigh the potential benefits.

If surgery is necessary, ask these questions:

- ✔ **Are less invasive or less risky surgical alternatives available?** For instance, can the doctor perform laparoscopic surgery (in which a small fiber-optic tube is inserted through a small incision in the belly)? The advantages of laparoscopic surgery include less pain, a smaller incision, a shorter hospital stay or even outpatient surgery, reduced cost, and a faster recovery.

 ✔ **Can you perform the surgery on an outpatient basis?** This option is less costly and not as stressful, reduces the risk of infection, shortens recovery time, and may allow you to go home the same day.

Get a second opinion

Consider a second opinion anytime your doctor recommends an invasive procedure such as a diagnostic test or surgery or even if you just want to confirm your diagnosis and how it's being treated.

Your insurance company may insist on a second opinion before paying for diagnostic or surgical procedures. Getting a second opinion is in your health's (and your wallet's) best interest.

Where do I go for a second opinion?

For an unbiased opinion, go to a doctor who's not a friend or colleague of your doctor. You also need to consider the source of the second opinion. A surgeon, for example, is less likely to recommend other treatments over surgery.

And for a totally independent second opinion, find a doctor on your own, which you already know how to do if you've read the previous section in this chapter.

Oops! The second opinion is different!

What do you do now? Seek a third or even a fourth opinion, if necessary. Make an educated decision by researching on your own at the library or on the Internet.

Informed Consent and What It Means to You

Informed consent means that your doctor must fully explain in simple terms the pros and cons of any proposed procedure, including surgery, that pose a threat to your life or continuing good health. Your doctor must also tell you why he feels that the procedure or treatment is necessary and any risks that accompany it.

Before you sign a written consent form, be sure that you fully understand what the doctor has said. If you don't understand, say no to the proposed treatment or procedure. Ask your doctor to explain the options until you do understand and can make a reasonable decision.

If you have an active partnership with your doctor, he should be willing to explain all procedures so that you can make an informed choice on what's done to your body. Your doctor will not feel threatened by your knowledge and autonomy. In fact, he should welcome it!

If you're hospitalized, you're asked to sign two types of consent forms: blanket consent and consent for a specific procedure.

Blanket consent

When you check in at the admissions desk, the clerk will ask you to sign a consent form. This form may be a "blanket" consent, meaning that if you sign it, you give the hospital permission to do with you as they see fit. Some forms may only apply to a specific procedure. Some hospitals may ask you to sign a consent form that includes a release against negligence on the hospital's part or that requires you to surrender your right to sue due to malpractice. However, these types of forms are not legally binding because they give the hospital an unfair advantage over you.

If you don't sign the consent form, chances are, you may not be admitted to the hospital. Here's what you can do if that happens:

- ✔ **Make changes to the form that you feel are necessary.** Write on the form that you are signing it against your will. This way, you can be admitted with the understanding that you consent only to the procedures for which you've been informed and for which you have already given consent.

- ✔ **Ask to speak with a supervisor if the admissions clerk tells you that you can't add to the form.**

- ✔ **Be prepared to move up the chain of command if necessary.** In the end, you most likely will get your way because hospital administrators know that your rights are being denied and want to ward off any legal action.

Consent for a specific procedure

The other type of consent form you sign gives your approval for a specific procedure or operation. You should be given a consent form for each procedure done, not a blanket consent form.

Make sure that the doctor who is performing a specific procedure — for example, a cardiologist about to do a cardiac catheterization — explains the procedure clearly and in terms you can understand. Before you give your consent, be sure that your doctor has explained the following:

- Your condition or diagnosis
- The benefits of the procedure
- The risks of the procedure
- The survival rates and effectiveness of the procedure
- Alternate treatments

Read the consent form carefully. If you don't agree to any of the items on the consent form, revise and amend it.

Things to watch out for regarding consent

The following are some common pitfalls to watch out for when signing a consent form:

- If you don't want videotaping, photographing, or spectators watching your procedure or body parts, write this on the form to reflect your wishes.

- Search the form for amend clauses that say the procedure will be performed "under the direction of" or by others "selected by him." You probably don't want anybody else (such as a medical resident) doing your surgery.

- Sign the consent form only if you fully understand what has been explained to you.

Chapter 3

Health Insurance and Other Important Choices for Your Future

∙ ∙

In This Chapter

▶ Making sense of insurance choices

▶ Managing managed care

▶ Understanding Medicare and Medical

▶ Choosing long-term-care options

▶ Dealing with death and dying issues

∙ ∙

*M*ention the words "health insurance" and you may get a reaction that ranges from a yawn to an "I'm so confused!" expression. We hope that this chapter cures your confusion as we clarify questions that you may have about health insurance and other choices.

What Is Health Insurance?

We hope you stay healthy — but because you or a family member will likely get sick at some point, you need to know about health insurance. You should choose the plan (within the limits imposed by your employer or other insurance provider) that will best meet your needs.

If you're like most people, you carry health insurance (if you can afford it) or your employer provides it for you. Perhaps your insurance plan covers most of your expenses and you pay only a few dollars out of your own pocket. Frankly, though, most coverage is not as extensive as it once was, which means that people pay more out-of-pocket expenses. And some employers who once provided cost-free health insurance now require employees to make premium contributions.

Confounding factors

Adding to these factors is the reorganization of the system from traditional "pay-as-you-go" insurance plans, called *fee-for-service* or *traditional indemnity plans,* to managed care. In fact, more than 140 million Americans today are enrolled in managed care plans — HMOs, PPOs, and other alphabet-soup entities.

Managed care's goals include studying and eliminating unnecessary, unproven, or not cost-effective health-care services, such as tests and surgical procedures, and increasing the role of preventive health-care services that help keep people from getting sick.

What insurance does for you

Whatever type of plan you're in (and we say more about the various types later), a sudden loss of coverage, a drop in protection, or any other dramatic switch in benefits can leave you and your family facing serious financial loss. Health insurance is designed to protect against such loss and against ruinous medical bills. But few policies pay all your medical bills all the time. So the guiding principle in shopping for insurance is this: The more comprehensive the coverage, the better. And whatever your plan, know what it pays (and doesn't pay) and how to the get the most out of your coverage.

Like you don't have enough to worry about, right? Staying healthy, paying for or sharing the cost of insurance, negotiating with doctors and hospitals to get the best care at the lowest cost. . . . When will it all end? Well, it begins with knowledge.

Types of traditional indemnity insurance

Traditional types of indemnity insurance work on a fee-for-service basis, which means that medical-care providers are paid according to the services they render. They include the following:

- ✔ **Hospital insurance:** This insurance provides coverage for inpatient and outpatient facility services. The policy usually specifies the number of days of hospitalization and the percentage of costs covered in a certain time period — or sets a dollar limit on the total benefits payable. After an initial deductible, the plan generally pays for all covered expenses.

✔ **Major medical insurance:** Sometimes called *catastrophic insurance,* this coverage protects you against high-cost medical care associated with serious illness or accident. Before benefits are paid, this type of insurance usually requires you to pay a yearly deductible, typically ranging from $100 to $500 (although some plans may have a $1,000 deductible). After you meet the deductible, major medical insurance pays up to a certain percentage of covered expenses, and you pay the remaining percentage.

✔ **Medical/surgical insurance:** This insurance is divided into two parts. The medical portion pays for doctor visits to the hospital and may pay for office visits that lead to inpatient or surgical care. It also pays for some drugs, X rays, anesthesia, and laboratory tests performed outside the hospital. The surgical portion covers the fees of the surgeon, assistant surgeon, and anesthesiologist, whether surgery was performed in the hospital or an ambulatory surgical center. There may be a dollar limit on benefits.

What Is Managed Care — and Why Should You Care?

Do you get the feeling that managed care is casting a shadow about as imposing as King Kong's over the industry? Well, you're not far from the truth. Although it's not a new concept, managed care is the biggest change in health care in the 1990s — and on into the next millennium, if all indicators hold true. Managed care is the "big gun" of health insurance in the United States, and even if you continue to be in a traditional indemnity insurance plan, chances are it has managed care elements.

Twenty years ago, if you were sick and went to the doctor, he probably didn't hesitate to order a whole battery of tests to figure out what was wrong with you. Then, when health-care costs began spiraling out of control in the early 1980s, everyone scrambled to find new, cost-effective ways to treat a person, without jeopardizing care.

Goals of managed care

All managed care is not the same, but managed care is a form of health insurance. No matter what the model of managed care is, the goals are the same: Provide only the health care you need, at a price you can afford. Physicians are paid either a salary or a monthly fee no matter how many visits or services you receive. Therefore, managed care removes the incentive to make more money by providing unnecessary services (a criticism leveled at traditional indemnity, or fee-for-service, plans). At the same time, managed care tends to be more prevention-oriented than traditional insurance. Simply put, managed-care companies make more money if you stay well.

Managed care directs you to use some providers and not others — for example, a primary care physician to manage high blood pressure rather than a cardiologist; and to use some services, such as one particular lab for blood tests, and not use others (for example, pharmacies that do not agree to dispense prescription drugs at the managed-care plan's rates).

Once you understand the fundamental philosophy underlying managed care, you can delve into the various types of managed care.

Types of managed care

Health maintenance organizations (HMOs) are the oldest and easiest type of managed care to understand. They are prepaid health-care plans that provide members, or enrollees, with medical care in return for a fixed monthly premium — paid by either you or your employer.

Preferred provider organizations (PPOs)

PPOs operate much like HMOs, offering what's called a closed panel of physicians. Typically, PPOs are large networks of doctors and hospitals organized and owned by insurance companies or doctors and hospitals in the PPOs. Usually, though, PPOs offer you more choices of doctors and hospitals than are available in HMOs, and members of PPOs generally have more freedom to see their doctors of choice whenever they wish. In other words, they're usually not required to visit a primary care physician for services or for referral to another practitioner. Instead, they're only required to stay within the designated groups, or networks, of providers.

If you use a provider outside the network or panel, you have to pay additional fees or higher copayments. And what's more — members must pay any difference between the covered fee of the PPO and the actual charges of the out-of-network provider.

Point-of-service (POS) plans

POS plans are a cross between an HMO and a traditional indemnity insurance plan. Confused? Okay, how's this? If you're in a POS plan and use the doctors or hospitals in the plan's network (the familiar HMO scenario), you either pay nothing or a small copayment for each visit. On the other hand, if you use a doctor or hospital not in the plan's network (as in traditional indemnity insurance), you pay a greater share of the cost.

Health maintenance organizations

HMOs usually cover physician's fees and services, hospital and surgical fees, home health care, outpatient surgery, some nursing home services, and preventive care such as routine checkups and immunizations.

In exchange for getting this wide range of services, you, as an HMO member, agree to use physicians and hospitals affiliated with or employed by the HMO. If at any time you use a hospital or doctor not affiliated with the HMO unless the HMO offers a *point-of-service option* — you will most likely pay for all or some of the cost of that service yourself. (Certain emergency situations may be exceptions to this general rule.) Some consider the limited choice of physicians the biggest drawback of HMOs.

In other words, an option for HMO and PPO members is that POS plans allow visits to participating or nonparticipating providers, but with different levels of coverage.

Physician hospital organizations (PHOs)

PHOs are a recent addition to the mix of managed-care plans. Typically, PHOs are owned by their member doctors and hospitals, who share resources such as administrative functions — processing claims and the like. A PHO can contract with an HMO to treat its members, or a PHO can — depending on state laws — compete directly with HMOs.

Getting the most from managed care

To make sure that you're getting the most for your money, do the following:

- ✔ **Review managed-care plans carefully:** Check out the company that owns/operates the plan. How long has it been around? Are the rules of the program clear and easily understood? Are you happy with the list of doctors and hospitals available? Know exactly what's covered and what's not.

- ✔ **Don't join a newly formed managed-care plan:** Wait until the plan has been up and running in your community for at least four years.

- ✔ **Know the plan's policy on emergency care:** Ideally, the plan wants you to use its emergency center, if it has one, or an affiliated hospital's emergency room. But emergencies don't often happen in convenient locations. Today, most HMOs and other managed care plans tell you to go directly to an emergency room. Usually, on the back of your membership card, there is a toll-free number for you or emergency personnel to call once you or your family member's condition stabilizes.

✔ **Know your rights when out of town:** Even though many managed-care companies are owned by major corporations and are national in scope, most programs have different rules in each locality. Knowing your rights in this regard becomes important if you travel on business or vacation out of what's defined as the local area. Also, be careful when you travel overseas. In most cases, your insurance or managed-care contract will not pay for care you receive outside the United States. You may need to buy traveler's health insurance before you depart.

Checking out doctors and hospitals

As a member of a managed care plan, you basically agree to use its doctors and facilities for a set monthly premium. If you go outside its network of providers, you will pay either a significant portion of the cost or all of it. So your comfort with the doctors and facilities is essential. These tips can help:

✔ **Make sure that the doctors are all board certified in their specialties:** Don't join a plan that has fewer than three doctors in any specialty or fewer than 10 primary care physicians. Be sure that you can pick any doctor on the list. (Sometimes, physicians limit the number of patients they take from any given managed-care plan, so check to see whether the practice or practitioner you're interested in is open to new patients.) Find out what happens when your doctor is unable to see you or is on vacation.

✔ **Be sure to interview your prospective doctor before enrollment (see Chapter 2):** Most managed-care plans don't encourage and may not even tolerate this practice, but stand your ground! Remember that the most important components of any managed-care plan are its doctors and its hospitals.

✔ **Be sure that all the hospitals in the plan are accredited by one of the following organizations:**

- Accreditation Association for Ambulatory Healthcare
  9933 Lawler, Suite 512, Skokie, IL 60077-3702; 708-676-9610

- Joint Commission on the Accreditation of Healthcare Organizations
  One Renaissance Blvd., Oakbrook Terrace, IL 60181; 630-916-5600

- National Committee for Quality Assurance
  2000 L St., N.W., Suite 500, Washington, DC 20036; 202-955-3500

✔ **Check to see that at least one of the hospitals has a department in the specialty areas you may use:** Find out whether the managed-care plan contracts with hospitals with national reputations for certain specialties such as cardiology outside your local area.

Pulling the ouch out of dental insurance

Just under half of the U.S. population has dental benefits, most often as part of their employers' benefits package, and as you may expect, the benefits are usually provided under either traditional indemnity (or fee-for-service) or managed-care plans.

Commonly, indemnity plans pay 100 percent of the cost of preventive services such as cleanings and examination; 80 percent of the cost of fillings and root canal therapy; 50 percent of crowns, bridges, and dentures; and nothing for orthodontics or cosmetic dentistry (trendy techniques such as bleaching and bonding). Of course, you may also have to meet an annual deductible, and you may have an annual maximum level of benefits.

Typical, too, of traditional insurance, indemnity plans do not limit your choice of dentist, although such plans often limit payments for certain types of procedures.

Although still by far the minority of dental insurance plans, dental managed-care plans are currently enrolling more new members than indemnity plans are. The two main types of dental managed-care plans are preferred provider organizations (PPOs) and health maintenance organizations (HMOs).

PPOs offer consumers a list of dentists who have agreed to provide services for a discounted fee, and as long as you go to one of the plan dentists, you receive benefits. Usually, you have no deductibles and no copayments on cleanings and other preventive services, but you do have copayments for fillings, crowns, and other, more expensive procedures.

As with a PPO, if you enroll in an HMO, you must select from a network of dentists who have agreed to provide care in exchange for an amount prepaid by the insurer monthly. Preventive services are usually covered in full, although some plans may have a small copayment such as $5 to $10 per office visit. Other covered services usually have a copayment, too.

✔ **Know how to appeal decisions:** A major complaint about managed-care plans is that doctors and consumers often don't have the final decision about treatments. By law, every licensed managed-care plan must have an appeals procedure that consumers can use to overturn — if they're lucky — a negative decision or at least have it reviewed.

✔ **Learn how to file a grievance:** Use any formal grievance procedure that your managed-care plan may have. Or you can file a formal complaint with your state insurance department. Find out your rights under the provisions in your state.

Medicare

Medicare is the federal insurance plan that covers people 65 years of age and older, those who are permanently and totally disabled, and those who have end-stage renal disease (kidney disease serious enough to require dialysis or a transplant).

The Medicare program is made up of two parts:

- **Hospital insurance.** Called Part A, hospital insurance provides coverage for hospital and related services, post-hospital skilled nursing care, home health care, and hospice services. Except for the deductible (which rises every year and which you pay out of your own wallet or through Medicare supplemental [called Medigap] insurance you may have), Medicare covers virtually all your hospital expenses. Supplemental insurance is available — for a fee, of course — to Medicare enrollees to help them cover Medicare's deductibles and copayments.

- **Medical insurance.** Called Part B, medical insurance is optional and provides coverage for doctors' fees, various outpatient services, medical laboratory fees, home health care, durable medical equipment, and the services of various therapists.

Medicaid

The Medicaid program provides health coverage to low income families and certain categories of aged and disabled individuals. Beginning in 1965, this program is jointly financed by the federal and state governments. The federal government establishes the regulations and minimum standards related to eligibility, benefit coverage, and provider participation and reimbursement. States have options for expanding their programs beyond the minimum standards but are subject to certain federal criteria.

Medicaid benefits are fairly comprehensive and include the services traditional in a commercial, group-health insurance package. As with eligibility, some benefits are federally mandated while others are optional.

States are allowed to have Medicaid recipients share nominally in the cost of their premiums, deductibles, copayments, coinsurance, enrollment fees, or other cost-sharing provisions. However, federal regulations do prohibit significant cost sharing. Check with your local state Medicaid office for more information.

Long-Term Care

According to the National Health Information Center, the number of Americans over age 85 is expected to triple to 8.5 million in the next 40 years, increasing the proportion of the population at high risk for chronic health problems. An estimated 7.2 million Americans age 65 or older currently need long-term care, as do 5.4 million children and working-age adults. Are they all in nursing homes or other such facilities? Not necessarily. Only about 2.6 million of these people are in nursing facilities. Efforts to create alternatives to institutionalization have resulted in an array of home- and community-based services designed to assist people with physical and mental impairments. Such services include everything from physical therapy to shared housing to skilled nursing to housekeeping.

Long-term care is not just nursing home care; rather, it is a continuum of services beginning with respite care (temporary relief to the primary caregiver) for the caregiver and home health care. Traditionally, families have provided most long-term care for those who need it, but demographic and social changes may reduce the amount of care family members are able to provide.

Long-term and degenerative illnesses can be costly, so you need to do some financial planning ahead of time. Whether you are the caregiver or the one needing care, you need to determine what type of care you want to provide and how you are going to pay for it. Long-term-care insurance (sometimes called nursing home insurance) may be a good option for you. If you're considering this kind of insurance, make sure that all parties — including patient, caregiver, practitioner, and maybe even attorney — discuss your plan, when you will need it, and how the plan will be carried out.

Death and Dying Issues

We don't want to be morbid, but you or someone you care about is going to die someday. And as difficult as facing that fact may be, making plans for the inevitable is in your and your loved ones' best interests.

Undoubtedly, many people owe their lives to advances in medical technology; however, high-tech medical care is also used frequently to prolong the last stages of life. And with this scenario, many issues surrounding death and dying have come to light: dying with dignity, the right-to-die issue, and even controversy surrounding the very definition of death.

With growing concerns over the quality of life and the quality of the end of life comes the matter of *advance directives*. These are written statements that state how you want medical decisions to be made should you become incapacitated. The two most common forms of advance directives are a living will and a durable power of attorney for health care.

Living will

A living will is a written statement that you do not want life-prolonging medical procedures when your condition is hopeless and you have no chance of regaining a meaningful life. Although called a "will," it has nothing to do with your property, but rather with yourself, and is intended to take effect when you are still alive.

A living will is a tool to control the extent and type of medical care you receive at the end of your life. It can also help reduce the emotional stress and strain felt by both your family and your doctor, who must decide whether to withhold, withdraw, or continue medical treatment that cannot cure or reverse your terminal condition.

Wait a minute: I have concerns . . .

Each state has its own laws regarding living wills, so if you have specific questions, you may wish to speak with your attorney (or state bar association) and physician.

Among other things, find out the following:

- ✔ Do I need more than the typical two witnesses to the document?
- ✔ Does the document have to be notarized?
- ✔ Does the withdrawal of life-sustaining treatment include artificial feeding and hydration? Many states prohibit the withdrawal of food and water, whereas others allow it.
- ✔ Can I add any personalized instructions, or must I stick to a particular form?
- ✔ If I'm traveling in another state, is my state's living will valid there?

Contact your state bar association or the organization Choice in Dying for a living will form.

Make sure that your physician, family, and attorney know that you have a living will — or even give them copies of it. Remember that you can revoke or change a living will at any time.

One important point to keep in mind: A living will has shortcomings. You have no guarantee that what you want will be carried out. Nevertheless, you are able to declare your wishes to your family and friends, giving them guidance in making health-care decisions for you.

A sample living will

Declaration made this ___ day of _____, 19___, [20___]

I, _____, being of sound mind, willfully and voluntarily make known my desire that my dying shall not be artificially prolonged under the circumstances set forth below, and do declare:

If at any time I should have an incurable injury, disease, or illness certified to be a terminal condition by two physicians who have personally examined me, one of whom shall be my attending physician, and the physicians have determined that my death will occur whether or not life-sustaining procedures are utilized and where the application of life-sustaining procedures would serve only to artificially prolong the dying process, I direct that such procedures be withheld or withdrawn, and that I be permitted to die naturally and with only the administration of medication or the performance of any medical procedure deemed necessary to provide me with comfort care.

In the absence of my ability to give directions regarding the use of such life-sustaining procedures, it is my intention that this declaration shall be honored by my family and physician(s) as the final expression of my legal right to refuse medical or surgical treatment and accept the consequences from such refusal.

I understand the full import of this declaration and I am emotionally and mentally competent to make this declaration.

Signed _____

Address _____

The declarant has been personally known to me and I believe him/her to be of sound mind.

Witness _____

Witness _____

Source: President's Commission for the Study of Ethical Problems in Medicine and Behavior Research, "Deciding to Forego Life-Sustaining Treatment," U.S. Government Printing Office pp. 314–15.

Do not resuscitate order

A do not resuscitate (DNR) order is another document that you can use to help gain more control over the circumstances of your death. It means that no one will start or carry out cardiopulmonary resuscitation (CPR) should your breathing or heartbeat stop. These orders also mean that your doctor will not place you on long-term, mechanical, life-support equipment.

Here are some tips to keep in mind:

✔ **Plan ahead:** Talk with your physician and know your hospital's policy regarding DNR orders before you may need help.

✔ **Make sure that your family (and whoever holds your durable power of attorney) knows your wishes.**

✔ **Document your wishes concerning emergency resuscitation and have your physician make it part of your medical record.**

Remember that if you change your mind, you can reverse a DNR order.

Durable power of attorney for health care

Another form of advance directive, a durable power of attorney for health care (sometimes called a DPA) is a written document that names an agent or surrogate who will carry out your wishes regarding medical treatment in the event that you become incompetent and are unable to make those decisions yourself. Although the living will is only about the final moments of life, the DPA can be drafted to give your agent the authority to make decisions about other areas of medical treatment.

You probably know durable power of attorney in its standard sense — that is, a way of authorizing another person to make decisions or take actions on your behalf in financial or property transactions. Indeed, all 50 states and the District of Columbia have durable-power-of-attorney laws, and these laws have been used as a basis for directives regarding health care. Despite that, some states have passed legislation creating a durable power of attorney specifically for health-care decisions. Check with your state bar association for details on these laws.

The person you choose to represent you to your doctors is called an agent, or *proxy,* and is legally able to speak for you. Clearly, you should choose carefully and consider someone who knows you and who will respect your wishes regarding treatment. Ask yourself: Who do I trust with life-and-death decisions? Who knows me best — my attitudes and values? Who would respect my wishes?

According to experts, your best strategy is to have both a living will and a durable power of attorney.

Part II
Righting the Wrongs

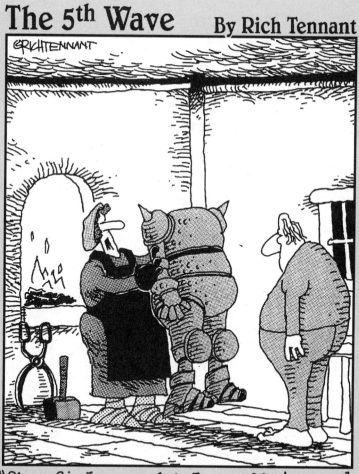

The 5th Wave   By Rich Tennant

"Okay, Sir Loungealot, I was able to pound out another inch in the waist, but you're gonna have to start taking care of yourself or buy a new suit of armor."

In this part . . .

*I*f something's wrong with your health, maybe reading this part can help you fix it. From lowering your weight to cutting stress to kicking a drug addiction, we show you ways to regain control of your life.

Chapter 4
Weight Reduction

● ●

In This Chapter

▶ Determining your ideal weight

▶ Eating smart for better health

▶ Using exercise strategies

● ●

*S*uddenly you discover that the comfortable old flannel shirt you haven't worn since last winter has magically shrunk in the wash. Okay, you can live with that. But when you glance in the mirror and see the buttons straining across your stomach, you think again. This scene clears your thoughts, especially now that you remember your shirt didn't shrink the multiple times you washed it before. That leaves only one choice — lose weight or hurt your health — and maybe you *can't* live with that.

We're not talking vanity here, guys (though if that helps to inspire you, all well and good). The real issue is common sense. Being overweight can be a matter of life and death because it increases your risk of heart disease and other serious conditions. The simple fact is that attaining and maintaining your proper weight is one of the most important aspects of good health.

This chapter is designed to improve your health, appearance, and overall feeling of well-being (not to mention that unfortunate wardrobe problem — you really did love that shirt). Look for your ideal weight, diet techniques, foods to avoid, ways to cook food and, more important, how to change your eating habits.

Calculating Your Healthy Weight

Perhaps you admit that you've been carrying around a bit more weight than is wise. But before we start talking about diet, exercise, and all those other concepts that can strike fear into the hearts of men (but don't have to), take a moment to check out some of the ways you can determine a proper and healthy weight range for yourself, based on your age and height.

A weighty issue

A survey by the National Center for Health Statistics in 1996 found that 59 percent of American men are overweight. And according to the medical experts, men who are overweight and who tend to put on weight around their stomachs (that "apple-shaped" look) are *especially* susceptible to such life-threatening conditions as diabetes, high blood pressure, coronary heart disease, and stroke.

The weight chart

One option, and the easiest one, is to look at the weight chart that appears in magazines and newspapers every now and then (often in conjunction with an article about the latest popular diet).

You can use Table 4-1 to find the suggested healthy weight for your age and height:

Table 4-1	Age-Adapted Healthy Weights for Men				
Height	*20-29 yrs*	*30-39 yrs*	*40-49 yrs*	*50-59 yrs*	*60-69 yrs*
4'10"	84-111	92-119	99-127	107-135	115-142
4'11"	87-115	95-123	103-131	111-139	119-147
5'0"	90-119	98-127	106-135	114-143	123-152
5'1"	93-123	101-131	110-140	118-148	127-157
5'2"	96-127	105-136	113-144	122-153	131-163
5'3"	99-131	108-140	117-149	126-158	135-168
5'4"	102-135	112-145	121-154	130-163	140-173
5'5"	106-140	115-149	125-159	134-168	144-179
5'6"	109-144	119-154	129-164	138-174	148-184
5'7"	112-148	122-159	133-169	143-179	153-190
5'8"	116-153	126-163	137-174	147-184	158-196
5'9"	119-157	130-168	141-179	151-190	162-201
5'10"	122-162	134-173	145-184	156-195	167-207
5'11"	126-167	137-178	149-190	160-201	172-213
6'0"	129-171	141-183	153-195	165-207	177-219

Height	20-29 yrs	30-39 yrs	40-49 yrs	50-59 yrs	60-69 yrs
6'1"	133-176	145-188	157-200	169-213	182-225
6'2"	137-181	149-194	162-206	174-219	187-232
6'3"	141-186	153-199	166-212	179-225	192-238
6'4"	144-191	157-205	171-218	184-231	197-244

Source: *National Institutes of Health*

All well and good, you say, but you don't like being lumped in with a group or being forced to fit into predetermined parameters. Well then, take out your calculator and use the do-it-yourself route instead. We describe it in the next section.

Fat or lean?

To determine your weight range, use the body mass index (BMI) and waist-to-hip ratio. These approaches won't give you a suggested weight per se, but they show if you have any reason to be concerned. BMI is a good indicator of how fat or lean you are, but BMI isn't useful for children, pregnant or breastfeeding women, serious bodybuilders, and the frail elderly.

1. **Multiply your weight in pounds by 703.**
2. **Divide the total by your height in inches.**
3. **Repeat the last step, dividing the new total by your height in inches.**

   That figure is your BMI.

If the final figure is 25 or less, you have a very low risk of the heart problems we briefly talk about earlier in this chapter. Between 25 and 30, the risk level is low to moderate; 30 or above, the risk shifts from moderate to high.

But even if your BMI is low, you can still weigh too much. If your waist measurement is high, you may still need to lose weight. Grab a tape measure and measure the circumference of your waist at its narrowest point (don't suck in your stomach; keep it relaxed — nobody is watching). After that, measure the circumference of your hips at their widest point. Divide the waist measurement by the hip measurement. If the ratio is less than 0.95, you're at low risk of heart disease; the risk increases accordingly for ratios above 0.95.

All finished? Okay, now that you know where you are and where you need to be, weight-wise, you need to figure out what to do about it.

Slimming Down and Shaping Up: Dietary Considerations

Slimming down is about eating less and exercising more. You have to commit to both. Despite what someone may tell you, though, exercise alone is not enough. If you're consuming more calories than you expend — and that's more likely to be true the older you get — you will put on weight. Factors such as genetic background (your parents were obese) and your metabolism (the rate at which you burn energy; it slows down after age 30) play a part, but these factors are usually incidental to the basic issue.

How to begin?

Before you begin a diet, visit your doctor for a complete physical examination.

Well, you've heard it all before, haven't you — especially if you read Chapter 1? Watch those calories. Avoid fat and cholesterol. No sugar, no salt. Eat more fiber. If you didn't know better, you'd swear the only answer is to stop eating entirely. And then you read that "national study" on the front page of this week's newspaper that tells you what you should or shouldn't eat, which totally contradicts itself in next week's newspaper. It's enough to make anyone say, "The heck with it" and gobble down a big bowl of ice cream.

Eating less doesn't mean you have to starve yourself. In fact, a "crash diet" designed to knock off pounds quickly is rarely the right thing to do. And besides, the weight loss you achieve this way usually isn't permanent. Most experts argue that a severe and drastic diet is about the worst way to drop those extra pounds. In many ways, they say, eating *less* really means eating *wisely.* So what's a poor guy to do if he wants to eat smart? Follow the upcoming suggestions for a healthier you.

Modify your eating pattern

Modifying your eating pattern is better than drastically changing it. In many ways, *how you eat* is as significant a factor as *what you eat.* For example, studies show that eating late at night can significantly contribute to excess weight because the body's metabolism tends to run slower at night.

If you have a hard time modifying your eating habits, seek help from a support group such as Weight Watchers or Overeaters Anonymous. They can provide information and moral support.

Use measured portions

A large helping is your worst enemy. To combat this foe, use a calorie counter, or look at the serving size recommendations on food labels. Accustom yourself to eating reasonable quantities at mealtime instead of gorging yourself. Aim to reduce your calorie intake slowly and steadily.

Eat slowly

What's the hurry? Is there a fire? The faster you eat, the more likely you are to overeat. Experts say that your mind takes several minutes after you've finished eating to realize that you're no longer hungry. When you finish your measured portion, sit back and wait a while before reaching for a second helping.

Drink at least eight glasses of water a day

Ever see a fat camel? You've seen this suggestion in a lot of diets, and it's a good one: Water fills you up and satisfies cravings for food. Water is good for ridding your system of toxins, and it is entirely free of those things that help add pounds (calories).

Reduce consumption

Although changing your eating habits is very important, you also need to control how much you consume. One of the main culprits of weight gain is eating more calories than your body needs to keep it healthy and strong.

Count calories and control your fat and cholesterol intake

Despite their bad press, fat and cholesterol are both essential for good health, so they can't and shouldn't be eliminated entirely from your diet. But as you may recall from Chapter 1, no more than 30 percent of the calories in your diet should come from fat, and what fat you do eat should be monounsaturated. Get a good calorie-counter and read those labels.

A simple way to cut fat and calories from your diet is to switch from whole milk to nonfat milk and other nonfat or low-fat dairy products.

Going low fat

Here are some tips for reducing the fat in your diet:

- Eat no more than 3 to 4 ounces of meat daily (which is about the size of a deck of cards).

- Substitute beans or peas for meats as your main source of protein.

- Choose lean cuts of meat, fish, and poultry.

- Avoid all foods fried or sautéed in oil, butter, or margarine.

- Choose low-fat or nonfat varieties of milk, yogurt, cottage cheese, and other dairy products.

- Eat at least five servings of fruits and vegetables daily. Scientific studies have shown that plant-based diets can reduce the risk of cancer, heart disease, obesity, and other health risks. Most vegetables are low in fat (except avocados and olives) and high in fiber. But don't be sneaky and add butter or oils!

- Avoid baked goods high in saturated fats such as doughnuts, pastries, croissants, and pie crusts.

- Avoid prepackaged foods and frozen dinners. What you gain in time you pay with added fat (sometimes twice as much fat as a home-cooked version!). And watch those processed foods; they're often loaded with sodium.

- Keep desserts low-fat. Gelatin desserts, sorbet, ice milk, angel food cake, and fruit are good choices. Low-fat versions of snacks and desserts are often high in calories, so limit them.

Table 4-2 shows the number of recommended daily fat calories for men (30 percent of total calorie intake). The number of calories that an individual needs varies, though, based on age and activity level. Generally, older men need fewer calories because they are usually less active than younger men.

Table 4-2	Recommended Daily Fat Calories	
Age	*Average Daily Calorie Needs*	*Maximum Fat Calories*
11-14	2,000-3,700	600-1,100
15-18	2,100-3,900	630-1,170
19-22	2,500-3,300	750-990
23-50	2,300-3,100	810-930
51-75	2,000-2,800	600-840
76+	1,650-2,450	495-735

Cook your food properly

Whether you or someone else does the cooking, the food that you eat should be prepared as healthily as possible. That means no fried foods because frying only adds excess fat and calories and leaches out nutrients. Cook your foods by broiling, steaming, baking, or microwaving instead, and don't add oil, butter, or margarine.

Eat a variety of foods, including high-fiber carbohydrates

A healthy diet includes grain products such as whole-grain breads and cereals, vegetables and fruits, as well as meat, fish, beans, and dairy products in order to provide the proper nutrients you need.

One way that you can help yourself is by choosing complex carbohydrates such as pasta, potatoes, rice, vegetables, and whole grains (avoid extra calories by not adding butter, margarine, or oil, or sauce and gravy made with fat). The body does not store complex carbohydrates as fat as quickly as other foods, and complex carbohydrates may also reduce cravings for fat.

Avoid alcohol

You've heard theories about how a small, daily quantity of red wine or beer can be helpful in avoiding heart disease and related problems. However, alcohol is also a source of empty calories and can slow down the body's metabolism. So when you're dieting, it's best to steer clear of beer (and other alcoholic drinks).

Get yourself to the point where you burn off as many calories as you consume on a regular basis. Dieting is a way of controlling the consumption end of the equation; exercise can play a part in determining what happens to those calories.

Slimming Down & Shaping Up: Exercise Strategies

Most people put on weight because their activity level slows as they get older. Having a job that entails too little activity (such as sitting behind a desk all day) or a long commute to work (which keeps you inactive) can contribute to weight gain. And too often after a hard day of work, "vegging out" in front of the TV for a couple of hours becomes a routine.

Middle-age spread

The American Heart Association reports that 25 percent of Americans over 18 do not engage in any physical activities during leisure time. Thirty-three percent of overweight men are not physically active in their leisure pursuits. And as people age, their *basal metabolic rate,* the speed at which the body consumes fuel, declines. As a result, the ratio of lean body tissue or muscle begins shifting to fat tissue. Because muscle burns energy but fat does not, fewer calories are burned, and you gain weight. However, you should keep in mind that muscle weighs more, and if you begin a strength-training program, you may gain weight. Weight gained by increased muscle mass is not detrimental to your health.

If you want to stop weight gain, a regular program of exercise is the answer. Ideally, you should combine aerobic and anaerobic exercises (see Chapter 1). Physical fitness has many benefits beyond weight control, including reduction of stress and increased self-esteem. You need to keep certain guidelines in mind, however, before you begin to exercise.

Consult your physician

As we told you before, if you've been a couch potato for a long period of time, or if you're overweight, talk with your doctor before beginning an exercise program. For that matter, you should absolutely see a doctor first if you are over 35, even if you think you're in great shape.

Start slowly

Just as with dieting, the best approach is to slowly modify your behavior rather than dramatically change it overnight. Choose an exercise program that is workable and enjoyable. If your primary criterion is burning calories, the list in the sidebar "Burn those calories" may help you decide what type of exercise program you need.

Burn those calories

The list of exercises below shows how many calories a 150-pound man burns doing any of the activities for 30 minutes. If you weigh more than 150 pounds, you burn more; if you weigh less than 150 pounds, you burn less.

Activity	Calories Burned per 30 Minutes
Aerobics, low impact	170
Aerobics, high impact	240
Baseball or softball	170
Bicycling, stationary	170
Dancing	150
Frisbee or bowling	100
Hockey or lacrosse	270
Jogging	240
Soccer	240
Skiing, cross-country	270
Tennis	240
Swimming laps	270
Walking (3 mph)	120
Walking (4 mph)	140
Weight lifting, light to moderate	100

Source: _Medicine and Science in Sports and Exercise_ 25:71, 1993.

Establish a routine

Find an appropriate time and place to exercise, and try to schedule it for the same time each day. Exercise periods should take place at least two hours after eating and no less than half an hour before your next meal. But don't push yourself if your muscles or joints hurt.

If you want to, consult an expert to package a comprehensive exercise program for you or research on your own to determine what is best for you.

For more information, contact the following organizations:

Aerobic and Fitness Association of America
15250 Ventura Blvd., Suite 200
Sherman Oaks, CA 91403-3297
800-466-2322

American College of Sports Medicine
P.O. Box 1440
Indianapolis, IN 46206-1440
317-637-9200

Chapter 5
Addictions

- -

- -

*M*ight as well face it — you're addicted to love. Some addictions, like the one in Robert Palmer's song, aren't so bad. But then again, too much of anything isn't necessarily a good thing. Defining what addiction is may be easier than explaining why one person can down cups of coffee and afterwards sleep like a baby, but another person takes a sip of coffee and can't sleep for a week.

Simply put, addiction is a chronic, uncontrollable, and compulsive behavior that happens when you continually use addictive substances such as alcohol, caffeine, nicotine, or other drugs. Because these substances are mood-altering and can make you feel good, the temptation to continue their use is strong. The trouble with addiction is that it can creep up on you so gradually that you don't know you're in its grip until your body begins to show symptoms.

This chapter is designed to help you recognize if you or someone you know has an addiction and offers advice on how to overcome it.

Alcoholism

Nobody wants to waste away in Margaritaville, but if you find yourself ordering one too many alcoholic beverages, you may have a drinking problem. You're not alone, however. According to the National Institute of Alcohol Abuse and Alcoholism, almost 14 million Americans are problem drinkers, and about two-thirds of these are men. An estimated 8.1 million problem drinkers are considered to be alcoholics. That's bad news. But the good news is you can get help if you want it. And with a little luck and determination, you may be able to kick a drinking problem.

What is alcoholism?

According to the National Council on Alcoholism and Drug Dependence, alcoholism is a disease characterized by the following:

- Periodic or continuous inability to control drinking
- Preoccupation with alcohol
- Use of alcohol despite its consequences (health risks and disruption of social life)
- Distortions in thinking, usually denial

Dependence on alcohol

Getting hooked on moonshine isn't all it's cracked up to be. You can be addicted to alcohol both psychologically and physically. An example of psychological addiction is needing a drink to calm yourself. Physical addiction doesn't show up until after you cut out the booze, unfortunately, and the withdrawal symptoms are severe. They include:

- Vomiting
- Sweating
- Diarrhea
- Trembling
- Cramps
- Seizures, coma, and death in severe cases
- Delirium tremens (DTs)

If you are physically dependent on alcohol and decide to stop cold turkey without medical intervention, you could suffer from delirium tremens (DTs). DTs are serious withdrawal reactions that happen to physically dependent alcoholics who stop drinking suddenly. Some of the symptoms include fear, anxiety, mental confusion, hallucinations (referred to as "pink elephants" in old-time cartoons), rapid heartbeat, loss of appetite, insomnia, fever, body tremors, sweating, and chest and stomach pain. DTs are a medical emergency that can last from three to six days. Medical intervention usually includes tranquilizers and sedatives to calm an incident of DTs. Deep sleep usually follows an incident.

Symptoms and signs of alcoholism

Dependence on alcohol is generally broken into four basic stages, which typically mix and overlap.

- ✔ **Stage 1:** You've developed a tolerance to alcohol (you need more and more to feel good).
- ✔ **Stage 2:** You forget what you did during a drinking binge.
- ✔ **Stage 3:** You crave the stuff and can't stop drinking whenever you want.
- ✔ **Stage 4:** You drink despite adverse effects on your mental and physical health.

Alcohol: What it is and how it works

Ever wonder why people began fermenting plants to make alcohol in the first place? Well, the reason is the way that alcohol acts. This section takes a look at what alcohol is and how it works.

Alcohol, also known as ethanol or ethyl alcohol, is a depressant that slows the central nervous system and acts like a mild tranquilizer and anesthetic. But alcohol also temporarily stimulates your body's brain chemicals — dopamine, serotonin, and endorphins — that cause you to feel good and happy with the world.

After you drink that glass of beer, wine, or other alcoholic beverage, the membranes of your mouth, throat, stomach, and intestines suck up the alcohol and transfer it through your blood system and into your brain. The stronger the percentage of alcohol, the quicker it gets in.

About 10 percent of the alcohol you take in "gases off" through your breathing and sweating (which is why drinkers often chew gum or use breath mints to cover the odor), and 90 percent is metabolized by an enzyme in the liver. Some studies show that men may have more of this enzyme than women and can break down the same amount of alcohol faster.

One bourbon, one shot, one beer: When one drink isn't enough anymore

The reason behind the fabled "hollow leg" of a longtime drinker lies in how the liver works. Think of your liver as a cleanup crew that mops up toxic waste spills. If you have a little spill (an occasional drink), the liver takes its time cleaning up the mess. You're more sensitive to the effects of alcohol at this time. But the more you drink, both in quantity and frequency, the quicker your liver works to break down the alcohol. As your liver gets better at cleaning up those toxic spills, you need to drink more to feel that buzz.

Drinking and driving

You should never operate machinery or drive after drinking. The following table is a general guideline on how long to wait after drinking before attempting to drive. Keep in mind that one drink equals 1.5 ounces of liquor, 12 ounces of beer, or 4 ounces of champagne or wine.

Body Weight (lbs)	1 drink	2 drinks	3 drinks	4 drinks	5 drinks	6 drinks
100 – 119	0 hrs	3 hrs	6 hrs	10 hrs	13 hrs	16 hrs
120 – 139	0 hrs	2 hrs	5 hrs	8 hrs	10 hrs	12 hrs
140 – 159	0 hrs	2 hrs	4 hrs	6 hrs	8 hrs	10 hrs
160 – 179	0 hrs	1 hr	3 hrs	5 hrs	7 hrs	9 hrs
180 – 199	0 hrs	0 hrs	2 hrs	4 hrs	6 hrs	7 hrs
200 – 219	0 hrs	0 hrs	2 hrs	3 hrs	5 hrs	6 hrs
Over 200	0 hrs	0 hrs	1 hr	3 hrs	4 hrs	6 hrs

Enough pussyfooting around

We've gone easy on you so far, but ignoring the grisly effects of alcohol abuse makes no sense. Check out this fact:

Drunken drivers cause more than 50,000 deaths every year in the United States, according to data from the National Highway and Traffic Safety Administration.

Alcohol abuse makes you susceptible to a laundry list of health problems:

- Gastritis, pancreatitis, and peptic ulcers
- Liver disease (including cirrhosis) and liver cancer
- Oral cancer
- Heart disease, high blood pressure, and stroke
- Kidney disease and kidney failure
- Nutritional deficiencies because you're getting so many of your calories from alcohol instead of from a normal, balanced diet
- Impaired sexual performance: Abusing alcohol decreases your testosterone level and hinders libido, erections, and orgasms

Had enough? Here's some hope!

The one bright spot in this picture of widespread alcohol abuse is the unbelievable amount of helpful resources — people, treatment programs, government programs, publications — all designed to help you out of alcohol-caused trouble. You may want to check out your local hospital because many hospitals have inpatient and outpatient clinics for the treatment of alcoholism.

Even though you may drink alone, you don't have to be alone in overcoming alcohol abuse. The way to stop alcoholism is through a medical facility called a *detoxification center,* where doctors, nurses, psychiatrists, social workers, and even other former drinkers help get you through this tight spot. Detoxification helps you get over withdrawal symptoms when you stop drinking. Three forms of long-term treatment follow detoxification. You may need one or more forms of treatment:

- **Psychological:** This therapy — usually done in a group setting — uses psychotherapy, a form of talk therapy that helps you to change your behavior and seek the emotional roots of the problems.

- **Social:** This therapy focuses on problems at work and home and includes family members as part of the treatment process.

- **Medical:** You need this type of therapy if you are suffering from severe withdrawal symptoms. If necessary, your doctor may want to try one of two drugs to help you stop drinking. One drug is Antabuse (disulfuram), and it works by making you sick if you sneak an alcoholic drink; another, newer drug is Revia (naltrexone hydrochloride). Revia works by reducing your craving for alcohol.

After you get out of a detoxification center (which typically requires you to stay there for several weeks), you may want to seriously consider attending meetings of Alcoholics Anonymous.

Nicotine Addiction

Perhaps you've never considered yourself a drug addict, but if you chew or smoke tobacco regularly, then maybe you should. Research shows that nicotine is as addictive as heroin and cocaine!

How could something that feels so good be so bad for me, you ask? The smoker knows there's nothing like the feeling of a much-needed smoke. But the "need" to smoke derives from the fact that nicotine is a powerful and addictive psychoactive drug that does some serious tinkering with your brain chemistry. Nicotine does the following:

✔ Gives you a feeling of reward

✔ Increases your concentration

✔ Raises your tolerance to pain

✔ Reduces your hunger

No wonder nearly 60 million people in the United States smoke, and out of this number almost 26 million of them are men. These minor benefits of nicotine, however, can't make up for the damage that smoking does. But before we look at what smoking does to your body, we want to take a closer look at the drug itself, nicotine.

What is nicotine?

Nicotine, a stimulant, is a clear to straw-color, oily liquid found naturally in tobacco. It's poisonous in high doses and is used to control crop-destroying bugs. Tobacco smoke contains 43 known *carcinogens* (cancer-causing agents) and more than 400 other toxins. Nicotine is the major "bad boy" in tobacco smoke because it's so addictive. And not only does nicotine influence your brain, but it also affects other parts of your body, such as your cardiovascular and endocrine systems.

The nicotine need

You already know that nicotine is addictive and that it's a psychoactive drug, but how, exactly, do you become addicted to the drug? The answer lies in how nicotine changes the way your brain exchanges information. When you smoke, nicotine enters your lungs and quickly gets absorbed into the bloodstream and carried to your heart and brain. When nicotine reaches your brain, it depresses your central nervous system by stifling the flow of information between nerve cells. But eventually your nervous system adapts to nicotine's effects. Therefore, you need to increase the number of cigarettes you smoke — thus upping the amount of nicotine in your bloodstream — just to feel good. The end result of this spiral is that you reach a target level of nicotine and have to smoke a certain amount to keep the drug level steady in your body or experience withdrawal symptoms.

What to expect when you kick the nicotine habit

Because nicotine is a highly addictive drug, giving it up won't be easy. So here's a list of some of the symptoms you can expect and how to handle them:

✔ **Coughing:** Suck on sugarless hard candy or cough drops.

✔ **Headache:** Try meditation or another relaxation technique. Take a warm bath or shower. Also, try an over-the-counter pain reliever that doesn't contain caffeine.

✔ **Irritability:** Exercise to keep your mind off smoking and to release your energy.

✔ **Insomnia:** Avoid caffeine, especially in the evenings. Meditation or another relaxation technique is usually helpful.

✔ **Constipation:** Drink 8 ounces of water daily and add high-fiber vegetables and fruits to your diet. You can also try a fiber supplement such as Metamucil.

✔ **Fatigue:** Don't try to do too much; remember that you're healing yourself. Try a nap during the day and go to bed early.

✔ **Sore or dry mouth:** Sip fruit juices or cold water. Chew sugarless gum.

✔ **Weight gain:** Don't worry too much about gaining weight while you quit smoking — experts say the average quitter gains about two pounds. Smoking increases your metabolism by a rate of 200 calories per day. When you quit smoking, your metabolic rate slows down and, over time, the 200 extra calories that smoking used to "burn off" begin to add up. Try eating low-calorie snacks, such as celery and carrots. Remember to drink water. Also, adding exercise (such as walking) can help to burn off calories.

The cost of smoking

Although smoking makes you feel good, you're enjoying that feeling at a great cost to your health. One dreadful cost may be lung cancer. Take any 10 men who died of lung cancer, and nine of them got the cancer because they smoked. Smoking also clogs your arteries and, in the process, raises the blood pressure in those clogged arteries. This condition helps to double the heart attack risk for smokers compared with nonsmokers. Smoking also thickens your blood and increases the risk of blood clots, which can result in a stroke. If you think these are the only potential consequences of smoking, read on.

If you value your looks, you should know that smoking can lead to wrinkles, weathered skin, and even hair loss! And last, but certainly not least, smoking can damage your sex life. Smoking contributes to heart disease and high blood pressure, both of which can result in erection problems. Smoking can also directly damage the small arteries — the ones needed to fill your penis with blood, and create and keep an erection. Studies, by the way, have revealed that most men with erection problems are smokers. And if you want to become a father someday, you should know that smoking may also reduce the number and vitality of the sperm you produce.

Looking at a smoker's lungs

Now we know you really don't want to take a peek inside of a smoker's lungs, but if you do, this is what you'll see. Instead of moist, pink, healthy tissue, you'll see something like oversmoked, dried fish. Smoking dries the tissues of your lungs and damages little helpful hairs called *cilia*. In healthy lungs, these hairs perform the essential function of carrying debris out of your lungs, as if on a conveyor belt. A busted conveyor belt means stuff builds up, causing you to catch more colds and lung infections.

Benefits to convince you to quit

We know that quitting isn't easy, but keep this crucial fact in mind: As soon as you stop, your body immediately starts to bounce back:

- ✔ Within 24 hours of quitting, your risk of heart attack drops.

- ✔ Within 48 hours, your senses of taste and smell improve because nerve endings in your mouth start to regenerate.

- ✔ Over time, the lung-cleaning cilia actually grow back, giving your body more oxygen and improving your lung function by some 30 percent.

- ✔ Within 10 years, your risk of dying is almost equal to that of a nonsmoker.

No matter the length of time you've been smoking, it's to your benefit to stop.

Tips for quitting

Here are a few things you can do to help yourself kick the nicotine addiction:

- ✔ **Enlist the aid of others:** Tell other people you are quitting, including people at work.

- ✔ **Change your habits so that you can avoid situations linked with smoking.** If you always smoked when watching TV, take a walk after dinner rather than switching on the tube.

- ✔ **Spend as much time as possible in places where you can't smoke:** movies, supermarkets, museums, schools, and libraries.

- ✔ **Avoid alcohol if you always smoked when you drank.**

- ✔ **Take it one day at time.** Don't think about the discomfort you'll feel in the beginning. The discomfort will not last.

Nicotine replacements: The patch and gum

Perhaps you're thinking that you simply can't quit smoking without gradually cutting down nicotine. If that's the case, you may opt for a form of nicotine replacement, such as a nicotine patch or nicotine gum. You can now buy the patch, once only available by prescription, over the counter. It works by delivering a steady low dose of nicotine right through your skin. You gradually taper off the dose by using weaker and weaker patches as time goes on through about a two-month period.

Generally, the patch is for heavy smokers. You know who you are. If you roll out of bed in the morning, and your first thought is, "Where are my cigarettes and lighter?" then the patch may be for you. If you need a specific number, smoking two packs a day is considered to be a heavy smoker. Nicotine gum, on the other hand, has the advantage of letting you decide when you need an extra dose of the drug. You are supposed to chew the gum for about 45 days until you no longer need it.

Never smoke while using the patch or chewing gum. You could be asking for side effects that include boosted blood pressure, nausea, dizziness, and even fainting.

If you smoke occasionally, you could inadvertently increase the amount of nicotine that your body is used to if you use an over-the-counter nicotine patch. In this case, it may be better to find an alternative nicotine replacement system or ask your doctor to prescribe a nicotine patch.

Other treatments

Following is a list of other methods and treatments that you may want to try if the patch or gum doesn't work for you:

- ✔ **Nicotine nasal spray:** This new product is available only by prescription. Your brain absorbs less nicotine when you send it through your nose than when you smoke.

- ✔ **Bupropion (Zyban):** This prescription antidepressant decreases withdrawal reactions. Bupropion works by affecting your brain chemicals that deal with nicotine craving.

- ✔ **Smoking deterrents:** These are over-the-counter oral drugs that — according to marketing claims — change the taste of tobacco in your mouth and control nicotine cravings.

- ✔ **Hypnosis:** This is a trancelike state that mimics sleep and makes you more open to suggestion. Hypnosis is used in psychoanalysis and psychotherapy to help change negative behavior. Sensitivity to hypnosis varies from person to person. You may want to ask your doctor to recommend a hypnotist for you — hypnotists are not licensed, so anyone can practice hypnosis.

Drug Abuse

Say the words "drug abuse" and you probably can name at least one person whose life was damaged by drugs. Drug abuse is a serious problem that destroys lives, removes self-control through addiction, and can kill through health complications such as AIDS, lung disease, and heart disease. Drug abuse is any deliberate misuse of a drug. All drugs — whether they be illicit street drugs, prescription medications, or legalized drugs such as alcohol or nicotine — are dangerous and have the potential of being misused.

Why use drugs?

The big attraction of drugs is the way they make people feel. People abuse illicit drugs for many of the same reasons that they do alcohol and nicotine: in order to relieve pain, intensify physical sensations, enhance certain abilities, and escape from reality (at least temporarily). As with alcohol abuse, illicit drug abuse is a widespread problem. A 1995 survey from the Substance Abuse and Mental Health Services Administration and the National Institute on Drug Abuse concluded that 7.9 million men in the United States had used an illicit drug within the past month, and 13.1 million had used one within the past year.

Types of drugs

People put drugs into their bodies in a number of ways: inhalation, ingestion, or injection. These different ways allow drugs to move through the bloodstream and, eventually, into the central nervous system. Inhalation or injection affects the user more quickly than ingestion.

Drugs are classified into four general categories:

- **Hallucinogens:** These drugs distort your senses or create full-blown hallucinations. They include cannabis (marijuana and hashish), LSD, ecstasy, mescaline, PCP, and psilocybin (from certain types of mushrooms).

- **Stimulants:** These drugs accelerate signals to the central nervous system and generate energetic, lively behavior. Amphetamines, cocaine, caffeine, and nicotine are stimulants.

- **Narcotics:** These drugs are essentially painkillers that also produce feelings of euphoria. Narcotics include heroin and opium.

- **Depressants:** These drugs slow down and relax signals going through the central nervous system. Alcohol, sedatives, barbiturates, and tranquilizers are all depressant drugs.

Addiction

If you abuse a drug, your need for it can take three different forms:

✔ You can crave a drug psychologically, thus needing it to feel good.

✔ You want the drug to avoid painful "withdrawal" symptoms. This is the classic physical dependence (or true addiction), such as that suffered by longtime heroin abusers.

✔ You can train one of your bodily functions to depend on the abused drug. For example, you could become functionally dependent on nasal sprays in order to breathe or laxatives in order to have a bowel movement.

Addiction isn't the only danger involved with drug use. Some drugs, such as cocaine, can kill you with a single dose.

Signs of drug abuse

Although symptoms and signs of drug abuse vary from person to person, general signs of abuse include the following:

✔ **Changes in behavior or personality:** Apathy, depression, change of friendships, violent mood swings, secretiveness, denial of problem. The drug abuser often lies, demands, or steals money.

✔ **A drop in school or work performance:** Poor attention at school or job, poor grades, or work effort.

✔ **Changes in physical appearance or habits:** Loss of appetite, weight loss, change in sleep habits, appearance of unusual skin lesions, puncture wounds, persistent cough, nasal congestion, bloodshot eyes, and physical exhaustion.

✔ **Withdrawal from parents, family, and friends:** Little or no contact with those around the user.

✔ **Appearance of drugs or drug paraphernalia:** Hypodermic needles, plastic bags, tubes, or other suspicious articles found around or on the user.

✔ **Frequent intoxication:** Watch for abnormal or dangerous behavior.

✔ **Withdrawal symptoms:** Drug addiction may also be suspected if lowering the dose or stopping the drug produces obvious withdrawal symptoms such as psychotic behavior, tremors, vomiting, weakness, aches and pains, anxiety, cramps, chills, convulsions, dehydration, dizziness, diarrhea, fever, and hot flashes.

Getting help

Ample services exist to dig yourself out of a drug-abuse hole. Many of the support agencies for alcohol abuse are also experts at addressing drug abuse problems because sometimes addicts overindulge in both drugs and alcohol.

Treatment can be drug-free or maintenance, residential or at an outpatient or inpatient treatment facility. Treatment is voluntary or involuntary or a combination of these methods.

Maintenance treatment involves detoxification by dispensing other drugs that prevent or relieve unpleasant withdrawal symptoms (Revia, for example, a drug that controls cravings for alcohol). Drug-free treatment involves no drugs.

Chapter 6

Stress and Your Body

• •

In This Chapter

▶ What is stress?

▶ Stress reduction

▶ Basic relaxation techniques

• •

*G*ot that "pressure cooker" feeling? The walls closing in around you? Have an elephant sitting on your chest? Uh huh, you have it bad. Stress is getting the better of you, but it doesn't have to. This chapter shows you how to manage stress and stop it from damaging your health.

Stressed-Out

Just to let you know, you're not alone. Stress takes a big toll on the nation's health and even the nation's finances. Studies from the National Institute of Mental Health and other surveys show that 70 to 80 percent of all visits to the doctor are for stress-related and stress-induced illnesses. Stress also contributes to 50 percent of all illnesses in the United States. And the cost of job stress in the United States is estimated at $200 billion annually, including costs of absenteeism, lost productivity, and insurance claims.

What causes stress?

Stressors — that is, anything that triggers a stress response — cause stress. And what is a stressor to one person isn't a stressor for another. For example, a busy executive may find a day at the beach — with no phone calls to make and no people to see — an aggravating waste of time. For the most part, though, people do share stressors, such as getting or losing a job, buying or selling a house, and experiencing the birth of a child or death of a loved one.

The stress response: Fight or flight?

No matter what you consider a stressor to be, your body reacts to stress the same way as everyone else's. Whether the cause of the stress is physical or emotional, real or imagined, the body reacts as if a physical threat is present. This instinctive response is as old as humanity. Long, long ago, when humans were one step ahead of toothy predators and other threats, stress was vital to survival because it gave people the *fight or flight response.* The body gets ready to either face the threat (fight) or run from it (flight). So in a way, stress played a positive role. Even today, stress can have a positive role. For example, it keeps you primed for that speech you have to make or it gives you the focus you need to solve a problem. But that's about the extent of the good stress does for you.

What stress can do to you

No doubt the stress response was well-suited to the environment of our ancient ancestors. Nowadays, though, the fight or flight response doesn't help many of the things that trigger a stress response — a speeding ticket or a traffic jam, for example. Sure, you could punch the police officer's nose (we don't advise it) or you could walk away and leave your car sitting in traffic (it probably won't be there when you come back), but behaving this way would only create more stress for yourself.

Unfortunately, the stress response doesn't offer a quick solution to modern day stressors, but your body doesn't know this. When your body stays in a state of readiness without physically fighting or fleeing to release the stress, this pent-up energy can lead to mental and physical problems. Anxiety, depression, heart palpitations, muscle aches, pain, and illness can develop.

Stress and your body

The body was not built for chronic or long-term stress. When stress hormones are not turned off after stress, overexposure to these hormones wears on the body. The chronic state of readiness shuts down functions such as metabolism, causing indigestion, heartburn, fatigue, weight gain, and decreased sex drive. Your immune system suffers because the cortisol produced during the stress response makes you more susceptible to infectious diseases, such as colds, flus, and tuberculosis.

Your cardiovascular system can suffer some of the most debilitating effects of chronic stress. You become more susceptible to heartbeat irregularities, chest pain called *angina,* high blood pressure, heart disease, and stroke. This sensitivity happens when your pulse quickens, your blood vessels constrict, and your blood thickens during a stress response.

FYI

Fight or flight

When faced with a stressor, the pituitary gland in your brain cues the adrenal glands to release several types of hormones, including epinephrine (adrenaline) and cortisol. Adrenaline, the "emergency hormone," prepares your body to deal with sudden danger or stress.

Adrenaline increases the rate of your heartbeat and breathing, raises your blood pressure, and increases the sugar in your blood (as an energy source). This energy source goes to the muscles. Because you're breathing faster, you have more oxygen in your lungs and muscles.

Glucose stored in your body is released to give extra energy-power to the muscles. Some of the blood and nutrients stored in your internal organs go to your heart, lungs, and muscles. Your brain switches to a "super-charged" state. Your senses are at their sharpest and you're aware of the slightest change around you (somebody switched the TV channel!).

These changes in your body give it the best chance for survival. You fight the best you can or you flee as fast as you can. After you've either fought or flown, your body returns to normal.

If you have asthma, a stress response can trigger an asthma attack. And you've probably had to make frequent trips to the bathroom during stress because your digestive system overproduces acids (which can aggravate an ulcer) and gives you bouts of indigestion or irritable bowel syndrome (see Chapter 14). You can also get headaches, backaches, and intense arthritic pain (if you have arthritis) because during stress, your muscles tighten. And last, but not least, stress can make your palms sweat, keep you up at night, and make you a real grouch.

Stress and your mind

Unfortunately, your mind isn't safe from stress. But what we're talking about here is more than just your attitude. We're talking about your brain, in particular, your memory center (the hippocampus).

Chronic stress can accelerate memory loss. One study showed that repeated doses of cortisol (a stress hormone) caused loss of cells in the hippocampi of animals. Because these are the cells involved in memory, researchers believe that there's also a negative effect on memory.

A Swedish study of 130 older men also showed that stress affects memory. In that study, the decline in memory and other mental skills was six times greater in those whose partner or child had died during the study. And other research shows that chronic stress sufferers are more inclined to depression because stress hormones overstimulate areas of the brain that trigger episodes of depression.

Relieving and Preventing Stress

You can't rid stress from your life completely, but you can reduce it. Know that it takes some effort because you may have to make changes in your attitude and lifestyle. Reducing stress requires that you know how you react to stress. If you know, you can change your behavior. Try to be more optimistic and assertive. See the glass as half full instead of half empty (and tell someone who disagrees that that's the way you see things). Also, develop a strategy for handling stressful situations. This way, you won't be caught off guard.

Add good nutrition and exercise

When your body is healthy, it can better stand up to stress. Keep your body healthy and strong with nutritious foods such as those found in the U.S. Government Food Pyramid (see Chapter 1). A low-fat diet helps slow the progress of some stress-related diseases. Avoid caffeine, nicotine, and alcohol.

Exercise, because it's physical activity and physical activity is what your body was built for in the stress response, is a good way to reduce any sudden increase in tension or stress (see Chapter 4).

Laugh

Studies show that laughter may be one of the healthiest antidotes to stress. When you laugh — or, according to some researchers, just smile — blood flow to the brain is increased, endorphins are released, and levels of stress hormones drop.

Be social

When you feel stress, your instincts tell you to isolate yourself. According to experts, nothing could be worse. When you withdraw, you allow yourself to concentrate more on the problem, which makes your stress level greater. Call friends. Be around young children, who can help make you forget yourself and your worries. Do volunteer work.

Know your stress personality

Do you know how you react to stress? Do you yell and kick the furniture? Or do you retreat into stony silence? Keep a stress diary for two weeks. Make note of any stressor; the time, place, and day it occurs; how you feel (angry, defeated, tired, overwhelmed); and what you do as a result. By knowing your own personality and triggers, you can learn to respond to stress before you reach crisis mode.

Make your job work for you

A recent survey found that the real cause of job-related stress is not over-work but lack of personal control. Interestingly, the most stressful positions are not at the top. One study concluded that workers in high-demand, low-control positions, such as computer operators and sales personnel, are more heart-attack prone than CEOs, who have a high degree of control in their jobs. Although you probably can't change your company's culture by yourself, you can change the way you react to stress at work.

Participate as actively as possible. Ask and answer questions, attend company meetings and events, and be sure you speak up in the workplace. Support your coworkers. Good relationships with peers and a respectful boss help you feel more in control of your job. But no matter how good things are at work, there's bound to be an upsetting event. What do you do then?

Try counting to ten before you react, which helps to avoid conflict. And the pause can help you regain a sense of control.

And finally, if you know you're in the wrong job, accept the fact and consider improving your skills so that you can change jobs.

Lose the anger: Gain some peace of mind

Anger itself isn't harmful, but the way you handle anger can be. Keeping anger bottled up inside of you isn't healthy, but neither is letting your anger make you hostile. Hostility is the single most damaging stress-related personality trait that precedes a heart attack.

What do you do then if you become angry? One approach says it's healthy to express your rage in order to get it out in the open. Another approach says you should acknowledge anger without resorting to open physical or verbal hostility. For example, discuss the conflict with the other person or sort things out on your own. The important point in either approach is to get the anger out of your system. Don't harbor a grudge, and don't let the anger build up until you explode. And after your anger has passed, let bygones be bygones, if only to reduce your stress level.

Get enough sleep

Probably one of the most important things that you can do for yourself is get enough sleep. Sleep helps your body replenish and maintain cells, fortifies your immune system, filters out toxins, and relaxes your muscles. Develop a daily sleep routine that signals your mind that it's time to sleep (for example, take a warm bath before bed). Don't drink alcohol or caffeine, and don't smoke because these substances contain chemicals that stimulate your mind (see Chapter 5).

TIP

Basic relaxation techniques

Teaching your body to flex and relax its muscles is a good way to release stored tension. Allot at least 15 to 30 minutes of relaxation time. Be sure to practice this relaxation technique when you know you will not be disturbed, and take the phone off the hook. You want to be comfortable, so wear loose clothing. Lie down on a mat or a bed in a quiet room with soft or no lighting, and place a pillow under your knees and head.

1. **Relax your mind.**

   Let it go blank. Inhale deeply for a count of four; hold your breath for a moment, then release it slowly for a count of four. Repeat this process a couple of times (don't make yourself dizzy!), and then keep your breathing easy and regular.

2. **Tense the muscles in your body.**

   Crunch your feet and toes; hold them for a few seconds and release. Move to each section of your body (calves, legs, hips and buttocks, stomach, chest, shoulders, arms, hands and fingers, neck, and face), and repeat the process.

3. **Breathe in and out evenly, saying to yourself that you are becoming more relaxed with each breath.**

   Your whole body should feel pleasantly numb and heavy, a sign that you are deeply relaxed. If you fall asleep, don't worry; you probably need it.

4. **After your session is over, gently stretch your body, allowing yourself to slowly come out of the relaxed state.**

   Do not jump up suddenly and dash out the door. Give yourself some time before you face the world again.

Chapter 7

Self-Care Techniques

*I*n a complex and often dangerous world, remember the Boy Scout adage: Be prepared.

Whether it's keeping track of your health or being prepared for an unexpected emergency, the more you know (and the more resources you have available to you), the more likely you are to do the right thing and meet the challenge.

This chapter tells you about some medical self-testing procedures you can use at home and some useful products you should have available to treat common health problems. And the chapter will help prepare you for dealing with sudden and unexpected medical emergencies. We won't show you how to win any merit badges, but you just may discover something that can one day save someone's life or your own.

Home Medical Tests

Home medical self-testing kits, once considered something of an oddity (high-tech was a basic thermometer), have become extremely popular today. This trend reflects the modern attitude that each person must be responsible for his own health care. These kits don't replace your doctor, of course, but they do offer you a sense of self-reliance and personal involvement.

Basically, home medical tests do one of two things: They determine whether or not a medical condition exists (such as a home pregnancy test, though if you're pregnant, this probably is not the book for you), or they monitor a condition you already know exists (such as glucose tests for diabetes or testing for high blood pressure).

Home tests are no substitute for professional medical advice, but home medical tests can help you decide whether you need to consult your practitioner. Most home medical tests are readily available in pharmacies, in some supermarkets, or through mail order. The following sections take a look at the most useful and important home medical tests available today.

Body temperature tests

This test is perhaps the most basic. It's also easy to do. Popular thermometers include the following types:

- ✔ **Oral glass bulb:** This thermometer is a thin glass tube filled with mercury or some other heat-sensitive chemical with a silver or red strip in the middle. You place it under your tongue.

- ✔ **Electronic thermometer:** This thermometer uses a heat-sensitive metal tip that you place in your mouth (or in the armpit or rectum). A computer chip reads and displays the temperature in digital form. But it's the most expensive type of thermometer.

- ✔ **Plastic strip thermometer:** This thermometer uses a plastic strip that you attach to your forehead. The strip displays the temperature or changes color. You can leave the strip in place for continual checking if needed.

- ✔ **Disposable thermometer:** You use this thermometer once and discard it. It works by using heat-sensitive paper that either displays the actual temperature or shows temperature by color change.

Pulse measurement and heart testing

You can check your pulse and heart rate with an electronic unit (about the size of a portable radio). The unit measures heart rate, not only in beats, but also in terms of oxygen intake and calories expended. Many models of these units can calculate target heart rates or even a fitness index based on your age, weight, and oxygen use.

Blood pressure monitoring

High blood pressure is called the "silent killer" and with good reason: Your body gives no clear outward sign that this potentially deadly condition exists. Checking your blood pressure regularly can be a true lifesaver. Home monitoring kits come with either a computerized or manually operated blood pressure cuff (a band that wraps tightly around your upper arm). The computerized version does all the work itself and displays the results digitally. The manual kit, which includes instructions, requires that you inflate the cuff, listen for your heartbeat, and read the blood pressure gauge. If you have difficulty using the kit, ask your health practitioner to show you how to use it correctly.

Vision testing

Things getting a bit blurry? If so, you can perform a vision test by using eye charts (like your optometrist uses) in the comfort of your own living room. You can check for visual acuity with a Snellen chart — the one with the big letters at the top and smaller ones at the bottom — check for astigmatism with a clocklike starburst chart consisting of parallel lines crossing in its center, or check for color blindness that hides a number within a multicolored chart.

Bowel cancer test

Colorectal cancer is another "silent" killer, mostly because people don't like to talk about it. The privacy that home testing provides, therefore, is a godsend. The cure rate for colorectal cancer increases dramatically when detected early. Three types of tests are available:

- ✔ **Stain test:** Requires a small stool specimen that you put on a specially treated piece of paper. You then add a staining solution to it to determine if *occult* (hidden from the naked eye) blood is present.

- ✔ **Toilet paper test (TPT):** TPT is similar to the stain test and checks for occult blood. The toilet paper turns blue when you spray it with a special chemical solution.

- ✔ **Pad test:** This test is the easiest of all. You drop the test pad into the toilet bowl after a bowel movement, and the pad changes color if occult blood is present.

Testicular self-exam

It's important for you to become familiar with your testicles by examining them monthly. A number of diseases can affect the testes, such as sexually transmitted diseases (STDs) and cancer. Most tumors found in the testicles are malignant and spread rapidly. Self-examination, however, can increase your chances of surviving testicular cancer by early diagnosis. You need no special equipment to do this test, other than your hands. After a warm bath or shower, test each testicle by using the following steps (and referring to Figure 7-1):

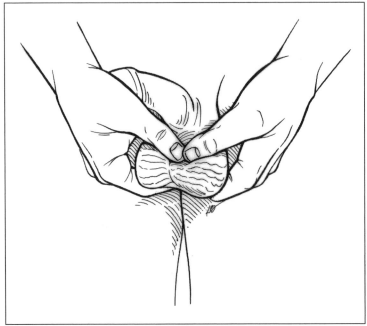

1. **Make sure that the scrotal skin is relaxed.**

2. **Roll each testicle between your thumbs and fingers of both hands.**

3. **Massage the surface lightly to check for any irregularities or anything that seems unusual to you.**

   Areas that are tender or swollen may indicate an infection. You may feel the *epididymis,* a structure along the back of each testicle, which is normal.

4. **Contact your doctor as soon as possible for more extensive testing if you find any irregularities, bumps, or hard lumps.**

5. **Most importantly, note any changes from month to month and alert your doctor immediately if you find any.**

Self-test for erection problems

Impotence (inability to achieve an erection) is every man's nightmare. The causes may be physical, psychological, or a combination of the two. The nocturnal penile tumescence stamp test (NPT) helps determine the nature of the problem. And, believe it or not, you can conduct the test by using postage stamps!

Generally, men have one to four erections during periods of deep sleep each night. For three consecutive nights, affix a strip of four to six stamps around your penis before going to bed. In the morning, if the stamps are perforated or broken in any way, chances are you had an erection during the night. This painless test may show that any erection difficulty you've been experiencing is primarily psychological. Either way, you have useful information to discuss with a trained sex counselor. If the only "mail" you want to put postage on is correspondences, special stamps and instructions are available for the NPT through most pharmacies.

Blood glucose monitoring

If you are a diabetic or have a history of diabetes in your family, you need to check your blood glucose. (Ask your practitioner how often you should check your blood glucose.) Two methods for checking glucose are reagent pads and glucose meters. In both cases, you begin by pricking your finger with a small lancet. Place a drop of blood on a test strip or on a treated sensor pad on a glucose meter. Some test strips change color according to how much glucose is in your blood. You compare this color change to a master chart. Other strips are inserted into the glucose meter and display digitally how much glucose is in your blood.

Cholesterol tests

Too much cholesterol can spell trouble. Most medical experts agree that high cholesterol is linked to the formation of *atherosclerosis* (plaque inside of the arteries), which can result in coronary heart disease and stroke. You can monitor your cholesterol by using a device that requires one drop of blood. The device separates the blood into its components, reads it, and displays the total cholesterol. Keep in mind that cholesterol levels can fluctuate daily in response to illness, stress, or weight loss. And be assured that your doctor will want to retest a home cholesterol test.

Emergency Care and First Aid

You're smart to be familiar with emergency care and first aid. First aid is immediate, on-scene care given to someone who is injured, struck with a sudden illness, or otherwise threatened. A family member, a friend, or often a complete stranger provides first aid while awaiting professional medical personnel to arrive. Ideally, the person administering first aid knows the basic fundamentals of both cardio-pulmonary resuscitation (CPR) and the Heimlich maneuver (abdominal thrust). Various course manuals are available to provide this information. Check the blue pages of your local phone book for the American Red Cross or the American Heart Association, both of whom offer training in first aid.

Learn first aid

Learn first aid so that you can act quickly and decisively in case of an emergency situation (the life you save could be a loved one's). The most devastating feeling in the world is to stand by helplessly while a loved one is suffering.

CPR training is good for one year and basic first aid for two years. At that point, you need to be recertified.

Evaluate the situation

If an emergency situation occurs, call for emergency medical help before you begin aid. After that and before you attempt first aid, take a moment to evaluate the situation for any existing danger to either the victim or yourself. It does no good if you rush in unaware and become part of the problem, rather than the solution. After you are satisfied that trying to help a victim is safe, quickly assess his or her condition and injuries. Check to see if the victim is breathing. If the victim has stopped breathing his or her life signs are faltering, CPR is probably going to be necessary. If the victim is able to communicate, ask if he or she wants your help before you attempt to give aid.

A useful medicine cabinet

Your medicine cabinet should always contain some basic self-care products. Store them in a dry place, but out of children's reach. Check expiration dates and discard and replace products. Here are some useful products:

- ✔ Pain relievers such as aspirin and aspirin substitutes (not everyone can use aspirin, which can interfere with prescription medicines)

- ✔ Antibiotic ointment, hydrogen peroxide, rubbing alcohol, and antiseptic preparations to cleanse wounds and prevent infections

- ✔ Gauze, bandages, cottons swabs, and similar basic items

- ✔ Antacids, antidiarrheals, and laxatives to treat stomach upset, diarrhea, and constipation

- ✔ Cough suppressant to keep you from coughing and expectorant to break up mucus

- ✔ Hydrocortisone cream for minor skin irritations

- ✔ Syrup of ipecac to induce vomiting for some poisons

- ✔ Tweezers to remove splinters

Also, keep a good, up-to-date, first-aid manual readily at hand, as well as essential phone numbers such as those for local police, fire, ambulance, your family physician, and your local Poison Control Center.

Common Conditions That May Require Emergency Care or First Aid

How can you tell if a situation is life-threatening? An obvious answer is when a person isn't breathing. But what if it involves something not as obvious, for example, an injury to the eye? The following sections take a look at some common conditions that call for emergency care or first aid, along with suggestions on how to deal with them or prevent them from happening.

Difficulty in breathing

If you're one of the 44 million Americans each year who suffer with breathing problems due to asthma, allergies, polluted air, or secondhand cigarette smoke, you know how frightening that can be. Sometimes difficulty in breathing is caused by allergic reactions to shellfish, insect bites, medication, or some other factor. This type of allergic reaction can be life-threatening if the victim suffers *anaphylactic shock*. Anaphylactic shock is a condition in which the airways narrow, the heartbeat races, and blood pressure drops rapidly. In such instances, you must obtain treatment immediately, as anaphylactic shock can kill in as few as 15 minutes.

Over-the-counter antihistamines can be helpful in alleviating the problem, but professional help is urgently needed. Obviously, you should know if you have allergies and avoid the things that trigger a reaction. And if you have asthma, avoid areas where there is heavy smoke or pollution.

Choking

If a person is grasping at his throat and not speaking, he is probably choking. To be sure, ask the victim, "Are you choking?" and point to or grasp your throat (the universal signal of choking). If he nods his head "yes," then perform the Heimlich maneuver until the victim coughs up the foreign body or becomes unconscious. If the conscious victim is pregnant or obese, use a chest thrust instead of the Heimlich maneuver (shown in Figure 7-2). Stand behind the person and put your arms under the victim's armpits to wrap around the chest. Press with quick thrusts until the foreign object is expelled.

If a person is unconscious and not breathing, call for emergency assistance. Check the inside of his mouth for food or a foreign body by sweeping with a hooked finger. After clearing the airway, attempt rescue breathing. If the airway is blocked, perform the Heimlich maneuver. Place the heel of your hand slightly above his navel and below the lowest part of his breastbone. Place your other hand on top of the first and press into the victim's abdomen with quick upward thrusts. Repeat the sequence until successful.

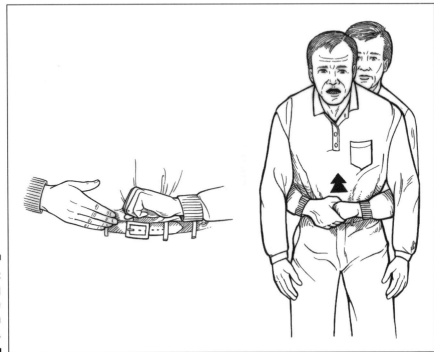

Figure 7-2:
Performing
the
Heimlich
maneuver.

Injuries to the eye

The human eye is easily damaged by physical blows, chemicals, bits of
foreign matter, insect bites, and even excessive exposure to the elements. In
the case of a severe blow, close the injured eye, apply a cold compress to
the injured area (not directly on the eye and without firm pressure) and lie
down until help arrives. If a foreign object gets stuck in your eye, do not rub
your eye. Cover the affected eye with a paper cup or other clean object that
does not touch it. If someone else is around to help you, also gently cover
the other eye with a bandage; doing so helps keep the affected eye from
moving. If a harmful chemical gets into your eye(s), flush it immediately with
warm water. If you are alone, do so by putting your face into a container of
warm water and rapidly blinking your eyelids.

Heat exhaustion or heat stroke

If you overexert yourself on hot days, your body temperature can climb to
dangerous levels. Heat exhaustion is the more common and less dangerous
problem and takes some time to develop during strenuous activity. Symptoms include cold or clammy skin, sweating, dry mouth, dizziness or
headaches, nausea, and muscle cramps. If you have any or all of these

symptoms, move to a cool place immediately, either indoors or in the shade, loosen your clothing, and begin taking fluids, either a sports drink such as Gatorade or cool water.

Heat stroke strikes suddenly, with very little warning, and can be life-threatening. Symptoms include a temperature of 104°F or more, hot, dry skin, no sweating, shallow breathing, and fast pulse. These symptoms are followed by shallow breathing and weak pulse, confusion or delirium, convulsions, and eventually loss of consciousness. A heat stroke victim is unlikely to be able to treat him- or herself and may even require CPR if not breathing. Lower the victim's body temperature by moving him or her to a cool place indoors or under shade. Raise the victim's feet slightly higher than his or her head. Loosen or remove the victim's clothing. Sponge the victim with towels or sheets soaked in cold water, or lightly spray the victim with cold water. Apply ice packs or cold compresses to the victim's neck, armpits, and groin area.

Neck and spine injuries

Most neck and spine injuries involve vehicle or sports-related accidents. Because such injuries can potentially cause paralysis, the victim requires emergency medical care. When administering CPR to a victim who has suffered such an injury, you must take care not to move the neck or spine. Make the victim lie still, immobilizing his or her neck with rolled towels or clothing.

Part III
All That Ails You

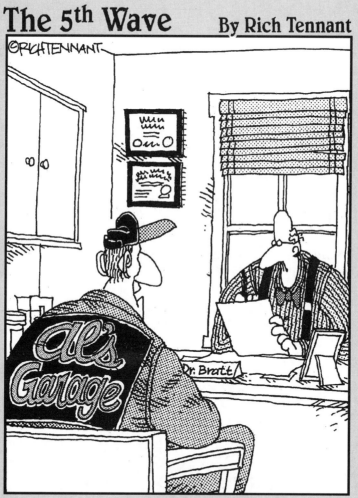

The 5th Wave   By Rich Tennant

"There's a 'thbump, thbump' when I walk up stairs and then I hear a low 'ka-chink, ka-chink' going around corners, and I'm having trouble getting my horn to work."

In this part . . .

This part is the largest in the book because it covers an awful lot of the diseases, injuries, and ailments that you may encounter in life. From something common like a headache to something serious like a heart attack, we discuss prevention, warning signs, treatement, medications, and much, much more.

Chapter 8

Passing Pains

• •

In This Chapter

▶ Treating and preventing colds and flu

▶ Heading off and treating headaches

▶ Relieving heartburn and hemorrhoids

▶ Relieving indigestion, nausea, and vomiting

• •

Sneezing, yawning, throbbing, burping, burning, itching, retching. Sound or feel familiar? If you're like most people, you've probably had your share of colds, flu, fatigue, headaches, and other passing conditions you could do without. And you're probably bound to face some of these conditions again. This chapter offers advice on how to treat and prevent such conditions.

Colds and Flu

Today, people are more mobile than ever, traveling with ease from coast to coast, city to city, meeting to meeting. With your many contacts and interactions, it's no wonder that colds and flu are transmitted easily and quickly. Unfortunately, neither condition has a cure.

Colds and flu are transmitted by viruses, nasty submicroscopic organisms that measure $1/2$ to $1/1000$ the size of the smallest bacterium. Bacteria are microscopic organisms. Some are beneficial and others are not. They do not cause colds and flu, although they can sometimes cause secondary problems such as bacterial infection. Viruses are never beneficial and cause disease, including colds and flu. They are parasites that can't reproduce on their own and need a host. Figure 8-1 shows a virus and a bacterium.

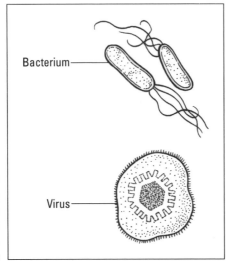

Figure 8-1:
A
bacterium
and a virus.

When a virus enters your body, it

- Invades the cells
- Breaks down the cells' molecular structures
- Changes and merges the cells' genetic information into its own
- Commands the revamped cells
- Destroys the cells during the virus's reproductive cycle

How bacteria and viruses make you sick

Bacteria produce poisons that hurt your cells. If they multiply quickly enough, the poisons overwhelm your immune response, and you get sick. On the other hand, viruses make you sick in one of several ways. Once a virus invades your body, your immune system may react symptomatically (resulting, for example, in a cough or sore throat) or with a disease process (producing antibodies that attach to the germs they're fighting as both travel throughout the body). Viruses can destroy or damage vital organs they invade, and viruses can mutate (change) the genetic character of some of your genes. Finally, a viral invasion can weaken your immune system to the point where you could fall prey to other infections that your body just can't fight simultaneously.

Colds and flu types

Of the 20 identified major virus families, most colds come from five. Three other viral families produce flu — identified as A, B, or C strains or types. Type B and Type C flu are generally mild in adults. Both can be confused with bad colds. After you have a Type C flu, you generally are immune to Type C for life. Type A flu is the least stable and most erratic when it comes to mutating (changing). Because it can change its genetic makeup so frequently, immunity to Type A is neither significant nor long lasting. Thus, Type A flu strains — which cause more severe symptoms than a cold — are the flu viruses of epidemics and pandemics (worldwide).

What are colds and flu?

As we've said, viruses cause colds and flu. They are highly contagious and spread through contact with an infected person (germs cling to hands and can also be spread through sneezing and coughing) or by touching objects harboring cold and flu viruses. Multiple cold and flu viruses exist, which explains why some colds and flu vary in duration and severity of symptoms.

A cold is known as an *upper respiratory infection,* which means it's restricted to your nose, throat, and surrounding air passages. Most colds don't produce fevers, chills, or the more severe symptoms associated with flu. However, they can produce slight aches and pains, some fatigue, nasal congestion, sneezing, sore throat, and mild to moderate coughing.

Flu, on the other hand, can be severe enough to land you on your back from 7 to 10 days. Flu is similar to colds, but arrives suddenly and is generally accompanied by high fever, chills, and extreme fatigue. It can also cause nasal congestion and coughing.

Typically, most colds or flu last 7 to 10 days. But if your symptoms worsen, or if your fever (anything above 98.6°F) lingers for more than three or four days, you probably have more than a cold or flu.

Is it a cold or flu?

Here's a quick checklist to see if your symptoms are cold- or flu-related:

Symptoms	Cold	Flu
Fever	Rare	High fever (101°F – 104°F or higher); lasts 3 – 4 days
Headache	Rare	Prominent
General aches, pains	Slight	Usual; often severe
Fatigue and weakness	Mild	Can last up to 3 weeks
Prostration (extreme exhaustion)	Never	Early and prominent
Stuffy nose	Common	Sometimes
Sneezing	Usual	Sometimes
Sore throat	Common	Sometimes
Chest discomfort, mild to moderate cough	Common	Can become severe hacking cough

Source: National Institutes of Health

Pneumonia: A nasty potential complication of colds and flu

Pneumonia is an inflammation of the bronchial tubes and air sacs of the lungs. (Inflammation is the response of your body's tissues to an intruder or injury. Typical signs are redness, swelling, heat, and pain.) Either bacteria or viruses can cause pneumonia. Both types (bacterial and viral pneumonia) are dangerous and can prove fatal for high-risk groups: people 65 or older; young children; and people prone to respiratory, heart, lung, or other chronic diseases such as diabetes and immune disorders. Pneumonia associated with colds or flu is called a *secondary infection* or *complication*. Bacterial pneumonia is treated with antibiotics, usually over a 10-to-14 day period.

Viral pneumonia is very dangerous, and occasionally lethal. This type of pneumonia strikes quickly and without warning, progresses rapidly, and is resistant to antibiotics. You should probably suspect viral pneumonia if you have a fever of at least 101°F that doesn't subside within two to three days and a dry, hacking cough that started simultaneously with the fever. Indeed, the kind of cough you have may be your only indicator of whether the condition is viral or bacterial: A cough that raises frequently foul-smelling mucus of a brownish or greenish color often signals bacterial pneumonia. Other signs of viral pneumonia include labored or rapid breathing, chest pains, wheezing, shaking chills, faintness, a sore throat, and extreme fatigue or irritability. Seek immediate medical attention if you have these symptoms. Timely treatment is critical.

Other things that can go wrong

In addition to bacterial and viral pneumonia, here are the most common complications of colds and flu:

- **Allergic rhinitis (hay fever):** A recurring inflammation (swelling) and irritation of the lining of the nose and upper respiratory tract as a result of an allergy — a reaction by the body against an invading foreign substance that it perceives as a danger. Hay fever does not always accompany a cold or the flu; it can be a stand-alone condition (see Chapter 19).

- **Asthma:** A respiratory condition in which the medium and small air passages in the head and chest cavity narrow, producing breathing problems (see Chapter 19).

- **Bronchitis:** An inflammation of the air passages of the throat and chest. The membranes become red and swollen, producing mucus that makes the chest feel tight and irritated. It may last from a few days to a few months.

- **Earache:** An infection, bacterial or viral, of the ear. If not treated, possible hearing loss and other complications can result.

- **Laryngitis:** An inflammation of the voice box, in which the voice becomes weak and hoarse.

- **Meningitis:** This dangerous, sometimes fatal, bacterial or viral infection attacks the membranes covering the brain and spinal cord.

- **Pharyngitis:** An inflammation of the throat, which causes the throat to become sore. If bacterial, it may be strep throat.

- **Sinusitis:** An inflammation and infection of one or more of the sinuses in the face and head.

- **Strep throat:** This type of throat infection is caused by streptococcus bacteria. A throat culture is necessary for proper diagnosis. If left untreated, complications of strep throat can lead to scarlet fever and kidney problems. Some signs of strep throat are chills, dizziness, red skin rash, pus on tonsils, and difficulty in swallowing.

Why you feel so bad when you get a cold or the flu

You can blame your own body for making you feel achy, exhausted, hot, chilly, and not hungry. Feeling rotten is your body's way of shutting down everything except the essential operations so that it can direct its energy to fighting the virus. Research shows that antibodies, called *interleukins,* trigger the release of hormones that block your body's normal storage of energy. Temporarily shutting off energy storage and sustaining the immune response takes a toll on your energy level, resulting in the fatigue you feel when you have a cold or the flu.

You may also notice when you have a cold or the flu that your muscles seem overly sensitive to pain. Scientists speculate that the achy feelings help to slow you down and conserve energy needed for waging war against viral attacks.

Making it better

Because excess mucus, coughing, sneezing, and a fever are the weapons that your body uses to fight illness, the best approach to treating a cold or the flu is not to medicate a symptom unless it's absolutely necessary. For example, a fever not only warns you that something is wrong, but it also shows that your body is trying to destroy an invader by increasing the body temperature. A fever circulates germ-killing blood proteins more quickly and effectively. Thus, you should probably endure fever's discomfort for a day or two to help your body fight off an illness.

Consult a doctor if you have a temperature of 101°F that lasts for longer than three days or if your temperature is 103°F or more. Consult your doctor immediately if any of the following symptoms accompany a fever: severe headache, stiff neck, severe swelling of the throat, or mental confusion.

If you feel you must have relief from your symptoms, remember this: The conditions caused by cold or flu have no cure. Even in the 24th century, Captain Picard of the U.S.S. Enterprise had a cold. *Star Trek* and other science fiction aside, treatment is focused to bring relief or shorten the duration of cold and flu symptoms. You should know that antibiotics can't fight cold and flu viruses. However, your doctor can prescribe an antibiotic when you have a secondary bacterial infection, such as sinusitis or strep throat.

Following are some common symptoms of colds and flu and suggested treatments. Be sure to follow directions on the labels of any medication.

Stuffy nose

Taking a decongestant helps clear your nose and improve breathing. Decongestants help to reduce swelling and inflammation in the sinuses and membranes that line your nose. If you use a nasal spray, limit yourself to three days of use because it's possible to become addicted and cause *rebound congestion* (the tiny muscles in your nose and throat become lazy and may require you to reopen nasal breathing passages with another shot of nose spray).

Don't take antihistamines for cold or flu symptoms. They dry out the mucous membranes, thus defeating your body's way of carrying out invading viruses. Antihistamines can also encourage mucus to thicken and slow down as it dries out, resulting in more congestion and an eventual cough.

If you find that the congestion is higher up in your nasal passages, you may need to gently shoot fluid into your nostrils. Try this: Fill a bulb syringe with a solution of $1/4$ teaspoon salt and $1/4$ teaspoon baking soda mixed in 8 ounces of warm water. Hold one nostril closed by applying light pressure while squirting the solution into the other nostril. Let it drain. Repeat two to three times, then treat the other nostril. You can also use a store-bought saline spray.

Blow your nose often (and the right way). Press a finger over one nostril and blow gently to clear the other. Blowing hard may force germ-carrying mucus back into the ear passages, which may result in an ear infection.

Try inhaling steam. Steam helps mucus to drain while soothing your nose and throat. Bring a pot of water to a boil. Remove from heat. Create a sauna by covering your head with a towel. Bend over the steaming water carefully and inhale. You may add pine, rosemary, eucalyptus, or thyme essential oil (four cups of boiling water to three or four drops of oil). Breathe in the vapor for 10 minutes. Repeat two to three times daily.

Cough

If your cough brings up mucus, drink warm or hot liquids to thin the mucus. If your cough is dry and hacking and produces no or little mucus (a nonproductive cough), you may need a cough suppressant, or antitussive. Use sparingly and, if possible, avoid an alcohol-based cough suppressant or one containing narcotics — such as codeine — because each can be addictive.

Sore throat

Suck on a lozenge that contains menthol, benzocaine, or phenol to slightly numb, soothe, and moisten your throat. You may also try mouthwashes and gargles containing phenol and sodium phenolate. All of these medications provide temporary relief. However, take care when using them to relieve a sore throat because they can mask strep throat.

Sinus infections

If you're prone to sinus infections, call your doctor immediately if you have any of the following symptoms: nasal congestion; a headache with pain or pressure around the face; very sensitive upper teeth; and/or yellow or green nasal drainage. Sinus infections that get too deeply ingrained before you start a course of antibiotics are harder to cure can develop into a more serious complication such as pneumonia or bronchitis.

Try gargling with warm salt water to moisten and soothe your throat. Make a mouthwash by adding a teaspoon of salt dissolved in 8 ounces of warm water. Use this mouthwash four times daily.

Fever and/or pain

You already know that a fever is your body's way of fighting off an intruder. But if fever or muscle aches make you too uncomfortable to get much-needed rest, take aspirin, ibuprofen, or acetaminophen to reduce fever or relieve pain.

Preventing colds and flu

Because you can only treat the conditions caused by colds or flu, prevention should be your goal. Many such tips come down to using common sense about your health.

- **Wash your hands frequently, preferably with a disinfectant, antibacterial soap.** If no soap is available, use plain hot water. Wash more frequently if you're around sick people. Most cold and flu viruses are spread by direct contact and self-inoculation (making yourself sick by touching a virus-contaminated object or person and then touching your nose, eyes, or mouth before washing your hands).

- **Don't cover your sneezes and coughs with your hands.** Although you may think you're just being polite, covering your hands with clinging viruses won't do anyone any good. When you feel a sneeze or cough coming on, turn your head away from people or look down while you expel your germs into the air. If you find yourself instinctively covering up anyway, use a paper tissue (handkerchiefs are catchalls for germs, so avoid them), dispose of it immediately, and wash your hands.

- **Use disinfectants on objects in your home and office that you frequently touch, such as telephones, faucets, and doorknobs.**

- **Don't share cups, silverware, toothbrushes, or any other item that may touch your lips or enter your mouth.**

Zinc lozenges: To suck or suck not?

Treating the common cold with large doses of zinc gluconate lozenges remains controversial. A 1996 study at the Cleveland Clinic found that cold sufferers who sucked on 13.3 mg of zinc every two hours appeared to have their symptoms subside in almost half the time of those who sucked on a placebo. However, a 1997 study reported in the *Archives of Internal Medicine* stated that evidence for the effectiveness of zinc lozenges in reducing the length of the common cold is still lacking. Doses above the recommended allowances may cause nausea, unpleasant taste, and low lymphocyte (a type of white blood cell that helps to fight infections) counts, and may lead to heart, cholesterol, and thyroid problems.

✔ **Drink plenty of fluids, such as water, natural juices, and noncaffeinated herbal drinks.** A typical healthy adult needs eight 8-ounce glasses of water or healthy liquids a day. You may need to drink more than this if you have a fever. To be sure that you're getting enough fluids, check your urine. It should look close to clear instead of a deep yellow.

✔ **Get fresh air.** Regular doses help to purge any airborne cold or flu viruses. Getting fresh air is especially important during cold weather when central heating dries you out and makes you more vulnerable to viruses. Open your windows and doors for a few minutes daily to circulate fresh air and help push out those freeloading airborne viruses.

✔ **Get a flu shot if you're in a high-risk group: 65 or older; prone to respiratory, heart, lung, or other chronic diseases such as diabetes and immune disorders.** Anyone can get a flu shot, and you may want to if you work in close proximity to large groups of people. Because some strains of viruses change so frequently, inoculations are good for one year. They are usually administered in autumn, just before the flu season begins, and generally take two weeks to become active.

✔ **Maintain a healthy diet.** Eating right ensures healthy cell and tissue reproduction, maintains strong muscle and bone systems, and provides your body with the fuels it needs to keep your immune system in top shape (see Chapter 1).

✔ **Take vitamin C.** Vitamin C stimulates a natural virus killer (interferon) and mobilizes the immune cells that patrol your body to attack invading cold and flu viruses. No one knows for sure if vitamin C actually prevents colds and flu. But most health practitioners accept that vitamin C can shorten the duration of colds and flu.

✔ **Get plenty of sleep.** If you're like most Americans, you cheat yourself out of at least one to two hours of sleep nightly. Studies say we need between seven and nine hours of sleep daily. As this sleep debt accumulates, it lowers the immune response, making it easier for cold and flu viruses to invade your body. Sleep is the primary activity that revitalizes cells and recharges your vital organs, muscles, and ability to think clearly.

Headaches

Just about everyone has felt that tiny vice clamp against his skull at one time or another. But if you had only a skull and brain inside your head, it's unlikely you would have headaches because neither the brain nor the skull is capable in itself of experiencing pain. Only nerves can experience pain, and in the case of headaches, these nerves are within the face, scalp, neck, and the brain's protective covering, known as the *meninges*. The type of headache you suffer depends on which of these nerves is being aggravated, and why.

Headaches come in two broad categories: tension, or muscular contraction, and vascular. Two distinct types of occurrences — blood vessel constriction and blood vessel dilation — cause most head pain. Constriction (tightening) causes a tension headache, whereas dilation (expanding) triggers a vascular headache (a migraine headache or a cluster headache). When tense muscles are the source of nerve aggravation — as is the case in some 60 percent of all headaches — the result is the dull, usually nonpulsating ache of what's known as a tension headache. If expanded blood vessels are the cause of nerve irritation, a vascular headache occurs, and the pain tends to be sharper and more throbbing, with pain frequently felt with every beat of the heart. About 30 percent of all headaches are in the vascular category, with migraine and cluster headaches being the most common.

Headaches may even be a combination of the two: tension and vascular. Only about 10 percent of all headaches are *organic* — symptoms or side effects of other conditions, such as tumors and head injuries, or diseases such as glaucoma.

In general, men suffer 16 percent fewer headaches than women. Tension headaches, the most common type of headache, strike two out of five Americans. The severity of any headache varies from person to person, with pain ranging from mild to incapacitating, and headaches can occur in any area of your head.

Although headaches are categorized as either tension or vascular, there are several types (sinus, organic, and psychogenic headaches) that don't fit so nicely into either group because they are caused by factors other than the constricting and dilating blood vessels. But before we look at these "misfits" of the headache realm, we're going to take a closer look at tension and vascular headaches.

Tension headache

Stress, poor posture, squinting, suppressing anger. What do these four things have in common? They all contribute to tension headaches by making you tighten the muscles in your shoulders, neck, jaw, face, or scalp. Tension in any of these areas causes your muscles to squeeze the blood vessels, constricting blood flow. Constriction has the following pain-producing effects:

- ✔ Cuts off the oxygen flow to the muscles, which increases muscle tension and irritates muscle nerves
- ✔ Prompts the nerves to send a pain-inducing message
- ✔ Prevents the circulatory system from flushing out the pain-inducing substance, which promotes even more pain, thus creating a cycle that has to be broken to relieve the pain

How do you know the pain in your head is a tension headache? Although tension headaches do have symptoms similar to other types of headaches, you can distinguish them by the following signs:

- ✔ Pain is moderate, steady, and dull instead of severe and throbbing.
- ✔ Both sides of the head tend to be affected equally.
- ✔ Pain or stiffness is felt in the shoulders and/or neck.
- ✔ Physical activity does not increase pain.
- ✔ Pain lasts from 30 minutes to several days.
- ✔ Pain flares up after long periods of sitting or driving.
- ✔ You may experience depression or loss of appetite but generally no nausea or vomiting.

Adapted from the "International Headache Society's Diagnostic Criteria and Freedom From Headaches," by Joel R. Saper, M.D., and Kenneth R. Magee, M.D., New York: Simon and Schuster, 1981.

Vascular headache

The nurse in Shakespeare's *Romeo and Juliet* is possibly feeling the pain of a vascular headache when she says, "Lord, how my head aches! . . . It beats as it would fall in twenty pieces." As you may have guessed, vascular head-aches are notorious for their severe, sometimes crippling pain — a sharp, piercing throb focused in just one part of the skull.

Vascular headaches, aptly named, are caused by the abnormal expansion or contraction of blood vessels both inside the skull (on the brain's surface and within its protective covering, the meninges) and outside the skull (in the tissues of the face, scalp, mouth, throat, sinuses, and neck). Overexposure to the sun, drinking too much alcohol, eating foods you're sensitive to, and even sleeping with your head under the covers can trigger vascular headaches.

Migraine headaches

The American Medical Association estimates that close to 30 million Americans suffer from migraine headaches, amounting to a 60 percent increase over the past 10 years. Migraines are of the vascular variety, and the pain of migraines has been described as everything from "a fiery poker twisted in the eye" to "a crushing sledgehammer." The pain can be so severe and debilitating that it can force even the hardiest soul into a dark, silent room.

Possible causes of migraines include food allergies, excessive hunger, change in altitude or weather, bright or flashing lights, excessive smoking, emotional stress, breathing noxious fumes or heavily polluted air, physical exertion, low blood sugar, emotional upsets, and heredity.

Migraines occur in two forms — "classic" and "common." Classic migraines (about 20 percent of cases) are preceded by an *aura,* a type of warning device. An aura warning episode lasts from 10 to 60 minutes and consists of bizarre visual disturbances (star bursts, black patches, zigzag lines), change in taste and smell sensitivities, slurred speech, tingling or weakness on one side of the body, bewilderment, and difficulty in concentrating. After the aura fades, pain begins.

Common migraines (about 75 percent) have no aura warning episode. Pain is severe, one-sided, and throbbing, frequently accompanied by nausea, vomiting, cold hands, tremor, dizziness, and a sensitivity to sound and light.

Cluster headaches

Cluster headaches also are of the vascular variety, but primarily affect men between the ages of 20 and 30. In fact, men are five times more likely than women to have a cluster headache. Scientists believe that this type of headache is connected with the male hormone testosterone.

Cluster headaches happen in groups between four and eight daily, and continue to strike every day or every other day for a period of one to three months. Normally, the headache sufferer is usually free of headaches except for the cluster episodes, and during attacks, nasal discharge or congestion occurs in the nostril on the same side of the face as the pain. Similarly, the eye waters on the same side of the face as the pain. Bending over can worsen the pain, and consuming alcohol, even in the smallest amounts, is thought to trigger attacks.

Rebound headaches

If you find yourself taking aspirin or other over-the-counter pain relievers regularly at the first sign of a headache, you could set yourself up for more pain than you bargained for. Regular use (more than two days a week) of any medication meant for headache relief — and especially medications containing caffeine — risks creating a *rebound headache* (a headache caused by the very same medication you take to relieve a headache). Don't take any medication for recurring headaches until you consult with your doctor. With so many types of headache medications working in different ways, it's important to find out which is the right one for your type of headache.

Making it better

Hundreds of medications — over-the-counter (OTC) and prescription drugs — attack headaches. And they do so in a variety of ways. Some are *abortive,* meaning they stop or reduce pain; others are *prophylactic,* meaning they prevent headaches from occurring. Abortive medications are drugs that work by numbing your body's ability to feel pain. Prophylactic medications are available by prescription only and work by treating the biological or emotional conditions responsible for causing headaches in the first place.

You can treat headaches in several ways. The best form of treatment for you depends on the types of headaches you have, the frequency, and the severity of the pain. If your headaches are relatively mild or don't occur more than twice a week, you may be a candidate for an analgesic (pain reliever) or some other abortive type of medication designed to stop pain after it starts. If your headaches are more severe, however, or occur more often than twice a week, you may need a prescribed prophylactic type of medication.

Abortive medications

These types of medication relieve headache pain. Here's an overview of the abortive medications currently meeting with the most success:

  - **Nonprescription analgesics and analgesic combinations:** These medications work by numbing your body's ability to perceive pain. They generally are safe and effective for the occasional relief of tension headaches and mild to moderate migraines. Examples of these medications are aspirin (with or without buffers), acetaminophen, and combination analgesics — those containing aspirin and/or acetaminophen in conjunction with caffeine to enhance absorption.

✔ **Prescription analgesics:** These medications are generally effective for all types of headaches that occur two or fewer times a week. They require a prescription because they contain ingredients that work on the central nervous system and are potentially addictive. Types include combination analgesics containing barbiturates, combination analgesics containing codeine, and analgesics containing narcotics.

✔ **Nonsteroidal anti-inflammatory drugs (NSAIDs):** These medications relieve pain by reducing inflammation within tissues as well as by inhibiting the production of *prostaglandins,* substances that make you more sensitive to pain. Available in both prescription and nonprescription forms, NSAIDs help to relieve both migraine and tension headaches of mild to moderate intensity. But you should use these drugs with caution if you suffer any of the following conditions: stomach ulcers, colitis, gastritis, kidney disease, severe high blood pressure, bleeding disorders, or aspirin-sensitive asthma. Nonprescription forms include ibuprofen and naproxen sodium. Some examples of prescription forms include fenoprofen and piroxicam.

✔ **Ergotamine derivatives:** These drugs are used for highly resistant migraines, chronic daily headaches, and cluster headaches. These drugs work by helping painfully swollen blood vessels of the head return to normal. An example is ergotamine tartrate.

✔ **Isometheptene:** These drugs are good alternatives for sufferers of moderate to severe migraines who cannot tolerate ergotamine derivatives.

✔ **Corticosteroids:** These drugs can be effective against cluster headaches and chronic and highly resistant migraines. Do not take corticosteroids with aspirin or any other nonsteroidal anti-inflammatory drug.

Prophylactic medication

These types of medications help to prevent headaches. You may be a candidate for them if your headaches occur more than two times a week and are severe, or if symptomatic relief medications no longer work or interfere with medications that you take regularly. Here is an overview of prophylactic medications:

✔ **Beta-adrenergic blockers:** These drugs (such as acebutolol, atenolol, labetalol, nadolol, and propranolol) are useful for migraines and cluster headaches. They work primarily by preventing dilation of cranial arteries.

✔ **Calcium channel antagonists:** These drugs (such as nifedipine, nimodipine, nicardipine, and diltiazem) are useful for cluster headaches. They work by reducing inflammation of vascular nerves as well as preventing vascular constriction.

✔ **Tricyclic antidepressants:** These drugs (such as amitriptyline, doxepin, desipramine, and protriptyline) are useful for migraines. These drugs are used to treat emotional disorders related to depression and to fight migraines by helping to stabilize blood levels of the brain chemical serotonin. Shortages of serotonin are thought to be responsible for painful vascular expansion during a migraine attack.

✔ **Fluoxetine:** This drug, commonly known as Prozac, is useful for all types of headaches. Fluoxetine works like tricyclic antidepressants.

✔ **MAO inhibitors:** These drugs (such as Nardil and Parnate) are used for extremely severe, persistent migraines, chronic daily headaches, and headaches associated with depression and panic disorders.

MAO inhibitors can be very effective, but because of their potential for adverse effects when taken with caffeine, alcohol, foods high in tyramine (cheese, vinegar, organ meats, pork, smoked meats, fish, spinach, citrus fruits, bananas, and figs) and certain drugs (antidepressants, appetite suppressants, asthma medications, decongestants, nasal sprays, and anticonvulsants), they should be taken only under the supervision of a doctor well experienced in their use.

✔ **Ergotamine derivatives:** These drugs (such as methysergide and methylergonovine) are useful for highly resistant migraines, chronic daily headaches, facial pain, and cluster headaches. Because of their potential for causing numerous side effects and rebound headaches, they should be used only under the close supervision of a doctor well experienced in their use. Avoid these drugs if you have high blood pressure, liver or kidney problems, cardiovascular disease, or phlebitis.

✔ **Anticonvulsants:** These drugs (such as phenytoin and carbamazepine) can be useful to treat migraines, daily chronic headaches, and cluster headaches.

✔ **Lithium carbonate:** This drug can be effective in treating cluster headaches and migraines that occur on a cyclical basis. Some side effects include tremor, thirst, water retention, mental changes, and excessive urination.

What you can do

You may be able relieve headache without drugs, too:

✔ **Get up and move around, preferably outside, if you've been sitting in one place (such as in front of a computer or in a car) for a while.** Doing so may also help to prevent a headache.

✔ **Try massage.** If you suffer from tension headaches, stimulate the scalp to help restore blood flow and relieve pain. Rub your scalp with your fingertips or use a hairbrush.

✔ **Apply heat or ice.** A heating pad, a hot shower, or a hot bath can help restore blood flow to the scalp in the event of a tension headache. For a vascular headache, apply an ice pack to your forehead to help restrict blood flow.

✔ **Relax.** Take a two-minute relaxation break. Sit comfortably in a chair, close your eyes, and consciously tense and relax your muscles, starting with your toes and working your way up to your head.

✔ **Try do-it-yourself acupressure.** Acupressure is a form of therapy that uses the fingers to apply pressure along energy points in the body. Stimulating the pressure points helps to release blockages. Gently, but firmly squeeze the web of skin (between your thumb and index finger) alongside the lower thumb knuckle between your other thumb and finger until you feel the headache fade away.

Preventing the pain

Because so many factors or combinations of factors can cause headaches, keep a headache diary. Record under what circumstances your headaches occur: when they occur, how long they last, the severity of the pain, foods and beverages consumed prior to headaches, emotional factors, and medications taken to relieve headaches. By recording this information, you may be able to identify what triggers your headaches and prevent them. Here are other strategies you can try:

✔ **Get enough sleep, in a regular pattern, on a supportive mattress and pillow.**

✔ **Don't skip meals.**

✔ **Use a good chair and sit up straight.** Good posture (besides making you look great) prevents muscle and nerve problems that may contribute to headaches.

✔ **Take regular breaks from working on computers, reading, or doing other close work.** Such work can bring on eyestrain and, with it, headaches.

✔ **Exercise regularly.** Research shows that exercise can reduce the frequency and intensity of headaches. In some cases, exercise may alleviate headaches. Experiment to see if it works for you.

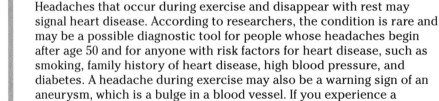

Headaches that occur during exercise and disappear with rest may signal heart disease. According to researchers, the condition is rare and may be a possible diagnostic tool for people whose headaches begin after age 50 and for anyone with risk factors for heart disease, such as smoking, family history of heart disease, high blood pressure, and diabetes. A headache during exercise may also be a warning sign of an aneurysm, which is a bulge in a blood vessel. If you experience a headache during exercise, call your doctor.

✔ **Learn to manage stress.** Relaxation is a strategy useful for both preventing and relieving headaches. Use time-management and stress-relieving techniques to resolve conflict in your daily life and practice relaxation frequently (see Chapter 6).

Heartburn

Face it, everyone pigs out once in a while, especially if the food is free or cheap. And it's still ingrained in the American psyche that you should eat everything that's on your plate, no matter if common sense tells you otherwise. Sometimes your reward for gluttony is heartburn.

Sixty million American men — the majority being middle-aged and older — experience heartburn at least once a month. The major cause is improper eating habits (eating too fast, too much, the wrong foods, and eating at the wrong time).

Knowing if you have heartburn

Heartburn is commonly felt as burning pain in the chest that begins behind the breastbone and radiates upward to the neck and as burning in the esophagus (throat) just below the breastbone.

Gastroesophageal reflux disease

Gastroesophageal reflux disease (GERD) is a digestive disorder that affects the lower esophageal sphincter (LES). At the point where your esophagus meets your stomach, the LES muscle keeps the esophagus closed. The pressure in your stomach is normally greater than in the esophagus, and the LES muscle keeps the stomach contents and stomach acid out of your esophagus.

When working properly, the LES muscle opens after you swallow to let food pass through and enter your stomach. It then quickly closes to prevent the return of the food and stomach juices into your esophagus. When the LES muscle isn't working properly, gastroesophageal reflux occurs. And like a volcano, pressure in your stomach forces stomach acid through the LES muscle and into your esophagus.

If this occurs on a chronic basis (more than twice a week), the condition is called GERD. Forty million Americans are affected with GERD, and it sends thousands each year to the emergency room because its symptoms closely resemble those of a heart attack (see Chapter 17). GERD is commonly treated with prescription drugs and dietary and lifestyle changes.

It is usually caused by contents of the stomach flowing back into the throat but can also be caused by too much stomach acid or a peptic ulcer. The burning sensation can last up to two hours, and lying down or bending over may make it worse.

Heartburn pain is sometimes mistaken for a heart attack. Likewise, men who think they are experiencing heartburn may be actually be having a heart attack. (See Chapter 17 for signs of a heart attack.)

Cooling heartburn with medication

Nonprescription antacids (see Chapter 2) provide temporary or partial relief from heartburn. New OTC medications such as Zantac and Pepcid AC (which belong to a class of drugs called H2 blockers) are designed to prevent the stomach from overproducing *pepsin* — an enzyme that digests food protein — decreasing the chance that acid will splash into your esophagus. If nonprescription drugs do not help relieve the symptoms of heartburn, see a doctor. He or she may refer you to a *gastroenterologist,* a doctor who specializes in digestive conditions and diseases.

Using antacids for longer than three weeks can result in side effects, such as diarrhea, altered calcium metabolism (the way your body uses calcium), and magnesium and aluminum retention. Some antacids are high in sodium, too, which may affect blood pressure and other conditions. People with high blood pressure should not use antacids that contain sodium bicarbonates because the sodium can promote high blood pressure and water retention. People with kidney disease should avoid antacids that contain aluminum or magnesium because their bodies cannot rapidly eliminate aluminum and magnesium, which may cause a toxic buildup of these substances.

Surgery for heartburn

If medications don't provide relief and your doctor has ruled out other diseases and conditions, then he or she may recommend surgery. During the operation, the surgeon wraps the top of the stomach around the bottom of the esophagus, which blocks the acid flow by constricting the LES muscle.

This procedure may sound extreme for a little heartburn, but untreated heartburn can be a serious problem. Consider this: Stomach acid that routinely overflows into your esophagus can hurt your vocal cords, irritate lung tissue and cause asthma-like wheezing (maybe asthma itself), and, according to the National Institutes of Health, contribute to cancer of the esophagus.

GERD is treated with prescription medicines (along with dietary and lifestyle changes) such as prescription H2 blockers, which are two times more potent than their nonprescription counterparts; *proton pump inhibitors* (Prevacid and Prilosec), which suppress stomach acid; and Propulsid, which quickens the pace that the stomach empties and, in turn, decreases the chance of acid causing a problem.

Preventing heartburn

With basic lifestyle changes, you can get heartburn under control. Try these tips:

- ✔ **Avoid foods that make your symptoms worse.** Foods that may cause heartburn are onions, garlic, chocolate, citrus fruits, peppermint, coffee, alcohol, tomatoes or tomato-based sauces, and fatty foods.
- ✔ **Don't smoke after eating.** Better yet, don't smoke at all.
- ✔ **Don't eat close to bedtime.** Lying down after eating can cause acid to overflow into your esophagus.
- ✔ **Elevate your head when sleeping or elevate the head of your bed about six inches.**
- ✔ **Decrease the size of your meals.** Try eating smaller meals more frequently because a full stomach is more likely to cause acid to overflow into your esophagus.
- ✔ **Wear pants that fit comfortably.**
- ✔ **Lose weight if necessary.**

Hemorrhoids

Hemorrhoids are more than the proverbial "pain in the derriere." The butt of many jokes, hemorrhoids are no laughing matter, as sufferers (about 75 million Americans) will quickly confess. A hemorrhoid, which means "flowing with blood," can cause you pain while sitting, standing, or lying down. The associated itch can prove almost unbearable. And frequently, it's no small task to eliminate the painful nuisance.

Caused by severe or repeated pressure in the anal area, hemorrhoids are inflamed or dilated veins of the anus. The anal veins drain blood away from the area, expand during a bowel movement, and return to normal size afterward. But if you repeatedly need to strain during a bowel movement (a common sign of constipation), the veins may bleed and become permanently swollen.

There are two types of hemorrhoids: internal and external. Internal hemorrhoids are located inside the anus in the wall of the rectum and may protrude through the anus outside of the body. This is called a protruding (or prolapsed) hemorrhoid, and it can become very irritated and painful. External hemorrhoids are located under the skin surrounding the anus. Sometimes a hard lump caused by a blood clot can develop. This condition is called a *thrombosed external hemorrhoid.*

Feeling and seeing the signs

The most common symptoms of hemorrhoids include the following:

- Rectal bleeding, itching, and tenderness
- Bright red blood covering the stool or toilet paper or appearing in the toilet bowl
- Discomfort or pain during a bowel movement
- Painful swelling around the anus
- A mucus discharge from the anus
- Itching around the anal opening
- A hard lump in the skin around the anus

Knowing for sure

Check with your doctor any time you have bleeding or blood in your stool for more than a couple of days, as these symptoms can be similar to the signs of other diseases such as colorectal cancer. Hemorrhoids are diagnosed through a physical examination.

Treating yourself

You can treat a mild case of hemorrhoids yourself. Popular OTC hemorrhoid medications vary in what they do. Some shrink the hemorrhoids; others merely treat the symptoms by easing the pain and itch. Some medications work to protect the area from further irritation. Preparations are available in ointment, cream, and suppositories.

If your hemorrhoids are small and not too painful, you may be able to treat yourself by taking the following measures:

- Insert a suppository or apply an over-the-counter hemorrhoidal cream or ointment to the affected area to help relieve itching and irritation.

✔ Soak in a warm bath of plain water several times a day to cleanse the area and soothe hemorrhoids. Be sure to dry the area thoroughly.

✔ Reduce swelling by applying an ice pack wrapped in a towel to the affected area.

✔ Gently clean the anal area after each bowel movement with a moistened towelette and then dry the area thoroughly.

Treating hemorrhoids with surgery

If self-care doesn't relieve hemorrhoids, you may need surgery. Internal hemorrhoids can be treated on an outpatient basis with *rubber band ligation,* a nearly painless procedure that requires no anesthetic. In this procedure, the doctor inserts a proctoscope into your rectum to view the hemorrhoid. Then, through the proctoscope, he or she places a tiny band around the base of the hemorrhoid. The band cuts off circulation, and the hemorrhoid withers away. After a few days, the band and the hemorrhoid drop off painlessly. *Sclerotherapy* is another procedure for internal hemorrhoids. The doctor injects a chemical solution around the swollen blood vessel to shrink the hemorrhoid. A protruding hemorrhoid is treated with *hemorrhoidectomy* (surgical removal).

External hemorrhoids that need surgery may be treated in one of two ways. Electrical or laser heat can be used to vaporize the tissue in a procedure called *laser coagulation.* Also, infrared light, called *infrared photo coagulation,* can be used to burn away hemorrhoids.

Preventing hemorrhoids

Prevent hemorrhoids by avoiding constipation. Exercise, plenty of fluids (at least eight 8-ounce glasses of water daily), and high-fiber foods (fruits, vegetables, beans, and whole grain products) help produce softer stools. Empty your bowels when you feel the urge to go, and avoid straining.

Indigestion

You just couldn't resist that second helping of Aunt Rosa's blueberry pie, could you? Now you're paying the price of greediness with indigestion.

A common occurrence known to most people at least once in a lifetime, indigestion *(dyspepsia)* is a term used to describe a feeling of discomfort under the breastbone and various symptoms associated with abdominal pain — especially right after eating — but it is not a disease.

Several factors can contribute to indigestion: smoking, swallowing air by chewing with your mouth open or gulping down food, drinking beverages with your meal (fluids can dilute the enzymes needed for digestion), eating foods (greasy, spicy, and refined foods) and drinking liquids (alcohol, caffeine, and vinegar) that can irritate the lining of the digestive tract, having food allergies, and emotional factors.

Indigestion may have a more serious cause, such as an intestinal obstruction, malabsorption, peptic ulcer, stomach cancer, and disorders of the gallbladder, pancreas, and liver.

Spotting the signs

Common signs of indigestion are

- Abdominal pain
- Belching
- Bloating
- Gas
- Heartburn
- Nausea
- Vomiting

Knowing for sure

If you suffer indigestion regularly and lifestyle changes or OTC medications don't bring relief, and/or if you've had problems for two consecutive weeks, you may have a peptic ulcer or other, more serious condition. Check with your doctor, who will probably ask you questions — such as when does your pain occur, what does it feel like, and where does it occur — to determine a pattern. Once your doctor detects a pattern, he or she may order tests, such as fecal occult blood tests and imaging tests (X rays, CT scans, magnetic resonance imaging, ultrasound) to determine the cause of your chronic indigestion.

Getting relief

Well, maybe you are to blame for eating that extra slice of pie, but if you usually have more self-control and find indigestion to be a rare occurrence, try these self-care tips:

✔ **Use antacids.** These drugs relieve indigestion by reducing gastric acid. They are fast-acting and provide short-term relief. Common over-the-counter antacids are Alka-Seltzer, Maalox, Tums, Tagamet, and Zantac.

✔ **Eliminate foods and drinks that provoke indigestion (such as greasy foods and alcohol).**

✔ **Eat smaller meals spread throughout the day.**

✔ **Don't smoke.**

✔ **Try to change the factors in your life that cause you stress (see Chapter 6).**

✔ **Drink an infusion of ginger tea.** Pour 1 cup of hot water over 2 teaspoons of dried or grated ginger root. Let it steep for 10 minutes, strain the grated root, and then drink the liquid.

Nausea and Vomiting

Almost everyone enjoys a ride on a roller coaster, but no one enjoys that roller-coaster feeling in the stomach. Nausea is like the anticipation of the first plunge of a roller coaster. Vomiting is the plunge. Put another way, nausea is the urge to throw up the stomach contents; vomiting is the act of throwing up. Several factors can cause nausea and vomiting: excessive eating or drinking, motion sickness (unusual or unfamiliar motion patterns can sometimes overstimulate the inner ear, which contributes to nausea and vomiting), headaches, dizziness, stomach viruses, food poisoning, or an adverse reaction to medications. Some more serious causes include stomach ulcers, hepatitis, meningitis, appendicitis, and brain tumors.

Feeling the signs

Nausea symptoms include an upset or queasy stomach, dizziness, stomach pain, and the feeling that you need to vomit. Vomiting has one symptom (one that usually keeps you chained to the toilet): forceful regurgitation of what's in your stomach.

Soothing the savage beasts

You can treat nausea with OTC medications called *antiemetics*. These drugs (for example, brand names Dramamine and Benadryl) relieve minor nausea and vomiting-related conditions (such as motion sickness) by affecting the inner ear. You can also try antacids, which can relieve nausea associated with heartburn and indigestion. You can also treat nausea with an herbal remedy. Add 1 to 2 teaspoons of powdered cinnamon to a hot cup of boiling water. Steep for 5 to 10 minutes, and then strain. Drink up to three cups daily.

Follow these steps to treat vomiting:

- Don't eat solid food until you stop vomiting.

- Drink clear liquids that are at room temperature. Take small sips, drinking only 1 to 2 ounces at a time. Suitable sources of liquids are water and sodas that have gone flat. Stir the soda to release all the bubbles before sipping it. Suck on ice chips if you can't keep anything down. You need to replenish lost fluids caused by vomiting.

- Eat clear liquid foods like gelatin and broths after you stop vomiting. If you can keep these liquid foods down, try the BRAT diet (bananas, rice, applesauce, and toast).

- Use an OTC oral rehydration medication like Emetrol. This type of medication restores your body's chemicals lost through vomiting. They work by using glucose to increase your body's absorption of sodium and encourage the rapid replacement of extracellular fluid.

- Don't smoke, and don't take aspirin.

- Call your doctor if you have been vomiting nearly continuously for more than 12 hours.

Preventing nausea and vomiting

Some vomiting is probably unavoidable, such as vomiting related to a stomach virus; however, here are a few things you can do to prevent most cases of nausea and vomiting:

- Refrain from eating or drinking to excess.

- Check for possible drug interactions with medications that you routinely take before taking additional medications.

- Throw away foods that have an unusual odor or color. Cook meats thoroughly.

- Take an OTC antiemetic before riding in a car or other vehicle if you are prone to motion sickness.

Chapter 9

Muscles, Bones, and Joints

• •

In This Chapter

▶ Treating strains and sprains

▶ Feeling and healing fractures

▶ Easing back pain

▶ Treating arthritis

• •

*O*uch! What is that pain? Is it a strain, a sprain, or worse — a broken bone? Maybe the pain you have is a joint disease, such as arthritis, or a bone disease, such as osteoporosis. And if the pain is in your back, stay tuned: We tell you what to do about it in this chapter, too.

The Musculoskeletal System

Your musculoskeletal system consists of muscles, joints, and bones. It allows you to move and acts as an armor to protect your internal organs. As marvelous as your musculoskeletal system is, breakdowns, such as strains, can occur at any time and from several causes. But before we talk about strains and other conditions, you need to be familiar with the various parts that make up your musculoskeletal system.

The muscles

Most people are not aware of how many muscles are in the human body until they catch a glimpse of bodybuilders. Even then you can't really tell that the body holds some 650 muscles. Your muscles are composed of elastic fibers that allow you to expand and contract them. This expanding and contracting motion creates movement at your joints (connections between bones).

Just about all your muscles are paired. In your upper arm, you have biceps and triceps muscles (located at the front and back of your arm, respectively). When you lower your forearms, or lower arms, your biceps extend (lengthen) and your triceps contract (shorten). Likewise, when you curl your forearms upward, your biceps contract and your triceps extend.

But not all the muscles in your body make you move. Movement is primarily the job of the skeletal, or striated, muscles (like your biceps and triceps). Muscles found in your internal organs, such as your bladder, stomach, and the walls of your blood vessels, are called smooth, or *nonstriated,* muscles. They are sometimes called involuntary muscles because you cannot consciously make them move. Another muscle you can't consciously control is your heart muscle, or *myocardium.* The smooth muscles and your heart muscle are not considered part of your musculoskeletal system because they are not directly connected to movement.

When you have pain in a muscle, you can probably attribute it to overexertion, or strain. For example, if you have been sedentary during the winter months and then in the spring enthusiastically find yourself digging a new garden, you will probably strain your unconditioned muscles. Or perhaps you decide to clean out the garage and end up with back pain instead.

The bones

Your body contains 206 bones (unless, of course, you believe you have one less rib than a woman). They are rigid parts made up of osseous tissue, which consists of proteins, bone cells, and minerals.

Although people commonly associate the skeleton with death (as Halloween decorations can attest), the bones, which make up your skeleton, are definitely alive. Forever changing, the bones support your body and act as a warehouse of sorts, storing up valuable minerals (such as calcium phosphate) to use as needed. Bones also contain *marrow* (soft tissue that fills the spongy inner spaces of the bone) where red blood cells are produced.

Pain in your bones is no laughing matter. It can occur as a result of bruising, a break, or dislocation. Sometimes the source of pain is from a more serious cause, such as osteoporosis or some other condition.

The joints

A joint is a type of hinge that allows your bones to move. It's made up of *synovial fluid* (lubricating liquid), ligaments (tough bands of fibrous tissue binding joints together and connecting bones and cartilage), a membrane, and a protective covering called a capsule. A joint is any place within your body where two or more bones meet. Joints allow movement and flexibility; you have hundreds of joints in your body. Your wrists, elbows, ankles, and knees are obvious examples of joints. Other examples of joints are found in your skull (the sutures between the plates of your skull that harden once your brain reaches its full size), your middle ear (which allows tiny bones to vibrate), and even where the roots of your teeth are embedded in your jaw.

Your muscles hold your joints together. Tendons connect the muscles to your bones. Ligaments attach bone to bone, wrapping the entire joint to keep it stable. When a joint is healthy, the ends of the bone are covered with cartilage, a smooth tissue that allows your bones to glide across each other easily.

Pain in your joints can come from several sources, such as simple overuse and sensitivity to temperature changes, or more serious conditions, such as osteoarthritis and rheumatoid arthritis. With *osteoarthritis,* a single joint becomes worn and torn — especially the cartilage. With *rheumatoid arthritis,* many or all of your joints become painful with inflammation in the synovial membrane and the cartilage. We discuss both types of arthritis later in this chapter.

Common Injuries

Your musculoskeletal system is strong but not infallible. Just about everyone has hurt a muscle, broken a bone, or sprained a joint. Too much stress can damage the most flexible muscle or rigid bone. Following are the most common types of injuries to your muscles, bones, and joints.

Strains

Strains are soft tissue injuries to your ligaments, but more usually to your muscles. You can strain a muscle through sports and exercise or through the simple activities of daily life. More usually, they occur when you fall, twist or turn suddenly, receive a blow to the affected area, or simply overuse an out-of-shape muscle.

Strains are especially common in the muscles of your feet and legs; however, they can occur at your back, shoulders, elbows, and wrists, too.

Strains are also common in your hamstrings and groin area. Your hamstrings, located behind your thighs, are the muscles that help you flex your knees and extend your thighs when you run. When you feel pain or weakness at the back of your thigh, suspect an injury to your hamstrings.

Your groin area is the part where your abdomen joins your thighs. Strains in the muscles of your abdomen, legs, and pelvic area comprise a groin pull.

Strains are classified into three categories or degrees depending on their severity:

- First-degree strains are mild or minimal injuries.
- Second-degree strains are more serious and involve a partial tearing of the muscle or ligament.
- Third-degree strains, the most severe, are those that involve the complete tearing of the muscle or ligament.

Recognizing the signs

Look for the following signs if you think you may have a muscle strain:

- Pain is localized, followed by tenderness and sometimes swelling and bruising.
- Stiffness can occur within 24 hours.
- If you can't use the injured muscle, it's probably torn.

Knowing for sure

If the pain is severe or persists for more than a few days, call your doctor. He or she will examine the injured area for signs of muscle spasms (painful contractions), swelling, and tenderness. Expect an X ray to rule out a fracture.

Treating a strain yourself

How you treat a strain depends largely on the degree of the injury. The following self-care treatment steps are commonly used to treat all strains, but serious strains require medical treatment:

- Apply an ice pack to the injured area for 10 minutes. After 10 minutes, remove the ice pack and let an additional 10 minutes pass. Repeat the ice on–ice off treatment for 60 to 90 minutes. Repeat this treatment several times in the first 24 hours following the injury. Place a towel over the area before icing to keep yourself more comfortable. If the swelling is extensive, continue to apply ice packs to the area through-out your recovery period (which may take several days).

  Fill a plastic lunch bag with crushed ice or use a bag of frozen peas or corn rather than ice cubes, which don't conform well to the injured area.
- Use a heating pad or hot water bottle or take a bath to soothe the pain.
- Compress (but don't tightly bind) the injury with an elastic bandage to help minimize swelling.
- Keep the injured area elevated.
- Stay off the injured area (or avoid lying on it in the case of an arm muscle pull), and try to rest and avoid using the injured area while it is still sore.

Treating a strain with medication

In addition to the preceding self-care techniques, you can try aspirin, acetaminophen (such as Tylenol), counterirritants (such as Ben-Gay), or some other nonprescription pain reliever for minor strains. If your strain is moderate (a second-degree strain), your doctor may prescribe an anti-inflammatory drug to reduce the swelling, a painkiller, or a muscle relaxant. You may need crutches or a sling to keep the injured area immobilized, which speeds up healing.

Treating a strain with surgery

If your strain is very serious, your doctor may recommend surgery to repair the tear. More than likely, your doctor will send you to a specialist such as a orthopedist. After surgery, expect to go through rehabilitation and physical therapy to restore strength and range of motion to your muscle.

Preventing a strain

You may not be able to prevent strains that are caused by accidents, falls, or blows to a muscle. But you may be able to prevent many injuries by warming up and stretching before exercise and cooling down afterward.

- **Warm up:** Warming up with slow, easy walking or jogging before vigorous activity increases your body temperature slightly — which makes your muscles more pliable and resistant to injury. Although you can warm up your muscles by applying a heating pad or soaking in a hot tub, warm-up exercises are more effective at preparing your muscles for vigorous activity, require no special equipment, and can be done almost anywhere.

- **Stretch:** After you warm up, stretch your muscles to lengthen them and give them a greater range of motion. To eliminate the possibility of injury, stretch no more than what you can comfortably hold for a count of 10 seconds.

- **Cool down:** Following vigorous exercise or activity, gradually slow down by slow walking or light stretching to prevent the pooling of blood in your muscles. If you suddenly stop vigorous exercise, the blood can collect in the dilated veins of your extremities and can cause dizziness or even fainting. Cooling down maintains proper circulation in your hands, arms, feet, and legs.

Sprains

The term "sprain" describes a variety of injuries, but technically speaking, sprains are injuries to the muscles, tendons, or ligaments around a joint. Sprains range from simply overstretching to tearing these bands. Your ankles, knees, and wrists are most prone to sprains.

Sprains occur when you overextend or twist a joint beyond its normal range of motion. For example, if you suddenly turn your foot sharply inward, you may sprain your ankle. If you suddenly twist your knee, or if it receives a blow, you may sprain your knee. And if you're not your usual graceful self and happen to fall, you may sprain your wrist.

Like strains, sprains are classified into three degrees or grades according to severity:

- ✔ A first-degree sprain is a mild injury that may cause some light swelling but no tearing of the ligament.

- ✔ Second-degree sprains are classified as moderate and are accompanied by obvious swelling and bruising. These moderate sprains can also result in painful or difficult joint movement.

- ✔ Third-degree sprains are the most severe and often produce swelling, bleeding, joint instability, or joint immobility.

Recognizing the signs

Remember that a sprain occurs at a joint location. With that in mind, here are the common signs of a sprain:

- ✔ Upon injury, the area rapidly swells and bruises.

- ✔ Over time, you have gradual difficulty using the injured joint.

- ✔ The injured area becomes tender and painful.

Upon injury, if you hear a popping sound at the joint and have immediate difficulty using the joint, apply ice and seek emergency medical care.

Knowing for sure

If you find that you can't use your joint at all, you probably have a fracture or a *dislocation* (the moving of any body part from its normal position). If you have pain and difficulty that doesn't go away within three days, call your doctor and expect an X ray to rule out a fracture or dislocation. In general, the more pain you feel, the more serious the sprain. Often, you can expect a sprained joint to be able to bear weight within 24 hours of the injury and be fully healed within two weeks.

Treating a sprain

How you treat a sprain depends largely on the degree of the injury. The following treatment steps are commonly used to treat all sprains, but serious sprains require medical treatment:

✔ Apply ice to reduce any swelling of the joint for the first 24 hours (see "Treating a strain yourself" earlier in this chapter).

✔ Wrap the joint with supportive elastic bandage and elevate. In the case of second-degree ankle sprains, you may need to wear a cast for up to three weeks to keep the joint from moving. Third-degree ankle sprains also require immobilization and perhaps even surgery.

✔ Don't treat a sprain with massage because ligaments heal more slowly than muscles and are not as pliable as muscle tissue.

✔ Move on to normal activity gradually after you have rested the joint for two or fewer days.

Treating a sprain with medication

You can take aspirin, acetaminophen, counterirritants, or some other nonprescription pain reliever to reduce minor pain and swelling. If necessary, your doctor may prescribe an anti-inflammatory drug.

Treating a sprain with surgery

When you have a third-degree sprain, surgery may be necessary to repair ligaments that have torn from the bone. Along with surgery, your doctor may want to immobilize the sprain with a cast. Following surgery, expect a period of rehabilitation (involving physical therapy and exercise) to make your joint strong again.

For injuries that are less serious, your doctor may order a procedure called *arthroscopic debridement*. In arthroscopic debridement, you are given a general or local anesthetic, and the surgeon makes a tiny incision along the side of your injured joint and inserts a tubelike device (consisting of magnifying lenses and fiber optics), called an *arthroscope,* in the incision. Once inside, the arthroscope allows the surgeon to view the joint and make repairs of minor tears. Recuperation time is quicker than with traditional surgery, and daily, normal activities can begin almost immediately. This procedure is usually done at the hospital but is sometimes done in outpatient surgery centers.

Preventing a sprain

As with strains, warming up before and cooling down after vigorous exercises can help prevent sprains. Here are other tips:

✔ Wrap your ankles, elbows, knees, or wrists with supportive elastic bandage (or first-aid tape) if you are prone to sprains.

✔ Use handrails on stairways for added safety.

✔ Use rugs with non-skid backing.

✔ Stick rubber mats on the floors of showers and the insides of tubs.

Fractures

Fractures are broken bones. Bone material is formed into latticelike structures that can support large amounts of weight. As you know, bones are rigid, but they can bend slightly under gentle pressure. If the pressure is more than your bones can take, however, they break.

Fractures are separated into two groups: simple and compound fractures. A simple, or incomplete, fracture occurs when a bone cracks but does not separate into two or more parts. A complete fracture is a bone that snaps into two or more sections. Fractures are further broken down into types based on three factors: the bone involved, the part of the bone, and the nature of the break.

The severity of a fracture is usually based on the amount and type of force that caused it. Bone breakage can range from a small crack in a bone to the protrusion of bone through the skin. Here are some examples of fractures, many of which are shown in Figure 9-1:

✔ A *comminuted fracture* is partially or completely shattered bone. Most are caused by automobile accidents and gunshot wounds. This fracture is quite severe and usually requires surgery.

✔ A *greenstick fracture* is an intact break limited to one side of the bone. It is common in young people.

✔ An *oblique fracture* is a break that runs on an angled course through bone.

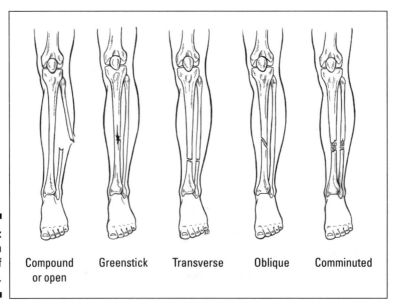

Figure 9-1:
Common types of fractures.

| Compound or open | Greenstick | Transverse | Oblique | Comminuted |

- ✔ A *transverse fracture* is a simple break that runs horizontally through bone.

- ✔ A *compound,* or *open, fracture* is a complete break that has an end piece of a broken bone protruding through skin.

- ✔ An *impacted fracture* is a piece of bone embedded into another piece of bone.

- ✔ A *pathological,* or *neoplastic, fracture* results from disease or illness, such as bone cancer and osteoporosis.

- ✔ A *stress fracture* is a hairline crack that is often missed on X rays because it usually doesn't become visible until six weeks after the injury.

Recognizing the signs

Here are the common signs of fractures:

- ✔ You see swelling and bruising over the injured bone.

- ✔ The injured limb may become deformed.

- ✔ You have localized tenderness and pain, which grows stronger if the injured area is moved or pressure is applied.

- ✔ The area of the injury does not function.

- ✔ Bone protrudes through skin in compound fractures.

Knowing for sure

Other than having bone protruding through skin, fractures are not always obvious. Also, severe sprains are sometimes mistaken for incomplete fractures. Your doctor will order an X ray to diagnose a fracture or a CAT scan in the case of vertebral (backbone) fractures, subtle stress fractures, and skull fractures.

It's not a good idea to move someone who may have a broken bone, especially if the injury appears to be in the neck or back area. Seek medical help.

Treating your broken bone

The basic idea behind the treatment of all fractures is to stop movement of the broken bone. If your bone moves following a fracture, additional damage may occur to the surrounding muscles and tissues. Therefore, a fracture must be treated with first aid and examined by a doctor.

Treating your broken bone with surgery

If the break is severe or comminuted, you may have to undergo invasive surgery (called an open reduction) that requires general anesthesia. During the procedure, your doctor makes an incision into the skin in order to set the bone in place. If the fracture is next to or extends into a joint, your doctor may use a pin, a plate, a special type of glue, or a screw to hold the bone in place. In some cases, especially in the long bones of your arms or legs, your doctor may insert rods through the center, or marrow portion, of the bone to properly align it.

Keeping your bone in place

Some fractures do not require additional immobilization. For example, in the case of broken ribs, the chest muscles surrounding your ribs act as a "natural" cast. Fractures to your toes and fingers may only require taping to an adjoining toe or finger. Following are several methods of keeping a fractured bone in place:

- ✔ **Casting:** The most common form of treatment for fractures, casts allow the fractured bone to heal while it's held together in the proper position and alignment. Before applying the cast, the limb is wrapped in soft gauze to protect the surrounding skin from chaffing.

- ✔ **Functional casting or bracing:** These casts hold the bone in place but still allow some movement of the limb or joint. Functional casts or bracing may be used in some fractures immediately following the injury or during the rehabilitation process.

- ✔ **Traction:** For bones more difficult to keep from moving, such as the thigh bone, traction is used. Traction involves the steady force of weights and pulleys to align and immobilize broken bone. Traction is applied through the use of skin tapes or through weights attached to metal pins inserted through the bone.

Getting better

Once your bone is properly set and attended to, don't expect to lie around in bed. You need to move within a day or two of treatment, even if you have a cast. Movement helps you heal faster by providing blood flow to your tissues and prevents potential harmful conditions, such as muscle and bone atrophy (wasting away) and blood clots. Moving around also helps to keep joints from becoming stiff.

Preventing a fracture

Your risk for a fracture is dependent on a few factors: age, activity level, medical condition, and risky behavior (such as mountain climbing or driving recklessly). As you age, your bones become more brittle and more likely to break. Following a healthy diet and getting adequate amounts of calcium are some ways to keep your bones healthy and strong.

Being physically active into your later years also helps keep bones strong. Regular, moderate exercise can make your bones denser, hence stronger. And if you think you're too old for exercise, a study has found that exercise by older people does not add to or cause joint pain.

Osteoporosis

Osteoporosis, sometimes known as *brittle-bone disease,* is a condition in which bones gradually lose their mineral content, becoming porous, thin, and fragile. In advanced stages, osteoporosis may cause pain, fractures, and loss of stature. It's usually considered a woman's disease; however, 20 percent of men have osteoporosis. One in eight men over the age of 50 will suffer some kind of fracture due to osteoporosis. One-third of men who suffer hip fractures as a result of osteoporosis die within a year of their injuries.

Are you at risk? Over the years, researchers have found that certain factors may lead to osteoporosis. Which possible risk factors apply to you?

✔ Caucasian, particularly with a northern European heritage or Asian race

✔ Underweight or a slender body frame

✔ Mother or father with osteoporosis

✔ Primary residence in northern areas of the country

✔ Diet low in calcium

✔ Cigarette smoking

✔ Excessive use of caffeine or alcohol

✔ Lack of exercise

✔ Use of certain medications, such as anti-inflammatory medications, sedatives, steroids, and thyroid hormones

✔ Chronic conditions of the kidneys, lungs, stomach, or intestines, or any disease that alters your hormone levels

If you think you are at risk of osteoporosis, talk with your doctor.

Indulging in risky behavior increases your chances of a fracture. When you drive, do so sensibly and wear a seat belt (whether you're the driver or passenger) even if your state doesn't have a mandatory seat belt law. Wear protective gear during sporting events and recreational activities — for example, wear a bicycle helmet while cycling.

Back Pain

Back pain, which is a very common problem, is usually a contracting pain near the lower back. Eighty percent of adults suffer from lower-back pain at some time in their lives, and most have more than one episode. Men tend to suffer more back pain than women, most likely because men tend to hold jobs that carry a high risk for back pain, such as construction and trucking.

The back is a complex integration of bone, nerves, and muscle. The spine, or backbone, consists of 33 cylindrical vertebrae stacked on top of each other to form a column (see Figure 9-2). The top seven vertebrae make up the *cervical vertebrae.* The 12 in the midback are the *thoracic vertebrae,* and the five in the lower back are the *lumbar vertebrae.* The nine remaining vertebrae at the very base the spine usually grow together by adulthood to form the *sacrum* and the *coccyx,* or tailbone.

Cushions known as discs separate the vertebrae from each other. These round, flat discs — made of collagen and filled with water — act as shock absorbers. The *facet joints* — paired connective joints that act as hinges between the vertebrae — hold the spine together (along with the nerves, muscles, ligaments, tendons, and cartilage). The spinal cord runs through a long, hollow canal formed by openings in the vertebrae.

Types of back pain

Back pain can occur anywhere in your spine; however, it's most likely to appear in your lumbar spine, or lower back. This area of the spine must endure more stress and strain than any other part of the back. Pain can also occur in the neck, or cervical spine. Acute back pain, which comes on suddenly and heals quickly, lasts fewer than three months — usually a few days to several weeks. Chronic back pain, which usually occurs slowly and is often caused by a condition or disease such as osteoporosis and certain forms of arthritis, may eventually become physically and/or emotionally disabling.

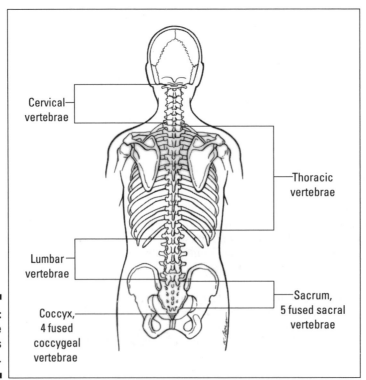

Figure 9-2:
The components of the spine.

Cervical vertebrae

Thoracic vertebrae

Lumbar vertebrae

Coccyx, 4 fused coccygeal vertebrae

Sacrum, 5 fused sacral vertebrae

Pain in your back is most often due to three factors: strained muscles, problems with a spinal disc, or problems with a facet joint. These factors can occur alone or together, making it difficult to pinpoint the cause of the pain.

More commonly, muscle strains, sprains, and spasms cause back pain. The terms strain and sprain are used similarly here in that both describe an overworked muscle, ligament, joint, or tendon. Sudden, unaccustomed exercise, a violent motion, or simply twisting your body the wrong way causes strains and sprains. A muscle spasm, usually a muscle's way of protecting an injured area, occurs when muscles painfully contract.

A herniated, or "slipped," disc is a condition that happens when the protective cushion bulges beyond its normal placement in the spine and presses on the spinal nerves (see Figure 9-3).

Finally, your facet joints can become worn or the synovial membrane can become inflamed — perhaps by arthritis (inflammation of one or more joints) or even gradual wear and tear caused by normal movement over the years. Facet joints can also be damaged if the adjoining discs become herniated because without that protective cushion, your vertebrae become compressed and rub together.

Other less common causes of back pain include osteoporosis, *scoliosis* (a sideways curve of the spine), infections (such as meningitis, an infection of the spinal cord), and other conditions.

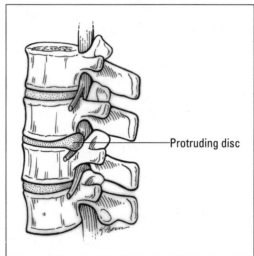

—Protruding disc

Figure 9-3:
A herniated
disc.

Recognizing the signs

The symptoms you may feel depend on the type of back pain you have. Back pain can occur anywhere in the spine, but it usually occurs in the lower back. Here are the common signs:

- Back strains and sprains produce a constant dull pain. Back spasms are sudden, painful muscular contractions. The pain can stop you from moving that muscle and therefore prevent additional damage. You can recognize the pain caused by muscular contractions, which is piercing upon movement.

- Pain from a slipped disc puts pressure on the sensitive nerve endings in the walls of the disc. In severe cases, the disc may rupture, causing the disc material to press on the nerves of the spinal cord or the spinal cord itself. When this occurs, the pain is excruciating, and you may feel it at the site of the rupture or anywhere along the route of the nerve — down to the lower back, even into your legs or feet. Unlike muscle or facet joint pain (see next bullet), disc pain may begin moderately and gradually grow worse. Disc pain sometimes lessens when you stand up and worsens as you lean backward.

Injuries to the vertebral discs can be serious and cause permanent damage to nerve function. Although these injuries are not as common as other back pain, seek medical attention if you suspect a disc injury.

- Pain due to the facet joints is hard to distinguish from muscle pain. In fact, disturbances of the facet joints can trigger muscle strain, sprains, or spasms. Facet joint pain is felt as spasms or, in the case of some degenerative situations, as a constant ache.

- Degenerative conditions of the facet joints may cause pain that shoots down the legs or buttocks. This shooting pain is called *sciatica*. The name sciatica refers to the sciatic nerve that runs down your spine and into your legs. When this nerve is pressed, you can feel pain in your back as well as your legs and buttocks. Pain worsens when you stand up straight and lessens when you lean forward.

If your back pain is characterized in any of the following ways or is accompanied by any of the following symptoms, seek professional care:

- ✔ Your back pain is constant and severe and hasn't improved after three days of bed rest.

- ✔ Your back pain is moderate but has persisted for more than a month despite efforts to relieve it.

- ✔ Your back pain disappears only to reappear on a regular basis.

- ✔ Your back pain is accompanied by a noticeable change in your bowel habits.

- ✔ Your back pain is accompanied by unexplained weight loss.

- ✔ Your back pain is accompanied by a fever that is not associated with a cold or flu.

- ✔ Your back pain is accompanied by swelling in your joints, such as your fingers, wrists, elbows, knees, or ankles.

- ✔ Your back pain is the result of a major fall or accident.

- ✔ Your back pain has been waking you up at night.

- ✔ Along with your back pain, you experience weakness in one or both of your feet.

- ✔ Along with your back pain, you have trouble raising the toes on one or both of your feet.

Knowing for sure

If you're like most people, you'll probably start with your primary-care doctor. An advantage to seeing a generalist is that a specialist, such as an orthopedist or a chiropractor, may not consider all the possible causes of back pain, including diseases or conditions that actually have nothing to do with the back. Of course, your doctor may send you to a specialist anyway.

The first thing most practitioners do — whether they're medical doctors, osteopaths, or chiropractors — is take a history to try to determine what triggered your pain. They conduct a physical examination to help determine the extent of your mobility, whether the pain comes from muscles, discs, nerves, or other sources, and what part of the back is involved.

For starters, you're asked to stand and walk. You will probably have to bend forward, backward, and sideways, twist in various directions, and walk on your heels and then your toes.

The doctor feels your spine for areas of heat, swelling, nodules, or tenderness, and palpates your back for painful muscle knots. He or she tests the strength of each muscle group, and may even measure the circumference of each thigh and calf to see if any muscle atrophy has occurred, which could indicate a disc problem. The doctor may also check your reflex by stroking the bottom of your foot. If your toes curl down, that indicates there's no damage to the spinal cord or brain.

If your doctor suspects cervical spine problems, he or she may test neck flexion (flexibility) by having you perform certain movements, such as trying to touch your ear to your shoulder. On the other hand, if low-back pain seems to be the problem, you have to take the straight-leg-raising test, in which you lie or sit on an examining table and raise each leg to see how far it can go before the pain becomes severe. This test helps determine whether spinal nerves are involved.

If your pain has persisted for longer than a month, your doctor may order diagnostic tests, including blood tests and imaging tests such as X rays, magnetic resonance imaging (MRI), and a CAT scan.

If your doctor wants to test for nerve damage, he or she may order an *electromyography,* a technique that measures the electrical impulses in your muscles. Tiny needles are inserted into the muscles being checked, and the electrical currents are viewed on a screen. During the second part of the test, electrodes are placed on the skin for studying the nerves, and a mild electric shock is sent down the nerve, revealing the speed at which nerve conduction ("message" transfer) takes place. Your doctor is likely to order the test if you feel numbness, tingling, or weakness in either of the arms or legs, which may suggest that muscles and nerves are affected.

Treating back pain yourself

Many back problems may resolve on their own. If doing nothing gives you no relief, try the following:

✔ A short period of rest (and we mean s-h-o-r-t) is usually recommended after the onset of severe back pain. Lying down for more than two days can weaken your muscles and bones, making your recovery longer. If you opt for bed rest, be sure to get up and walk around every few hours, even if your back hurts.

✔ During the first 48 hours after your back pain begins, apply a cold pack or ice pack to the area for 5 to 10 minutes at a time every few hours to numb the area and reduce inflammation. After 48 hours, use a heating pad or take a hot shower or bath up to three times daily to increase blood flow to the area.

✔ Nonprescription painkillers, such as acetaminophen, aspirin, and ibuprofen, may give some relief.

✔ Until your back feels better, avoid heaving lifting and sitting for extended periods of time. Gentle exercises such as T'ai Chi stimulate the production and release of endorphins, your body's natural painkillers, and improve the flow of blood and oxygen throughout your body.

Treating back pain through other ways

If self-treatment doesn't work, you may need to seek professional help. The first step is to see your family doctor who can properly assess the nature of your injury. He or she may recommend nonprescription painkillers or prescribe *corticosteroids,* drugs to reduce inflammation and pain, such as cortisone and prednisone. These drugs are usually used only for a short period of time due to potential side effects that include weight gain, nervousness, insomnia, increased body hair, muscle wasting, lowered resistance to infection, and mood swings.

Once diagnosed, you may want to seek treatment in the form of chiropractic therapy, physical therapy, and *spinal manipulation* — the use of hands to apply pressure to your spine in different directions and locations in order to adjust your spine. Rand, a research organization based in Santa Monica, California, conducted a study and concluded that spinal manipulation can be effective for patients with certain types of low-back pain. The study said the best candidates were people whose pain had lasted less than three weeks, who had no signs of spinal nerve damage, and whose spines appeared to be normal in X rays. Other types of treatments include massage therapy, which can stretch and loosen muscles, and acupuncture, which uses needles placed at strategic points to relieve pain. In addition, back braces, traction, and ultrasound are sometimes used, though their benefits are not proven.

In some cases, you may require surgery. There are two general types of back surgery: *decompression* (done to relieve pressure on a nerve or other spinal structure) and *fusion* (done to fuse a spinal structure together to prevent painful or damaging movement). People with nerve problems, fractures, or dislocations are the most common candidates for surgery.

Many experts maintain that much of the back surgery done in the United States is unnecessary. Seek a second opinion, and get all the information on the risks and benefits of a recommended procedure before consenting to it (see Chapter 2).

Preventing back pain

Although some forms of back pain cannot be eliminated, such as the effects of normal aging on soft tissues and bone, they can be slowed. Here are tips for preventing back pain:

- **Exercise correctly and regularly:** Obesity, poor muscle tone, and poor flexibility are all risk factors for back pain — and all factors that exercise can help remedy. Also, regular exercise keeps the muscles that support your back strong and flexible. Experts recommend a combination of aerobic exercise and strength training. But remember to warm up before each workout to avoid pulling a muscle.

- **Lift weights that you can handle and lift correctly:** As shown in Figure 9-4, place your feet shoulder-width apart to create a solid base of support. Bend at your knees, not at your waist. Let your spine curve naturally. Tighten your stomach muscles and lift with your legs, not your back. Be careful not to twist your body. Instead, point your toes in the direction you want to move and pivot in that direction. And most important — don't try to be Hercules. If the object you're trying to lift is too heavy, get some help.

- **Maintain your recommended body weight:** Estimates claim that every extra pound that goes to your abdomen adds five pounds of pressure to your back.

- **Use good posture:** Bad posture, such as slouching, puts extra stress and pressure on your spine than sitting up straight.

- **Stop smoking:** Studies have found that smokers can have three times the risk of developing disc problems in the lower back and four times the risk of having pain due to disc problems in the neck than nonsmokers.

- **Take advantage of ergonomics:** Use a chair, possibly one that reclines slightly, with good lower-back support. This is especially important if you sit for long periods. If you stand all day, try resting one foot on a small stool to take pressure off your back. Also, as the United States grays, more back-friendly tools are becoming available to prevent back pain. Shovels with specially designed handles, strange-looking chairs with huge lumbar supports, and special gardening chairs that allow you to sit while weeding your garden are only a few of the new devices on the market. Long-term clinical studies on the effectiveness of these items are lacking, but any item that can prevent back pain may be worth a try.

- **Adopt a proper sleeping position:** Most experts recommend sleeping on your back with a pillow under your knees or on your side with a pillow between your bent knees. Don't sleep on your stomach. A firm mattress also does your back good.

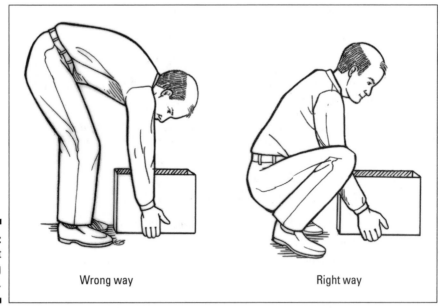

Figure 9-4:
The right
and wrong
ways to lift.

Wrong way   Right way

Arthritis

Arthritis is a term used to describe more than 100 different conditions that affect and cause pain to your joints. Arthritic disorders affect some 14 million American men. *Ankylosing spondylitis* (a rare form of inflammatory arthritis that primarily attacks the spine), gout, osteoarthritis, and rheumatoid arthritis are among the forms of arthritis that affect men. The most common form of arthritis, osteoarthritis, appears to affect both genders equally. In fact, the disease is more common in men than in women before the age of 45; after that, it's more common in women than in men. Women are three times more likely than men to develop rheumatoid arthritis, another common form of the disease that most often occurs between the ages of 35 and 50.

Gout

Gout can strike at any age, but you're more likely to have the first bout of gout when you are in your 40s.

Gout flares up when an excess of uric acid — a product of protein metabolism in your blood (called *hyperuricemia*) — causes tiny, needle-shaped crystals to form in a joint. The crystals cause the joint lining to become inflamed. If you don't treat gout, you could end up with a buildup of lumpy crystal deposits, called *tophi,* under your skin. These lumps can accumulate in other areas of your body such as the fingers, elbows, and the outer edges of the ears. If tophi are not treated, they can damage your joints.

Hyperuricemia occurs when the body makes too much uric acid or when the kidneys can't eliminate it fast enough. Even if you have hyperuricemia, you may not develop gout; however, you do have an increased risk of kidney stones (see Chapter 14). But when you do have excess uric acid in your blood, influencing factors such as joint injuries, severe illness, chemo-therapy, or an eating or drinking binge can trigger an attack of gout.

Recognizing the signs

Here are the common signs of gout:

- ✔ You experience severe, sudden pain in one joint only — usually the big toe.
- ✔ Intense pain is accompanied by swelling around the joint.
- ✔ The affected joint may appear red.
- ✔ The pain may last for several days and gradually subside within two weeks.

Knowing for sure

Along with observing the characteristic pain and swelling of gout, a blood sample to measure the levels of uric acid in your blood is necessary to diagnose gout. Your doctor may also take a sample of your synovial fluid (lubricating liquid) and examine it under a microscope for uric acid crystals to rule out pseudogout, or infectious arthritis, a condition that sometimes mimics gout.

Treating gout

Gout has no cure — you may have to be on medication for the rest of your life to prevent symptoms. But some experts recommend treating acute attacks only with medication. Drugs commonly used are colchicine (an antigout medication that seems to work by reducing inflammation), NSAIDs such as ibuprofen or naproxen, or corticosteroids — drugs to reduce inflammation and pain — such as cortisone and prednisone. Your doctor may also prescribe allopurinol, a drug that slows your body's production of uric acid. To prevent uric acid deposits in your joints and dissolve the ones already in your joints, your doctor may prescribe the drugs probenecid or sulfinpyrazone. Probenecid and sulfinpyrazone are also used to prevent and dissolve tophi.

Preventing recurrent attacks of gout

Once you're diagnosed with gout, you can do a number of things to prevent recurrent attacks. Try the following tips:

- ✔ **Drink plenty of liquids — at least 10 to 12 eight-ounce glasses of water, juice, and other nonalcoholic fluids daily.** The liquid helps your kidneys eliminate excess uric acid.

- ✔ **Maintain a healthy weight.** Obesity has been linked to high blood levels of uric acid.

- ✔ **Avoid drinking alcohol, which can contribute to gout.**

- ✔ **Don't eat foods rich in substances called *purines,* which increase uric acid production.** These include organ meats (such as liver and sweetbreads), sardines and anchovies, mushrooms, and all meat broths and gravies.

Osteoarthritis

The most common type of arthritis, osteoarthritis results in damage due to the "wear and tear" on the cartilage of your bones (see Figure 9-5). Healthy cartilage is smooth — which allows your joints to move freely — and tough, to act as a shock absorber between your bones. But in osteoarthritis, the cartilage breaks down in slow stages:

1. It becomes soft, frayed, and less elastic.

2. Large sections wear away completely, letting the ends of bones rub together.

3. As a result, your bone ends thicken, and the joints may change shape, grow spurs (bony growths), and develop fluid-filled cysts.

No one knows for sure what causes osteoarthritis or even if it's actually age-related, but heredity, obesity, injury, and overuse all appear to play roles in osteoarthritis. For example, a long-term study from the Johns Hopkins School of Medicine found that men who are 20 pounds overweight in early adulthood are nearly four times more likely than those who are not over-weight to develop osteoarthritis of the knee and hip by age 65.

Osteoarthritis can affect any joint in the body, but it's mostly found in the knees, spine, fingers, big toes, and hips. Men are especially likely to suffer from osteoarthritis of the hip.

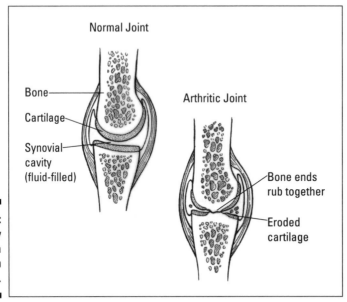

Figure 9-5:
A healthy
joint and a
joint with
osteoarthritis.

Recognizing the signs

Here are common signs associated with osteoarthritis:

- ✔ In the early stages of osteoarthritis, you may experience pain as an ache or stiffness after you do exercise that you normally don't do or during times when you are inactive.

- ✔ As the disease progresses, the pain becomes severe and throbbing but often differs from joint to joint.

  - If you have osteoarthritis in your knee, you may feel the sensation of catching or grating, compared with spinal arthritis, which may cause aching or numbness in your legs.

  - If your fingers are affected, osteoarthritis can cause the formation of large nodes in your knuckles.

Knowing for sure

Generally, your doctor diagnoses osteoarthritis by your medical history and a physical examination of the painful joints. An X ray can access the amount of damage in your joints. In addition, he or she may draw fluid from a joint by using a needle to rule out other causes of arthritis. You may also have blood tests to rule out the possibility of rheumatoid arthritis.

Treating osteoarthritis

The bad news: Osteoarthritis has no cure. The good news: You can treat its symptoms. Acetaminophen is often recommended because it relieves pain with the fewest side effects. Over-the-counter NSAIDs such as aspirin and ibuprofen reduce inflammation as well as pain and may be helpful. However, these drugs can irritate the stomach. To prevent irritation, try coated aspirin or take medications with meals.

If the pain is severe, your doctor may prescribe stronger NSAIDs and, rarely, corticosteroid injections, shot directly into your joints. Topical therapy, with creams that contain aspirin compounds or capsaicin (the hot element in chili peppers), may also relieve pain. Along with drug therapy, exercise, and physical therapy, alternative arthritis treatments (covered later in this chapter) may also bring relief.

Recently, the FDA has approved injections of hyaluronic acid (brand names are Hyalgan and Synvisc) for the treatment of osteoarthritis. Hyaluronic acid, originally developed as a treatment for lame race horses, has been used as an arthritis treatment in people in Europe and Asia for more than 10 years. Hyaluronic acid, which is made from purified rooster combs, supplements the synovial fluid of the diseased joint and has been shown to reduce pain as effectively as other drug treatments on the market. However, the long-term safety of this drug hasn't been determined at present.

Treating osteoarthritis yourself

Self-care is also a valuable tool in treating arthritis. Learning to pace yourself during the day and getting enough rest at night are two of the most important ways to help yourself if you have osteoarthritis. Rather than think about what you can no longer do, focus on what you can do instead. Take advantage of the 12-hour self-help course offered by the Arthritis Foundation (call your local chapter or call 800-283-7800 or access their Web site at www.arthritis.org). Useful devices available for the home, such as automatic can openers, are also helpful. Two other items that can make you more comfortable are a firm mattress and comfortable, well-fitting shoes.

Regular exercise increases joint protection by stimulating the production of synovial fluid, which coats the ends of the joints. Like oil, this thick substance lubricates your joints and may help prevent further damage. Gently moving the joints and stretching the muscles and tendons are the best ways to relieve strain on painful joints, improve body alignment, and help you feel more relaxed and in control of your disease. You should do a few simple, carefully controlled mobility and stretching movements once or twice daily, even when your joints are swollen and painful.

Rest is also important because it can lessen inflammation. The key is balance. Adjust the amount of rest and exercise according to the stage of your disease and how you feel each day. Too much inactivity makes the condition worse, but too much exercise puts you at risk for exhaustion, injury, and more pain. Experts now advise you to exercise as much as you can to increase movement and strength, improve the functioning of the joints, and create better all-around physical well-being. Learn to listen to your body and know when it's telling you to take things easy.

Treating osteoarthritis with surgery

Your doctor may recommend surgery if your joints are severely damaged. One procedure, called *osteotomy,* corrects bone deformity by cutting the bone and repositioning it. Osteotomy is usually done on the knee, as is arthroscopic debridement (see the section "Treating a sprain with surgery" earlier in this chapter). Total joint *arthroplasty* involves resurfacing, or relining, the ends of the bones so they can move more freely against each other; this term is also used for total joint replacement in which the joint is removed and a metal, ceramic, or plastic device is inserted in its place.

Preventing osteoarthritis

You can do several things to lower your risk of developing osteoarthritis:

- ✔ **Exercise.** It can be your best tool against osteoarthritis because exercise strengthens your muscles and works to keep your joints flexible. Exercise can also help you maintain a healthy weight (or lose weight if necessary). Obesity is often considered a factor in some types of arthritis. However, be sensible: Don't overdo high-impact aerobics such as running. And if a particular joint (for example, those in your knees, ankles, and feet) starts to suffer from overuse, change your exercise regimen. Try low-impact exercises such as walking and swimming and stretching exercises to loosen your joints, increase your range of motion, strengthen your muscles, and more important, relieve arthritis pain.

- ✔ **Protect your knees against injury during sports, starting in your teens.** Wear protective gear such as knee and elbow pads when playing contact sports or other, riskier sports such as in-line skating.

- ✔ **Sit straight and don't slump.** Your mother was right! Good posture, whether sitting or standing, can help reduce the pressure on the joints, especially those in your spine.

- ✔ **Learn to perform your job without stressing your joints.** If your job requires repetitive movement (such as typing) or movement that stresses your joints, be sure to vary your activities and working position as much as possible.

- ✔ **Wear a seat belt to prevent injury to your knees (and other body parts) in case of a car accident.**

Rheumatoid arthritis

Rheumatoid arthritis (RA) is a less common form of arthritis that causes inflammation in the joints and other parts of your body, including the connective tissue that surrounds organs such as your heart and lungs. This form of arthritis is very debilitating, inflaming the synovial membranes. The affected membranes thicken and become tough and fibrous, causing pain when you move the joint. Because RA can cause deformities in the joints, it can lead to loss of mobility.

RA differs from osteoarthritis in that it occurs in younger people between the ages of 20 and 40. It is also more painful than osteoarthritis and can cause joint inflammation and severe breakdown. If you have RA, you can also experience fatigue, loss of appetite, weight loss, fever, and general malaise, whereas osteoarthritis symptoms are limited to joint pain. The disease is usually chronic (long-term) but tends to cycle between active and inactive periods called flare-ups and remission.

No one knows what causes RA; many think it is an autoimmune disease — a disease in which your body's immune system malfunctions and attacks its own tissues. RA also has a genetic factor — if a parent or sibling has the disease, you're up to five times more likely than the rest of the population to have it. If you think you may have RA, seek treatment as soon as possible because the sooner you begin treatment, the better your chances of recovery.

Recognizing the signs

Here are the common signs of RA:

- ✔ You experience swelling, pain, and warmth in the joints, especially in the smaller joints of the hands and feet.
- ✔ You have an overall feeling of aching and stiffness in the joints.
- ✔ The stiffness is pronounced after a period of inactivity, such as when watching a movie or sleeping.

Knowing for sure

As with osteoarthritis, you can expect your doctor to ask about your medical history and perform a physical examination to diagnose RA. Your doctor may also order blood tests such as a CBC (which measures the amount of red and white blood cells and platelets in your blood), a *sedimentation rate test* (which shows how fast your blood cells cling together), and a test for *rheumatoid factor* (a protein that shows the presence of inflammation).

Treating rheumatoid arthritis

As with osteoarthritis, treatment focuses on relieving your symptoms rather than curing the disease. Your doctor may prescribe aspirin and other NSAIDs for pain relief because of the anti-inflammatory properties of these drugs. Corticosteroid drugs such as prednisone and cortisone are sometimes prescribed for the treatment of RA. If your doctor prescribes steroid drugs, you may be on them for a short period of time only because of potential side effects that include weight gain, nervousness, insomnia, increased body hair, muscle wasting, lowered resistance to infection, and mood swings.

Other drugs, called *remittive agents,* are thought to slow the progression of RA. These include gold salts (taken orally or as injection), Plaquenil (a malaria drug), penicillamine, and methotrexate. These drugs work slowly, over a few weeks or more, to bring about a remission or partial remission. However, little scientific evidence shows that they are effective, despite the fact that they sometimes work.

Treating rheumatoid arthritis yourself

In addition to drug therapy, exercises that strengthen your muscles and normal activity can restore some function to your joints. However, because RA cycles between flare-ups and remission, you need a balanced approach of rest and exercise in treating the disease. During flare-ups, avoid exercising the affected joints, and during remission, return to exercise and normal activities. Know your limits and follow the advice of your doctor or physical therapist.

Treating rheumatoid arthritis with surgery

As with osteoarthritis, surgery may be used as a last resort. Procedures include *synovectomy,* in which the thickened lining of the diseased joint is removed. Other procedures flush out debris caused by the wearing down of joints. An affected joint may also be fused or changed (for example, the angle or length of your bones changed), or your entire joint may be replaced. Joint replacement, a complicated technique, is another procedure that may be done when other medical treatments have failed and the painful joint is beyond repair.

For a knee replacement, done under general anesthesia, the surgeon usually makes one long incision on the front of the joint. He or she cuts through the joint capsule and synovium and then pushes aside the kneecap to get at the joint. Special surgical tools are used to carefully measure the joint and cut, shape, and drill both the femur and the tibia (the larger calf bone) so that they can accept the artificial joint. The bottom half of the knee joint is a metal plate with a slight depression in its center. The top half is a metal cap that fits over this rounded bone. The metal cap rests in the bottom plate. Part of the back of the kneecap is cut away to give a flat surface and then drilled to accept the kneecap part of the joint.

Alternative arthritis treatments

Along with medication and exercise therapy, here are several therapies you can try when treating osteoarthritis and rheumatoid arthritis:

- **Physical therapy:** This form of therapy restores or keeps the range of motion in your joints and strengthens the surrounding muscles. A physical therapist can help you learn how to use supportive devices, such as crutches, canes, and braces, and also teach you to do everyday tasks with as little pain as possible.

- **Heat and cold therapy:** Apply heat to your joints to increase blood flow and loosen the joints. Apply cold to your joints to relieve pain.

- **Hydrotherapy:** Not only is soaking in a whirlpool or hot tub pleasurable, but it may also help to loosen tight joints and reduce some of the pressure on your aching joints by providing heat and buoyancy.

- **Diet therapy:** Some experts believe that certain foods are linked to arthritis symptoms. In some studies, milk and cheese were found to cause symptoms. Other research shows foods in the nightshade family (chili and bell peppers, eggplants, tomatoes, and potatoes) trigger arthritis flare-ups.

  Other studies show that foods containing omega-6 fatty acids (vegetable oils such as safflower, soy, sesame, and sunflower) can produce inflammatory chemicals in the body. On the other hand, foods that contain omega-3 fatty acids (salmon, sardines, and mackerel) may have an anti-inflammatory effect.

- **Antioxidants:** There may be some evidence that not having enough *antioxidants* (molecules that help fight against *free radicals* — destructive molecules made in the body by a chemical process called oxidation), such as vitamins E and A and beta-carotene, could be a precursor to rheumatoid arthritis. In an article reported in the *Annals of Rheumatic Diseases*, researchers identified 21 people with rheumatoid arthritis who had developed the disease within 2 to 15 years of donating blood. These people were matched up with 108 healthy people who had also donated blood simultaneously. Blood samples revealed that the people with rheumatoid arthritis had lower levels of several types of antioxidants, including beta-carotene and vitamins A and D at the time they donated blood than the 108 healthy people. Additional studies have found that vitamin E may help ease swelling, pain, and morning stiffness associated with osteoarthritis and rheumatoid arthritis. For proper amounts and good sources of antioxidants, see Chapter 1.

- **Dietary supplements:** Supplements such as chondroitin and glucosamine, two compounds found in healthy joints, have shown promise in relieving pain and improving mobility. In European tests, they have performed at least as effectively as currently prescribed medications.

They are taken separately or in combination — either in a pill or as a powder that can be mixed with a liquid. Because these are sold as dietary supplements in your local health food store, they are not monitored or tested for safety and efficacy by the FDA.

✔ **Herbal therapy:** Some herbs that may help to relieve arthritis pain include arnica, feverfew, devil's claw, meadowsweet, cayenne pepper, and stinging nettles. However, because not all herbal therapies are effective or safe for everyone, you should speak with your doctor.

Chapter 10

Hair Loss

*A*long with losing sexual potency and being audited, hair loss is a major fear for men. For most men, hair loss is eventual. More than 66 percent of all men will experience some hair loss, or *alopecia,* during their lifetime. Those who become bald usually have significant hair loss by age 35. Even as topical solutions such as Rogaine have grown in popularity in recent years and science has helped diagnose causes for hair loss, no cure is available at this time. Fortunately, you do have options, and this chapter shows you what they are if you're concerned about hair loss.

What's Going On Up There?

Although the average person loses about 100 hairs a day — not to worry, the human head contains about 100,000 hairs — men are more likely to lose their hair than women are. According to a study by the American Hair Loss Council in Chicago, 19.5 million women lose hair in some form, but that number jumps to 33 million for men.

Many factors can cause hair loss, including stress, heredity, chemotherapy, medical conditions (such as ringworm), hormonal changes, and old age. Male-pattern baldness (MPB), the most common type of hair loss, can begin in men in their late teens or early 20s. By the age of 35 to 40, about 66 percent of Caucasian men will show some signs of hair loss. Men who begin to lose hair at a younger age are more likely to suffer severe baldness than men who begin to lose hair at an older age.

If your mother's father or her male relatives went bald, you're more likely to eventually have a hair-free scalp. Hereditary male-pattern baldness usually passes through the mother's genes.

How hair is lost

Understanding how hair is lost can help you and your doctor deal with the problem. *Androgenetic alopecia,* or male-pattern baldness (MPB), begins when an enzyme called *5-alpha reductase* in a hair follicle (the place where hair grows) combines with testosterone. The enzyme changes testosterone into a hormone called dihydrotestosterone (DHT). Researchers believe that DHT causes the hair follicles to shrink until hair grows thinner and smaller and eventually forms what looks like the fuzz on a Georgia peach.

Hair loss types

In addition to MPB, which accounts for 95 percent of all hair loss, other types of hair loss include the following:

- *Alopecia areata:* With this condition, hair falls out in patches or clumps, as the result of some immune disorder.

- *Alopecia totalis:* A rare, advanced from of *Alopecia areata,* this condition is total loss of hair on the head.

- *Alopecia universalis:* Another rare, advanced form of *Alopecia areata,* this condition is a complete loss of all body hair.

- *Anagen effluvium:* With this condition, hair falls out due to chemotherapeutic agents used in treating cancer that poison growing hair follicles.

With the exception of *Anagen effluvium,* call your doctor if you experience any of the above types of hair loss.

Signs of hair loss

Don't expect to find clumps of hair fall into your sink, because hair loss normally doesn't happen overnight. Hair loss caused by MPB can happen so slowly that you may not notice it until the sun's rays begin to glint off your scalp. MPB usually progresses as follows (see Figure 10-1):

1. The hairline recedes, forming what is known as a "widow's peak."

2. The hair on the crown also thins, eventually causing a bald spot.

3. Sometimes the receding hairline and the expanding bald spot connect, leaving a ring of hair around the sides and back of the head.

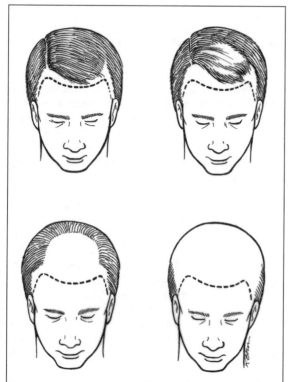

Figure 10-1:
The progression of male pattern baldness.

Myths about hair loss

Of course, there are some things you don't need to worry about when it comes to your hair. For example, did anyone ever tell you that wearing a hat or washing your hair frequently will hasten the loss of your hair? Those are myths. Eating right doesn't guarantee you'll have a thicker head of hair, either. Nor does dandruff speed you along the road to Telly Savalas-ville.

Treating Hair Loss

Sorry, guys. You won't be able to stop inevitable hair loss that comes with age and genetics. However, if the process is too quick or problematic for your liking, consult your doctor or dermatologist, who may be able to prescribe medical treatment or other alternatives.

Pharmacological treatment

The first word in drug treatment for hair loss today is topical minoxidil (Rogaine), manufactured by Pharmacia & Upjohn. Minoxidil is an agent that saves hair follicles from shrinking by tackling the testosterone in the follicles. Available only by prescription before 1996, minoxidil is now sold over the counter. Initially, minoxidil was designed to reduce high blood pressure, which it did effectively, but one of its side effects was the "awakening" of dormant hair follicles — and not just on the top of the head. The exact way minoxidil works is unknown. It doesn't create new hair follicles, but it does stop the shrinking process of existing ones and encourages regrowth of hair that tends to be very fine, like that of a newborn's. Researchers also believe that minoxidil opens potassium channels that may increase circulation to the scalp or even stimulate hair follicles directly.

Minoxidil, a colorless solution available in various strengths (2 or 5 percent), must be applied to the scalp twice daily for best results. But don't expect results until after four to six months of daily use. Unfortunately, one disadvantage of using minoxidil is that you commit yourself to it for life. Otherwise, if you stop treatment, any hair that was previously saved or regrown due to the treatment falls out. Possible side effects associated with minoxidil include irritation, rash, itching, and dry or flaking skin.

This drug works its magic best at the top of the head. You're more likely to see good results with minoxidil if you have a mild case of hair loss and/or have lost your hair recently.

If you don't like the idea of applying medication to your scalp daily, you may want to try a new oral pill instead. Propecia, cleared by the U.S. Food and Drug Administration in December 1997, blocks the enzyme responsible for hair loss and inhibits the conversion of testosterone into DHT. Manufactured by Merck, Propecia is the brand name given to finasteride (1 mg strength). Finasteride, in a stronger strength (5 mg), is used to treat *prostatic benign hypertrophy* (enlargement of the prostate gland) and is sold under the name Proscar.

Propecia, unlike Rogaine, is for men only and is currently only available through a prescription. Possible side effects include a decrease in semen, difficulty in achieving erection, and a diminished desire for sex. Men with liver problems should avoid using this medication.

Because of the risk of birth defects to the fetus, pregnant women and women of childbearing age should not come in contact with Propecia. During intercourse, wear a condom to avoid passing the drug to your mate via the sperm.

Studies have shown that Rogaine and Propecia can be effective in treating MPB. As with any medicine, however, successful results vary from person to person. The 5 percent solution of Rogaine appears more effective than the 2 percent solution for overall hair regrowth and thickness. However, itchiness and dryness occur more frequently with the 5 percent solution. At present, there are no direct comparison studies between Rogaine and Propecia, but clinical trials comparing the two drugs with placebos show that 50 percent of the subjects reported an increase in hair growth for both drugs.

If you don't want to use drug treatment or if it fails to give you the results you want, then surgery may be an option.

Surgical treatment

Hair replacement surgery is an alternative for men who find that self-care measures (which we cover later in this chapter) or drug treatments (which we cover earlier) don't help in their fight against hair loss.

Hair replacement surgery consists of three main types of techniques, which are shown in Figure 10-2:

- ✔ Hair transplants
- ✔ Hair flap surgery
- ✔ Scalp reduction

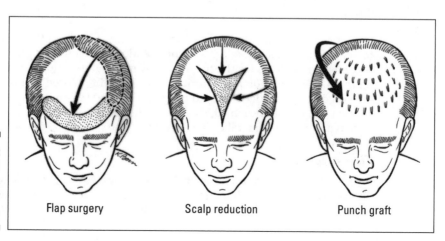

Figure 10-2: Surgical treatments for hair loss.

Flap surgery   Scalp reduction   Punch graft

It is not uncommon for a doctor to perform more than one of these techniques on one man for best results. And don't worry, guys — anesthesia is used.

Hair replacement surgery can enhance your looks, but don't expect to come out of it looking like Fabio. First, discuss your expectations with the surgeon and then decide if surgery is for you. Keep in mind that this type of surgery works with your existing hair located at the back and sides of the head. Also, the surgery is likely to be more effective if your hair is thick and curly.

Hair replacement surgery rarely requires an overnight stay at the hospital; it is usually performed on an outpatient basis.

Hair transplants

If you're looking for modest changes in the thickness of your hair, then hair transplants may be a good choice. This surgical process, also known as *grafting,* removes small portions of hair-bearing scalp grafts from the donor site (the sides or back of the head) and relocates them, about $^1/_8$ inch apart from each other, to the bald or thinning areas. (Don't worry: The grafts taken from the donor sites will not leave you bald in those areas.) Grafts vary in size and shape and range from a micro graft (1 to 2 hairs) to a strip graft (30 to 40 hairs).

Before surgery, your hair in the donor area is trimmed short to make the grafts easier to remove. The surgeon may either use a special tubelike instrument to punch a small, round graft (called a *punch graft*) out of the donor area or a scalpel to remove tiny sections of hair-bearing scalp. When the surgeon takes the grafts, he or she may inject small amounts of saline solution into your scalp to keep the skin strong. The donor site holes are usually closed with stitches and are usually hidden within the surrounding hair. After the grafting session is complete, your scalp is cleansed and covered with gauze. (You may have to wear a pressure bandage for two days.)

Expect several surgical sessions (which usually last about three hours each) to achieve best results, and it's recommended that you take a few months off between sessions for the healing. How much coverage you need depends on the texture and color of your hair. Coarse, light-colored hair offers better coverage than fine, dark-colored hair. Don't forget to bring your wallet: One session can cost between $3,500 and $8,500. Considering that the entire transplant process can take as long as two years, start saving now.

Flap surgery

If you're looking for a dramatic change, then flap surgery may be a good choice. This procedure has the advantage of covering large areas of baldness rather quickly (one flap can cover an area comparable to 350 or more punch grafts). It involves cutting out a section of bald scalp and lifting off a flap of hair-bearing skin still attached at one end. The hair-bearing flap is moved into its new position and sewn into place, while staying connected to its original supply of blood. The scar resulting from the surgery can be covered up by the relocated flap of hair. Flap surgery is more extensive than other procedures: Expect to pay between $3,500 and $10,000.

Scalp reduction

This procedure also offers dramatic change and is best for covering bald areas at the back and crown. Sometimes called *advancement flap surgery,* this procedure pulls sections of hair-bearing scalp forward to fill in a bald crown. Almost all scalp reductions are done in combination with either grafts or flaps.

In this process, a piece of skin from the scalp is cut out. If a large amount of coverage is the goal, the surgeon removes a segment of scalp shaped like an inverted "Y." Excisions can be other shapes as well, such as a "U" or a pointed oval. The surrounding edges are pulled together and stitched, and the process can be painful due to the extensive tugging and pulling of the scalp. Several sessions may be necessary, and the average cost is $1,600 per procedure.

Alternatives to surgery

If you elect not to go the surgical route to treat your hair loss, you can try other alternatives.

Nonsurgical hair addition is an option. Examples include hair weaves, toupees, and wigs. Check your local hair salon and wig store to find hair additions or ask your doctor for a reference. Keep in mind that the quality of hair additions varies (just as hair replacement surgery is only as good as the surgeon performing it). Hair additions consist of human or synthetic hair, or a combination of both, and give the appearance of fuller hair. They can cost between $750 and $2,500.

- ✓ **Hair weaves:** Weaves are made by weaving or braiding human or synthetic hair (or a combination of both) into your existing hair. Hair weaves are not without problems because they make it difficult to keep the hair and scalp clean. Also, because they are woven into existing hair, they can stress the existing hair, which may possibly cause more hair loss. Another downside is that as your natural hair grows, the extensions must be repositioned every four to six weeks. Expect to pay up to $2,500.

- ✔ **Toupees:** These items are made from either human or synthetic hair and are kept in place with adhesives or clips. Toupees vary in quality, and the really bad ones are easy to spot. Human hair toupees look very natural but tend to break down sooner and can cost around $1,000. If you're active, synthetic toupees are better because they are easier to keep clean and last longer. Expect to pay $150 or more for a synthetic one.

- ✔ **Wigs:** Like toupees, wigs are made from either human or synthetic hair and cover the head more fully than other options. Prices are comparable to that of toupees.

If you do choose a hair addition, make sure to maintain proper hygiene. Keep your hair and scalp clean. Adhesives (such as two-sided tapes) are safe to use, but because the possibility of an allergic reaction exists, you may want to have a patch test done before using one.

Self-care

You can do some things on your own to battle hair loss, but remember, you can't prevent eventual hair loss. Your goal is to protect your hair follicles from damaging chemicals, styling techniques, and other products. Hair products that change the color (dyes and bleaches) or texture (perms and straighteners) of your hair can damage hair follicles. What you do to your hair can also damage the follicles — drying your hair with a hair dryer or braiding and cornrowing your hair, for example. If your scalp is sensitive, stick to gentle shampoos and conditioners, such as those used for infants.

Avoiding stress is also a good way to help keep your hair in place, but avoiding stress today is about as possible as avoiding a late-night infomercial. Rather, deal with stress through exercise, rest, and other mechanisms that help both your sanity and your hair (see Chapter 6).

Try a new hairstyle if you have partial hair loss. Cut your hair short or blunt because either style makes hair look thicker and less patchy. Stay away from gels, as they tend to clump hair together, emphasizing thinning hair.

For something more simple, try a completely bald look. Michael Jordan is bald, and he's one of the richest, most well-liked guys on the planet. Bald is trendy!

Chapter 11

Skin Disorders

• •

In This Chapter

▶ Understanding your skin

▶ Treating irritating skin conditions

▶ Keeping your skin healthy

• •

*B*eauty is only skin deep or so the saying goes. Whether or not the skin reflects who we are on the outside, it's more than just a thing of beauty: The skin is an organ — a rather large organ. Weighing in at six pounds and covering about 25 square feet of area, the skin is the largest and most visible organ of your body. But as big and tough as it may be, the skin is also your most vulnerable organ — routinely exposed to chemicals, bacteria, ultraviolet rays, and other damaging entities.

You may think that taking care of your skin is merely a cosmetic concern, but it's much more than that: Keeping the skin healthy boosts your immune system, helps your body regulate its temperature, and helps in the production of vitamin D. The skin is rather fascinating, isn't it? Keep on reading because we have lots to say about it.

Anatomy of the Skin

Although it measures only 6 millimeters thick on the soles of the feet and a mere $1/2$ millimeter on the eyelids, the skin is well equipped to perform its many functions (see Figure 11-1). An average square inch of the skin contains some 600 sweat glands, 100 fat glands, 100 oil glands, 65 hairs, 20 blood vessels, and thousands of nerve endings. These structures are contained within the three layers of the skin — the epidermis, the dermis, and the subcutaneous tissue.

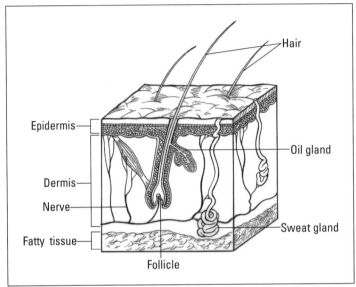

Figure 11-1:
A cross
section of
skin.

Labels on figure: Hair, Epidermis, Oil gland, Dermis, Nerve, Sweat gland, Fatty tissue, Follicle

The epidermis

The epidermis, the topmost layer of the skin, is only 0.1 to 1.5 millimeters thick. It's made up of five layers: the basal cell layer, the squamous cell layer, the stratum granulosum, the stratum lucidum, and the stratum corneum. Working together, these layers continually rebuild the surface of the skin from within, maintaining the skin's strength and helping to prevent wear and tear. Also found in the epidermis are *keratinocytes* (producers of keratin), *melanocytes* (producers of melanin, the skin's pigment), and Langerhans' cells, which are linked to immune system function. The epidermis not only regulates bodily water loss (through openings called the pores), but it also serves as a barrier against the environment for the rest of the internal organs. It also produces new skin cells.

The dermis

The dermis, which lies just beneath the epidermis, is 1.5 to 4 millimeters thick — the thickest of the three layers of the skin. It's also home to most of the skin's structures, including sweat and oil glands (which secrete substances through openings in the skin called pores, or *comedos*), hair follicles, nerve endings, and blood and lymph vessels. The main components of the dermis are *collagen* (a tough, insoluble protein found throughout the body in the connective tissues that hold muscles and organs in place) and *elastin* (a similar protein that keeps the skin flexible).

In addition to collagen and elastin, the dermis contains water. In fact, the dermis stores much of the body's water supply. When the amount of stored water increases — for example, when you're retaining water — the skin becomes tight and expands to accommodate the surplus. The dermis also contains scavenger cells from the immune system. If intruders (such as bacteria) pass through the epidermis, these cells engulf and destroy the uninvited guests.

The subcutaneous tissue

The subcutaneous tissue is the deepest layer of the skin. It is missing on parts of the body where the skin is especially thin — the eyelids, nipples, genitals, and shins. Subcutaneous tissue acts both as an insulator, conserving body heat, and as a shock absorber, protecting internal organs from injury. It also stores fat as an energy reserve in the event that you need extra calories to power the body. The blood vessels, nerves, lymph vessels, and hair follicles also cross through this layer.

Common Skin Problems

More than a thousand conditions can affect your skin. These problems are too numerous to describe individually, so we'll take a look at some common skin problems.

Skin conditions range from the mild to the very dangerous. Keep in mind that something as simple as a skin rash may be a sign of some other, deep-rooted problem and may require more intensive medical treatment to bring the symptoms under control.

Athlete's foot

Athlete's foot *(tinea pedis)* is a fungal infection of the feet. It's caused by a group of fungi called *dermatophytes,* commonly known as ringworm. These fungi can be passed by people, animals, soil, or an artificial humid environment such as a shower stall or locker room. Fungi thrive in warm, moist environments, such as those created by perspiration. Socks can soak up perspiration, providing the perfect breeding ground for fungi if they are not changed daily. Athlete's foot is most common among teenage and adult males.

Recognizing the signs

Here are the common signs of athlete's foot:

- ✔ The area of the toes may burn and itch.
- ✔ The skin may peel and crack, especially around the toes.
- ✔ Minor bleeding may accompany cracked skin.

Knowing for sure

Athlete's foot is fairly easy to spot because the signs are so specific and confined to the feet. However, if self-care and medical treatment (which we discuss later in this chapter) do not bring relief, your doctor may have to examine your feet. Most likely, he or she will scrape a tiny section of the affected area to send off to a laboratory for analysis.

Treating athlete's foot

Numerous over-the-counter (OTC) antifungal creams, solutions, and powders treat athlete's foot. Examples of antifungals include Lotrimin AF, Absorbine Jr. Antifungal Foot, and Tinactin. You must apply the medication for the entire length of time directed even if the symptoms subside. The medication may take up to six weeks to clear up the infection. In addition to treating your feet with medication, wash them twice daily, making sure to dry the feet completely before applying medication. Change your socks at least once daily and, if possible, your shoes. Expose your feet to light and air as much as possible. Should the symptoms continue past six weeks, stop self-treatment and seek the advice of a physician.

Preventing athlete's foot

You can prevent athlete's foot by following these easy instructions:

- ✔ Wash your feet at least once daily.
- ✔ Keep your feet thoroughly dry. After showering or bathing, apply cornstarch or powder to the toes to absorb moisture.
- ✔ Avoid tight shoes, especially in warm weather. Sandals are the best summer footwear.
- ✔ Keep your feet dry by wearing dry shoes and absorbent cotton socks or by dusting the feet with absorbent powder. White socks are better than colored socks because they reflect sunlight and don't contribute to heat buildup inside shoes.
- ✔ Expose your feet to light and air as much as you can. Go barefoot at home if possible. However, if you're prone to athlete's foot, don't go barefoot in locker rooms or around swimming pools where you may come in contact with fungi.
- ✔ Sprinkle an antifungal powder into your shoes during the warm months.

Jock itch

Jock itch *(tinea cruris)* is a fungal infection of the groin. It's caused by the same fungus responsible for athlete's foot. Likewise, it spreads in the same manner as athlete's foot (by people, animals, soil, shower stalls, or anything else that holds moisture). Because fungi thrive in warm, moist environments, such as those created by sweating, jock itch is common in men who wear jock straps (athletic supporters) or spandex shorts.

Recognizing the signs

Here are the common signs of jock itch:

- The genitals and inner thighs may burn and itch.
- Red, scaly lesions or rings on the genitals and inner thighs may accompany burning and itching.

Knowing for sure

Like athlete's foot, jock itch is usually easy to spot because it's confined to the groin area and the signs are so specific. However, if you need confirmation, your doctor can examine you and if necessary, send a sample of the affected area to a laboratory for analysis.

Treating jock itch

Even though jock itch can be irritating and annoying, it's usually not difficult to treat. To get rid of jock itch, apply a topical OTC antifungal ointment, such as Cruex, Lotrimin, or Tinactin, to the affected area for two weeks after symptoms disappear to make sure that the fungi are gone for good. Sometimes, the fungi can affect other parts of the body, such as the scalp and the nails. If this should happen, your doctor can prescribe an oral antifungal medication such as griseofulvin.

Preventing jock itch

To avert a future infection, make the groin area inhospitable for the fungi by following these tips:

- Keep the skin around your groin area clean and dry.
- Wear absorbent cotton underwear.
- Use drying powders and products that reduce sweating.
- Change out of sweaty or wet gear as soon as possible after athletic activity.
- Use a clean towel from home if you plan to shower at the gym — a breeding ground for fungi and other germs — and dry off from head to toe, not vice versa.

Acne

Acne, the most common skin condition, is the reason behind 25 percent of all visits to the dermatologist. In acne, a sebaceous gland within a hair follicle overproduces oil, which irritates the follicle's lining. The excess oil also causes *Propionibacterium acnes* bacteria trapped in the follicle to produce a substance that causes cells lining the follicle to clump together. Pressure builds in the pore, pushing up a plug of trapped oil and debris to the skin's surface. If the follicle is open, a blackhead, or open comedo, occurs. If the pore is tightly closed, a whitehead, or closed comedo, occurs. If a follicle ruptures, a pimple develops. If the oil continues to build up and the follicle does not rupture, cysts — large, movable lumps — may develop under the surface of the skin.

Acne is common in teenagers, especially boys. However, as your mirror may reveal, acne isn't restricted to this age group and affects men into their 40s. Although *androgens* (hormones that stimulate the development of male sex characteristics) play an important role in the development of acne, heredity is a factor.

Recognizing the signs

Here are the most common signs of acne:

- Raised swellings, usually located on the back, chest, face, neck, and shoulders.
- Pus-filled plugs that break open and release fluid (in severe cases).
- Soreness, pain, and itching in the affected area.

Knowing for sure

Acne is usually easy to identify. However, pimplelike, pus-filled sacs without blackheads or whiteheads may be another disease. To be sure, make an appointment with your family doctor or dermatologist who can examine you.

Pimple-producing foods?

You've probably heard that certain foods, such as chocolate, can trigger acne flare-ups. However, there's little scientific proof that this is the case. But if you notice that certain foods seem to worsen your acne, you may want to avoid such foods. Discuss this issue with your doctor.

Treating acne yourself

Be patient: Dealing with acne may require consistent and long-term treatment. First, identify factors that trigger acne flare-ups and eliminate them if possible. For example, if stress seems to worsen your acne, practice relaxation techniques (such as deep breathing). Second, don't pick at pimples; instead, follow your doctor's advice about removing blackheads and pimples, or have your dermatologist remove them. Third, use cleansers or soaps that dry out the skin to promote minor flaking, which helps flake off clogged follicle plugs. Fourth, use OTC products that contain benzoyl peroxide to dry acne and slow the growth of skin bacteria. You can use products that contain salicylic acid, sulfur, or resorcinol to dry existing acne, though they can't prevent new blemishes. Finally, avoid the sun if possible because sunlight can cause acne to darken, making it look worse.

Treating acne with medication

Topical or oral antibiotics (commonly tetracycline) may be used to kill bacteria within the follicles. The drug tretinoin (brand name Retin-A) alleviates acne by increasing the production of the cells that line follicle walls, which release trapped oils from the pores. Isotretinoin (Accutane) shrinks oil glands to relieve acne. Azelaic acid (Azelex), a newer drug, works by fighting bacteria.

Treating acne with surgery

Your family doctor or dermatologist may surgically drain cysts if necessary, using minor surgery and a local anesthetic. Your doctor can perform the surgery in his or her office.

Dermabrasion and chemical peeling are techniques used to lessen scars left by acne. Dermabrasion is usually reserved for severe scarring and involves rubbing the skin with a rotating wire brush or sandpaper. Your doctor will use a local or topical anesthetic. Chemical peeling involves the application of powerful exfoliating chemicals to remove the surface of the skin, revealing the new, undamaged skin beneath.

Shaving and acne

If you have acne and you shave, try both an electric and a safety razor to see which is more comfortable. When using a safety razor, soften your beard with warm soap and water and then shave as lightly as possible over the skin. Always use a sharp blade.

Preventing acne

Try washing with a mild soap, such as those used for infants. Use oil-free, noncomedogenic skin-care products. Avoid abrasive cleansers and masks, and if your hair is long, wear it away from your face.

Dermatitis

Dermatitis, or eczema, is a general term used to describe any inflammation of the skin. Examples of eczema include *atopic dermatitis, allergic contact dermatitis,* and *seborrheic dermatitis.*

✔ **Atopic dermatitis** is a chronic inflammation of the skin, which is believed to be caused by allergies. Typically, those who have this condition usually have a family history of allergic diseases, such as hay fever and asthma. This condition often develops early in life, usually disappearing by age 15. Though related to allergies, atopic dermatitis has no known cause — and no cure.

✔ **Allergic contact dermatitis** is an allergic reaction that occurs when the skin comes into contact with an *allergen* — a substance, such as chemicals, detergent, poison ivy, or wool, that triggers an allergic reaction.

✔ **Seborrheic dermatitis,** or dandruff, is a condition in which dead skin flakes from the scalp or face (bridge of the nose). It is caused by an overly oily scalp.

Recognizing the signs

Atopic dermatitis has the following signs:

✔ Affected area itches and blisters and is sometimes accompanied by a crusting rash.

✔ The patient usually has a family history of allergies, such as hay fever and asthma.

✔ Sometimes skin eruptions accompany allergies.

Allergic contact dermatitis has the following signs:

✔ Affected area itches and is accompanied by a red rash.

✔ Affected area blisters and swells.

✔ Sometimes scaling and thickened skin follow rash.

Seborrheic dermatitis has the following signs:

- ✔ Scalp may have greasy scales and patches of dried skin that are yellowish, pinkish, and brownish in color.
- ✔ Scalp is itchy and inflamed.
- ✔ Flaking of dead skin accompanies itching and inflammation.

Knowing for sure

Most of these conditions are fairly easy to identify through a self-exam, but if you're unsure, see your family doctor or dermatologist. For atopic dermatitis, your family doctor or dermatologist examines your skin and asks questions about your family history. For allergic contact dermatitis, the doctor examines your skin and may do allergy tests to pinpoint irritating substances. For seborrheic dermatitis, your doctor or dermatologist examines your scalp and also the sides of your nose, behind your ears, between the eyebrows, and over your breastbone.

Treating dermatitis yourself

For atopic dermatitis, drink plenty of water and use a non-irritating, alcohol-free moisturizer. Avoid contact with irritating substances, such as wool and harsh detergents. Skip frequent hot or long showers or baths because water can dry the skin. Use OTC hydrocortisone cream or calamine lotion to soothe the itch, or soak in a bath that contains colloidal oatmeal (contains starch, protein, and oil). Some believe that supplements of evening primrose oil taken orally may help, but scientific studies conflict.

For allergic contact dermatitis, take regular baths to soothe irritated skin. Apply calamine lotion, hydrocortisone cream, or a similar OTC product.

For seborrheic dermatitis, wash frequently with a mild shampoo. If that is not effective, use a dandruff shampoo that contains sulfur, salicylic acid, selenium, or tar as needed. Be sure to rinse thoroughly after shampooing. When your dandruff clears up, shampoo as needed and occasionally use a dandruff shampoo to keep mild cases of dandruff under control. Antifungal creams and shampoos also help.

Treating dermatitis with medication

For atopic dermatitis, your doctor may prescribe antibiotics, antihistamines, or topical corticosteroids. For allergic contact dermatitis, your doctor may prescribe cetirizine (Zyrtec) or topical corticosteroids. For severe cases of seborrheic dermatitis, your doctor may prescribe lotions or shampoos.

Preventing dermatitis

Around 70 percent of people with atopic dermatitis have a family history of the disorder. However, atopic dermatitis is a passing condition, which you can treat with OTC products and prescription drugs.

In allergic contact dermatitis, avoid contact with known allergens. Use a *barrier cream,* a specialized product that you apply to your skin to help protect it from allergens. Wash your skin thoroughly with soap and water as soon as possible if you think you've come in contact with an allergen.

If you're one of the unlucky ones born with a tendency to have seborrheic dermatitis, you may never be able to be completely free of it. However, you can keep dandruff under control by washing frequently with a mild shampoo or dandruff shampoo.

Nail fungus

Nails consist of the protein keratin, and they grow from the *lunula,* the white area at the base of the nail. Nails become susceptible to fungi when they are traumatized. When the nail is repeatedly injured, it can become dislodged from the nail bed. The result is no contact with the skin and loss of its only blood supply. Without blood, the nail becomes food for fungi. Nail fungus can affect fingernails and toenails.

Nail fungus is commonly caused by fungi responsible for athlete's foot and jock itch.

Recognizing the signs

Here are the common signs of nail fungus:

- The nail turns white after trauma occurs and blood supply is lost.
- Eventually, the nail yellows.
- The nail thickens and changes color.
- The nail may become brittle or thickened or may be completely destroyed.

Knowing for sure

To diagnose nail fungus, your doctor may take clippings or scrapings of the affected nail for examination under a microscope.

Treating nail fungus

Your doctor may prescribe an oral antifungal medication such as griseofulvin, which takes 6 to 12 months to be effective, or he or she may prescribe two newer drugs, called itraconazole (Sporanox) and terbinafine (Lamisil), which can work in 3 to 4 months. However, if you are taking astemizole, non-sedating antihistamines, do not take Sporanox — the combination can cause severe cardiac side effects. Anyone with liver damage should avoid both Sporanox and Lamisil.

Another treatment includes grinding the surface of the nail to make it porous and then applying an antifungal cream. At home, apply the cream daily, and file the nail every two or three weeks with an emery board.

Preventing nail fungus

Avoid damaging your fingernails and toenails. Don't bite your nails or cuticles because an infection may develop. If your nails tend to be fragile, coat them with a clear nail polish to help strengthen them. Because the fungi responsible for athlete's foot can cause nail fungus, avoid walking barefoot around swimming pools and public shower stalls. Keep your nails trimmed. Use sharp manicure scissors or clippers to trim your nails and an emery board to smooth out rough edges.

Moles

Moles appear in many shapes and sizes, on all parts of the body, alone, or in groups. Over the years, moles change. Some seem to just fade away, some hardly change a bit, and some become so raised that they eventually fall off or are rubbed off. Exposure to the sun and certain steroid drugs used in therapy can cause moles to darken. The average mole "lives" for about 50 years.

Recognizing the signs

Here are the common signs of moles:

- Moles begin as flat circular spots on skin.
- Moles usually appear as brown, black, and blue in color.
- Over time — each mole has its own growth pattern — moles usually change, becoming raised and lighter in color.

Moles and skin cancer

Studies have shown that some moles have a higher-than-average risk of developing into a form of skin cancer known as malignant melanoma. Moles that appear at birth, known as *congenital nevi,* are more likely to become malignant than those that appear later in life. A congenital nevus larger than eight inches in diameter poses the greatest risk for skin cancer. Moles called *dysplastic nevi,* or atypical moles, are usually larger than a pencil eraser, irregularly shaped, and unevenly colored. People with these moles, which tend to be hereditary, may have an above-average chance of developing malignant melanoma. The majority of moles and other blemishes, such as freckles, are not cancerous. Only those that suddenly change size, shape or color, or those that bleed, itch, become painful, or first appear when a person is over 30 warrant medical concerns. See Chapter 18 for warning signs of skin cancer.

Knowing for sure

If you notice that a mole changes its shape or color, becomes itchy, painful, inflamed, or bleeds, consult your doctor. Moles are usually harmless; however, they can become cancerous. Consult your family doctor or dermatologist.

Treating a mole

If a mole seems suspicious, a dermatologist removes all or part of it for examination. If it turns out to be malignant, the dermatologist removes the mole completely. Most mole-removal procedures are quick and can be done in the dermatologist's office. Moles in the beard area can be quite annoying. The most common methods of removal are shave excision and cutting out the mole and stitching the area closed.

Shaving over a mole will not cause it to become cancerous. Hairs that grow out of moles can be clipped close to the surface of the skin, or a dermatologist can remove them permanently.

Psoriasis

Psoriasis is an overproduction of skin cells causing scaly red patches that usually affect the elbows, knees, groin and genitals, arms, legs, scalp, and nails. About 3 million Americans have psoriasis and 100,000 of these people have severe cases. The cause of psoriasis is unknown. However, there may be a genetic link. It usually occurs in people between the ages of 10 and 30. Psoriasis cycles between flare-ups and remissions.

Recognizing the signs

The severity and form of psoriasis differ from case to case. Here are the common signs of psoriasis:

- ✔ It usually begins with little red bumps that slowly grow and form silvery scales.
- ✔ The scales usually don't itch but flake off easily.
- ✔ Bleeding may occur when scales are removed.
- ✔ Nails infected by psoriasis show pitting, thickening, and crumbling.

Knowing for sure

Your doctor examines you for visible signs. He or she may also take a sample of the affected area for microscopic examination to rule out fungal infection or another disorder.

Treating psoriasis with self-care

An important way to treat psoriasis is by staying healthy. For example, maintaining a normal weight lessens irritation between the folds or creases of your skin. Try not to pick, scratch, or rub at the patches — doing so may thicken the patches. Use moisturizers, especially during the dry winter months, and cool them in a refrigerator before applying. The coolness helps to soothe itching. Bathe in hot water to reduce scaling. Adding baby oils, bath powders, and table salt to the water can help soften scales. Soak in hot water for 20 minutes, and gently wash away softened scales before applying any medication because the scales can block the penetration of the medicine. Avoid contact with harsh soap and chemicals.

Treating psoriasis with medication

Your doctor may prescribe topical medications such as corticosteroids, coal tar applications, anthralin, vitamin D3 (Dovonex), and retinoids. Systemic treatments include ultraviolet light B (UVB) therapy; psoralen, and ultraviolet light A (PUVA) therapy, in which the photosensitizing medication psoralen is given prior to a dose of UVA; and the oral prescription drugs methotrexate (Rheumatrex), etretinate (Tegison), acitretin (Soriatane), and isotretinoin (Accutane). PUVA therapy may increase the risk of skin cancer; however, many experts believe the benefits outweigh the risk. As of yet, no treatment offers a permanent cure for psoriasis; however, many treatments, either alone or in combination, can clear up or greatly improve its nagging symptoms.

A University of Michigan study found that psoriasis treatments are far less effective in men who consume a great deal of alcohol — a six-pack of beer or five shots of whiskey daily — than in moderate drinkers.

Rosacea

Rosacea, sometimes called "adult acne," is a chronic, progressive skin condition that affects the face. It differs from acne in that no oiliness or blackheads are present. In severe cases, the nose may become bumpy and swollen, and the eyes may become inflamed. Rosacea affects 13 million Americans, usually after age 30.

Although the exact cause of rosacea is unknown, most cases are thought to be inherited. You're at a greater risk if you tend to blush easily or have Eastern European, English, Irish, Scottish, or Scandinavian ancestry. Rosacea is more common in women but usually more severe in men.

Recognizing the signs

Here are the common signs of rosacea:

- Affected areas of the face show redness, bumps, and inflammation.
- Cheeks are red and ruddy.
- As rosacea progresses, tiny pimples — both solid and pus-filled — may appear, and enlarged blood vessels may be visible (a condition called *telangiectasia*).
- Advanced rosacea may develop into *rhinophyma,* a condition characterized by a bulbous nose, puffy cheeks, and thick bumps and lines on the skin's surface.

Knowing for sure

Because you may confuse rosacea with acne, consult your doctor to be sure. Prompt treatment is best because rosacea rarely heals itself, and without treatment, it worsens over the years.

Treating rosacea with self-care

To help relieve the symptoms of rosacea, stay out of the sun as much as possible, and avoid extreme hot and cold temperatures. Also, avoid rubbing or massaging the face, which can irritate the skin. Too much alcohol, spicy foods, hot drinks, and smoking may aggravate the redness of rosacea. The condition has been wrongly linked to alcoholism (in part because comedian W.C. Fields, a heavy drinker, had a severe case of rosacea and resulting rhinophyma). Though alcohol may worsen rosacea, symptoms can be just as bad in someone who abstains from drinking.

Treating rosacea with medication

Because OTC skin creams and ointments may irritate rosacea, you're better off seeing a dermatologist if your skin's redness does not improve in a few weeks and if pimples or enlarged blood vessels appear. He or she will most likely prescribe a topical medication in gel or cream form, which should result in noticeable improvement within two months of use. Your doctor may prescribe oral antibiotics, too. Sometimes laser surgery can treat tiny blood vessels visible through the skin, as well as excess tissue on the nose.

Warts

Warts are round, pale, harmless growths that affect the uppermost layers of the skin. Warts are caused by a virus, and they can be spread both from person to person and to different areas of the body. For the most part, warts are similar except for their location on the body. They are categorized according to the area of the body where they occur. Warts commonly appear on the hands, feet, knees, and face.

Recognizing the signs

Here are the most common signs of warts:

- ✔ Warts are usually round and small lumps on the skin.
- ✔ Warts tend to be colorless, but they may also be white or pinkish. Warts on the feet look like black dots.
- ✔ Warts that are flat-looking or have a flat top tend to occur at the wrists, arms, legs, and face.
- ✔ Warts that appear at the bottom of the feet (called plantar warts) are flat and can make walking painful.
- ✔ Warts can occur on the genitalia (called genital warts), around the anus, and within the rectum. Genital warts tend to be soft, pink, cauliflower-like bumps that grow extensively.

Knowing for sure

If you've never had a wart before, you must see a dermatologist for diagnosis and treatment because what looks like a wart may be something else, possibly a sign of skin cancer.

Treating warts through self-care

You can treat properly identified warts with OTC wart removers that contain salicylic acid, a mild corrosive. Don't apply wart removers to the healthy skin around warts, however. Wash your hands before and after touching warts to prevent their spread to elsewhere on the body.

Pamper your skin

Here are some tips to keep your skin healthy:

✔ **Drink at least eight glasses of water daily.** Plenty of water helps keep the skin flexible and elastic.

✔ **Eat right.** A balanced, low-fat diet ensures that you're getting all the substances your body needs to build healthy skin. In addition, high-fat intake has been associated with an increase in risk for precancerous lesions (abnormalities of the skin).

✔ **Use a mild, moisturizing soap.** Harsh deodorant soaps can dry your skin and make it more vulnerable to disease by stripping its protective outer layers. Applying a moisturizer after a shower can help to minimize dry skin. Avoid scented products, which can be drying or irritating to the skin.

✔ **Treat your skin gently.** Avoid rubbing your skin vigorously while washing and try not to dry off too roughly after a shower, which can stretch and damage your skin. Wash gently — especially your face, where skin is most delicate — and pat yourself dry.

✔ **Skip the long, hot shower.** Hot water (and excessively cold water) harms the skin, and long showers can remove protective oils from your skin's surface. Stick to a temperature of about 95°F to 100°F, and don't stay in longer than 10 minutes. Be watchful in a hot tub, bathtub, or sauna.

✔ **Fight wrinkles.** To help prevent wrinkles, don't smoke. Smoking deprives the skin of blood and much-needed nutrients. By some estimates, smokers are likely to have five times as many premature wrinkles as nonsmokers. Also, try to sleep on your back. When you sleep on your side with your face pressed against a pillow, you're more likely to develop wrinkles than if you sleep on your back.

✔ **Get your daily vitamins and minerals.** Certain vitamins can benefit the skin and help protect it against bacteria and other damaging forces. For example, a B-vitamin deficiency can leave the corners of your mouth cracked and leave large pores on your nose. Some other valuable nutrients include vitamins C, E, and beta-carotene and the mineral selenium, which are *antioxidants,* substances that may help neutralize free radicals that may lead to the development of wrinkles.

✔ **Protect yourself against the sun everyday.** Though most people associate a deep tan with health, ultraviolet rays damage the skin, contribute to the risk of skin cancer, and may cause premature aging and wrinkles. Screen out the ultraviolet rays by using a sunscreen with a sun protection factor (SPF) of at least 15 and avoid exercising or working outdoors between 10:00 a.m. and 2:00 p.m., when the sun's rays are strongest.

✔ **If you have a skin condition or infection, avoid using a washcloth, the perfect breeding ground for germs.**

✔ **Conduct a monthly skin examination, using a mirror to be aware of any changes in your skin.** (See Chapter 18.)

Treating warts through medication

A dermatologist can remove warts with liquid nitrogen, corrosive agents, or surgery. *Electrosurgical destruction,* or burning away the wart, is also an option. This treatment can be painful and leave some scarring. Genital warts may be treated with the drug podophyllin. Sometimes a rectal exam is required to locate all the genital warts so that they can be treated effectively. A practitioner can also remove genital warts with acid or freezing; periodic office visits may be necessary because genital warts are difficult to treat. All warts may recur because the virus remains in the body indefinitely.

Preventing warts

Use a condom during sexual contact to prevent transmission of genital warts.

If you have been diagnosed with genital warts, tell your sexual partner. Women with genital warts have an increased risk of cervical cancer and need effective treatment immediately.

Chapter 12

The A B Zzzs of Sleep Disorders

• •

In This Chapter

▶ Recognizing sleep disorders

▶ Treating sleep disorders

▶ Getting a good night's rest

• •

Did you sleep well last night? If you're like millions of other men today, the answer is probably a resounding "no." According to the National Commission on Sleep Disorders and Research, one in three Americans doesn't get enough sleep, and at least 40 million people suffer from chronic sleep disorders.

Although most consider sleep a normal body function, too many people take this activity for granted. The amount of sleep you get each night has a significant effect on how your body functions during the day. Too little sleep can weaken your immune system, affect your memory, increase stress, and result in traffic and work-related accidents.

Just about anything you do can play a significant role in how you sleep. Your sleep habits and environment, diet and nutrition, exercise, stress, smoking, alcohol, caffeine — even your personality type — can all affect your sleep. So stay awake for a little while and we'll tell you how to get a good night's rest.

What Is Sleep?

Sleep is a period during which your body repairs itself, consolidates memory, removes wastes from its systems, and collects energy for the next day. The average person spends about one-third of his life asleep — approximately 205,000 hours in a 70-year lifetime.

Ticktock ... your body's clock

Your body operates a lot like a clock. The night-time, or *circadian clock,* promotes sleep; the daytime, or *homeostatic clock,* promotes arousal. Together, they control the body's sleep-wake cycle.

The circadian clock refers to the body's rhythm patterns — or *circadian rhythm* — of about a day (usually 25 to 27 hours), which has been adjusted to 24 hours to coincide with the Earth's daily revolutions into daylight and dark, thus synchronizing us with the rest of the world. The circadian rhythm controls the body's temperature, which greatly affects the sleep-wake cycle. When your body temperature is highest, you're most alert and function best. When your body temperature is lowest, you become drowsy. The average adult experiences two temperature peaks — one in mid-morning, the other in mid-evening.

The second internal timekeeping mechanism is the homeostatic clock, with a cycle of 28 hours. Some researchers theorize that the homeostatic clock prompts us to go to sleep in the late evening and, without circadian coordination, would cause us to wake up in only three to four hours. But the circadian clock kicks in late at night to allow us to sleep longer.

The circadian rhythm and homeostatic clock work hand in hand, allowing your body to get a good night's sleep. At various stages of your life, your normal circadian rhythms change, running longer or shorter than the self-imposed 24-hour patterns. For example, older people tend to run on a shorter cycle — the reason many older sleepers wake early in the morning.

When you sleep, your body has a chance to rejuvenate. Sleep allows your body to repair itself, test its internal systems, strengthen memory, and reserve energy for the day ahead. When you don't get a good night's sleep, you're likely to wake up feeling tired and irritable, have difficulty concentrating and making decisions, and become forgetful; and you are more likely to have a traffic or work-related accident.

Sleep is generally broken down into two phases: REM (rapid eye movement) and NREM (non-rapid eye movement), which alternate in 90-minute cycles during a typical seven-to-eight-hour night. REM sleep is the shallower sleep cycle associated with dreaming. As your body temperature and blood pressure rise, your breathing becomes shallower and faster, and your brain function remains active just as if you were awake. During NREM sleep, the brain becomes less active, which leads to deep, restorative sleep.

The typical amount of sleep recommended for the average adult is seven to nine hours per night — but most people get fewer than seven hours.

Sleep Disorders

Sleep disorders can occur when your internal clocks or neurotransmitters are out of sync (for example, work shift changes or the use of excessive caffeine). At these times, unless you're vigilant, you start running "out of sync" with the rest of the world. And the more you try to catch up on lost sleep, the harder stabilizing your sleep-wake schedule becomes. There are more than 200 known sleep disorders, which generally fall into four categories:

- ✔ Difficulty falling or staying asleep
- ✔ Difficulty staying awake
- ✔ Difficulty maintaining a proper sleep-wake cycle
- ✔ Difficulty with various types of disruptive behavior during sleep, such as snoring and sleepwalking

Brain chemicals

Brain chemicals, or *neurotransmitters* — hormonelike chemicals manufactured by your nervous system — play a key role in how you sleep. These include cortisol (hydrocortisone), melatonin, serotonin, epinephrine (adrenaline), norepinephrine (noradrenaline), and dopamine.

Cortisol helps you get to sleep. The amount of cortisol in the body usually peaks at 6 a.m. and runs down around midnight. As the amount of cortisol decreases, body temperature falls and the mind winds down, becoming less alert, preparing for sleep. Drowsiness results.

Melatonin also promotes sleep by helping to control the circadian (light-dark) rhythm.

Darkness stimulates the brain's production of melatonin.

Serotonin appears to control states of consciousness, as well as mood and sensitivity to pain. Like cortisol, serotonin affects body temperature changes and also plays a role in the sleep-wake cycle.

Epinephrine, norepinephrine, and dopamine work to keep you awake. These brain chemicals are most active during times of stress or emergency, and they stimulate the brain to make you more alert, attentive, motivated, and mentally energetic.

Insomnia

Insomnia — the inability to fall asleep or stay asleep — is the most common sleep disorder reported today. According to the National Commission on Sleep Disorders and Research, 20 to 30 million people suffer intermittent insomnia serious enough to put themselves or others at risk of injury or illness. Although more common in women and the elderly, insomnia affects men, too, and all age groups.

Insomnia generally comes in three forms:

- ✔ **Transient** (short-term), lasting a single night to a few weeks, often due to excitement or stress
- ✔ **Intermittent** (on and off), usually due to stress, illness, jet lag, or shift work
- ✔ **Chronic** (constant), lasting a month or more, due to a variety of factors

Insomnia has a number of causes, including psychological factors, such as stress, depression, and anxiety disorders; behavioral factors, including unhealthy sleep or lifestyle habits; other sleep disorders; allergies; poor sleeping conditions (noise, light, cold, and so on); pain; urinary problems; and circadian rhythm disorders.

Chronic insomnia may also be linked to medical conditions such as arthritis, kidney disease, heart failure, asthma, sleep apnea, narcolepsy, restless leg syndrome, Parkinson's disease, and hyperthyroidism; or behavioral factors such as the misuse of caffeine, alcohol, or other substances; or environmental factors such as a disrupted sleep-wake cycle caused by night-shift work or jet lag.

Sleeping too long can also lead to insomnia. When you stay in bed longer than usual to make up for lost sleep, you only make your sleeping problems worse. In addition, if you often worry about not being able to fall asleep or constantly think about work and other worries before going to bed, you may fall into a pattern of irregular or unpredictable sleep-wake schedules or begin spending excessive amounts of time in bed — which ultimately leads to the prolonged inability to fall asleep.

Insomnia can also be hereditary, so if you're having trouble sleeping, chances are high that an immediate family member has or had a similar problem. Discovering a pattern of sleeplessness in your family can help lead to a solution to your own problem.

Insomnia: Is it all in your head?

More than 75 percent of America's chronic insomnia problems have a psychological basis, and many are curable with professional help. Your doctor may recommend counseling or behavior-modification treatment if he or she concludes that psychological problems are the root of your insomnia. You also may consider seeing a psychiatrist with experience in treating sleep disorders.

Recognizing the signs

The most common signs of insomnia include the following:

- ✔ Inability to fall asleep at regular scheduled bedtime
- ✔ Waking up in the middle of sleep and not being able to return to sleep
- ✔ Fatigue
- ✔ Irritability
- ✔ Lack of energy
- ✔ Impaired memory
- ✔ Difficulty concentrating

Knowing for sure

A wide variety of health-care providers, including general practitioners and specialists in neurology, pulmonary medicine, psychiatry, and psychology, can diagnose and treat sleep disorders.

Before your physician can treat insomnia, he or she has to identify the underlying problems that are causing your sleeplessness. Your doctor usually begins by evaluating both your medical history and sleep history. You can determine your sleep history by keeping a sleep diary to record your daily sleep patterns and problems, or by having your physician interview your bed partner concerning the quantity and quality of your sleep. Your doctor may recommend a specialized sleep study if he or she suspects that you have a more serious sleep disorder, such as *sleep apnea* (a brief absence of breathing during sleep) or narcolepsy (excessive sleepiness).

Treating insomnia through medical means

If self-care techniques don't bring relief, you may need to see a specialist. An ear, nose, and throat (ENT) specialist or an internist with a background in breathing disorders or in pulmonary diseases can treat problems related to snoring or sleep apnea. A neurologist can treat sleep problems related to the central nervous system.

Sleeping pills are intended for short periods only to reestablish good sleep, either with self-help measures or after other causes of insomnia have been ruled out. Over-the-counter sleeping remedies usually contain antihistamines, drugs with sedative side effects that are mainly used to relieve allergies. Few doctors, however, find them effective as sleep inducers.

Prescription sleep medications work by suppressing nerve-cell activity within the brain. They include two major classes of drugs: benzodiazepines and tricyclic antidepressants.

Benzodiazepines are prescribed to treat short-term insomnia caused by emotional stress or travel. They relieve anxiety, promote sleep, and are effective for short periods — about two weeks. Side effects include sweating, nausea, rapid pulse, and depression. Benzodiazepines, which include Valium, can be addictive.

Tricyclic antidepressants are prescribed for insomnia related to chronic pain or nonrestorative sleep. They are effective in very small doses, and their side effects are usually mild — dry mouth, constipation, urinary problems, and tremors. Common tricyclic antidepressants are Elavil, Desyrel, and Tofranil.

Snoring

Snoring is no laughing matter. Most people who snore can't help it, and the noises made are usually a sign of obstructed breathing, which can be serious (not to mention annoying to those who sleep with a snorer). The noise of snoring is produced by the soft palate, the uvula (small tissue projecting in the middle of the palate in the throat), or the vibration of both against the back of the throat or at the base of the tongue. The vibration results from a rapid alternating opening and closing of the air passage, which makes inhaling more difficult.

It's estimated that approximately 90 million Americans over the age of 18 snore occasionally, and about 37 million are habitual snorers. The majority of snorers are men who are overweight. And snoring tends to worsen with age.

Snoring may signify significant problems, such as high blood pressure and heart disease. And extremely loud, raspy breathing followed by gasping or choking sounds may be a sign of sleep apnea (see the following section), in which breathing is obstructed during sleep, causing the person to awaken numerous times during the night.

Although you often don't hear yourself snore, the noise may disrupt the sleep of others. Although often embarrassing, snoring is not usually life-threatening and can be treated.

Many factors contribute to snoring, including the following:

- **Poor muscle tone in the muscles of the tongue and throat.** This condition allows the tongue to fall back into the airway or allows the throat muscles to draw in from the sides into the airway. This problem usually occurs when your muscles become too relaxed from alcohol or through the use of certain medications, or when you fall into the deep NREM sleep stages.

- **Excessive bulkiness of tissues in the throat, such as large tonsils and adenoids, a big uvula, or a long soft palate.** People who are over-weight also tend to have bulky neck tissues.

- **Obstructed nasal airways.** An obstruction in the nasal airways can force airways to become smaller, as a result of stuffy and swollen mucous membranes. The obstruction causes you to breathe with exaggerated force to move the air through the narrow passageway.

- **Deformities of the nose or nasal septum, such as a deviated septum (center section of the nose moves to one side).**

- **Obesity.** Weighing 20 percent more than your ideal weight makes you three times as likely to snore than if you're at a normal weight.

Treating snoring yourself

Here are tips to reduce the likelihood of snoring:

- Lose excess weight.

- Exercise regularly.

- Sleep on your side.

- Avoid smoking, drinking alcohol, or eating heavy meals right before bedtime.

- Increase the humidity in your bedroom to avoid dry, swollen mucous membranes.

- Avoid tranquilizers, sleeping pills, and antihistamines before bedtime.

- Get proper treatment for allergies.

- Elevate the head of your bed.

- Try improving nasal breathing through the use of nasal sprays and breathing strips.

Treating snoring through medical means

For more serious snoring problems, or when snoring becomes disruptive to your sleep or the sleep of others, seeking medical advice is important. Your doctor can examine your nose, mouth, palate, throat, and neck to determine the cause of your snoring, and studies performed in a sleep lab can help determine how serious your snoring is and what effects it is having on your health.

The treatment recommended depends on your diagnosis and may be as simple as managing a nasal allergy or sinus infection or as complicated as surgically correcting a nasal deformity or removing the tonsils or adenoids. In more serious cases, surgery can be done on the throat and palate to tighten up flabby tissues and expand your airways.

Some oral devices worn in the mouth during sleep have been proven to eliminate snoring in certain cases. These oral appliances work by pulling the lower jaw forward, thereby opening the airway. And some also bring the tongue forward and out of the way.

Another treatment that's still being tested uses radiofrequency energy. The technique involves inserting a radiofrequency energy-generating electrode into the excess soft tissue blocking the upper airway to gently heat and destroy the obstructive tissue. Once the wound heals, scar tissue (which takes up less space than the original tissue) replaces the old tissue. The doctor performs the procedure in an outpatient setting. The procedure requires two to three treatments over a three-week period.

Sleep apnea

Snoring can also be a sign of a more serious sleep disorder called sleep apnea, which is characterized by loud snoring and periodic lapses in breathing that cause a person to awaken numerous times throughout the night. The disorder gets its name from the Greek word *apnoia,* meaning "want of breath" or "lack of wind."

Sleep apnea affects men in their 30s, 40s, and 50s, many of whom are overweight. Although most patients with sleep apnea snore, not all snorers have sleep apnea. About one in three male snorers has sleep apnea, compared with one in five female snorers. The National Commission on Sleep Disorders and Research estimates that 38,000 people die every year from heart complications of sleep apnea.

The two types of sleep apnea are *obstructive* and *central.* Some individuals suffer a combination of both, which is called *mixed sleep apnea.*

Obstructive sleep apnea, or OSA, the more common condition, occurs when air cannot flow into or out of a person's nose or mouth, despite the body's efforts to keep breathing. During episodes of OSA, the muscles of the upper airway — including the tongue, throat, and pharynx — relax during sleep, causing the throat to collapse, which blocks breathing. OSA affects approximately 4 percent of middle-aged men and is the most common cause of excessive daytime sleepiness.

Central sleep apnea, which is relatively rare, occurs when the brain tells the diaphragm to stop moving air in and out with each inhalation and exhalation, which halts breathing altogether.

In both types of sleep apnea, falling oxygen levels and increasing carbon dioxide in the blood cause "arousals," which awaken the sleeper in order to restart the breathing process. These involuntary breathing pauses, or apneic events, can occur hundreds of times nightly, and the cessation of breathing may last 10 seconds or more. The individual usually doesn't know he is awakening.

Recognizing the signs

The most common symptoms of sleep apnea include the following:

- ✔ Snoring, often associated with gasping and choking that cause the sleeper to wake up and begin breathing again
- ✔ Excessive daytime sleepiness or fatigue
- ✔ Restless sleep
- ✔ Morning headaches
- ✔ Impaired concentration and memory
- ✔ Depression, irritability, and anxiety
- ✔ Night sweats

You're more likely to have or develop sleep apnea if you snore loudly, are overweight, have high blood pressure, or have some physical abnormality in the nose, throat, or other parts of the upper airway. The condition may also be genetic.

Knowing for sure

You may be aroused from sleep often enough or completely enough to notice gasping or snorting, but your sleep partner is likely to be the one who notices a problem. The first step is to consult your family doctor, who will study your medical history, conduct a physical examination while checking for indicative symptoms, and possibly consult your sleep partner.

If your doctor suspects sleep apnea, he or she may refer you to a sleep disorder center. The most common diagnostic test available is an overnight sleep study called *polysomnography*. The test records a variety of body functions during sleep, such as the electrical activity of the brain, eye movement, muscle activity, heart rate, respiratory effort, air flow, and blood oxygen levels. This test can also help determine the severity of the condition.

Another diagnostic test, called the Multiple Sleep Latency Test (MSLT), measures the speed of falling asleep. People without sleep problems usually take an average of 10 to 20 minutes to fall asleep, but individuals who fall asleep in less than 5 minutes are likely to be diagnosed with a sleep disor-der. The MSLT can also be used to measure the degree of excessive daytime sleepiness associated with sleep apnea and rule out other types of sleep disorders. Most often, these diagnostic tests are performed in a sleep disorder center.

Treating sleep apnea

Behavioral changes are an important part of the treatment program for sleep apnea patients. You can help mild sleep apnea by using self-care techniques. Otherwise, a variety of treatments are available depending upon the severity of the sleep apnea. One nonsurgical option is continuous positive airway pressure, in which a mask connected to a compressor is worn during sleep. The mask forces air through the nasal passages and into the airways, keeping them open.

Oral appliances, which include tongue retainers and jaw-advancement devices, are sometimes used to treat mild cases of sleep apnea. Tongue retainers hold the tongue in place so that it doesn't block the airway; jaw advancement appliances change the position of the lower jaw.

Your practitioner may prescribe Protriptyline, an antidepressant drug. This drug works by reducing or inhibiting REM sleep, the phase when sleep apnea is most likely to happen. The drug may also help increase the tone of the throat muscles.

Treating sleep apnea with surgery

If the preceding treatments don't help or if a physical abnormality such as enlarged tonsils or a deviated septum is the cause of sleep apnea, you have several surgical options.

Uvulopalatopharyngoplasty (UPPP) can be performed to overcome an upper airway obstruction. The surgery involves removing excess tissue at the back of the throat, including part of the soft palate, tonsils, and uvula.

Laser-assisted uvulopalatoplasty (LAUP) is a new procedure that uses a laser to remove part of the soft palate and uvula. LAUP is done as an in-office procedure and requires several sessions.

Other procedures to open the airway include *inferior sagittal mandibular osteotomy (ISO)* and *geniohyoid advancement with hyoid myotomy (GAHM)*. In ISO, the lower bone of the jaw is brought forward. In GAHM, the hyoid bone (the u-shaped bone that holds your lower teeth) is attached to the windpipe. The success rates of these surgeries depend on your weight and jaw structure.

Another procedure, *maxillomandibular advancement,* involves moving both the upper and lower jaw forward. After surgery, the jaw is wired shut for four weeks, requiring a liquids-only diet. Orthodontic work may be neces-sary after the procedure to realign the teeth.

A less common surgical alternative is *tracheostomy*. This procedure involves making a small hole in the windpipe and inserting a tube into the opening to bypass the upper airway obstruction and allow air to pass directly into the lungs. During the day, the tube is plugged to allow the individual to breathe and speak normally.

Treating sleep disorders yourself

You can often treat sleep disorders with simple lifestyle changes. Here are tips for getting a better night's sleep:

✔ **Establish good sleep habits.** It's important to go to sleep and wake up at the same time each day — even on weekends — to help stabilize your sleep-wake schedule and enhance your ability to get the amount of sleep you need.

✔ **Avoid excessive physical and mental stimulation too close to bedtime.** Exercising, watching action-adventure movies, working, or reading just before going to sleep may stimulate instead of relax you. Your body needs adequate time to disengage from physical and mental activity before you can relax enough to fall asleep.

✔ **Try relaxation therapy.** For good sleep, you need to relax away your stress throughout the day, not just before bedtime. See Chapter 6 for relaxation tips.

✔ **Take a short daytime nap if you are sleepy.** Napping in the late morning or early afternoon — no longer than 20 to 30 minutes — may help you feel more alert during the afternoon, but minimize longer or more frequent napping to avoid excessive daytime sleepiness or the inability to fall asleep at night.

✔ **Exercise regularly.** Active people sleep better and more easily; but don't do strenuous exercise right before bedtime.

✔ **Watch what you eat or drink.** Caffeine, alcohol, and foods high in protein may inhibit your ability to fall asleep or stay asleep if you consume them too close to bedtime. Cheeses and other foods containing tyrosine (an amino acid) stimulate the release of dopamine and noradrenaline to energize your mind and heighten your alertness. Tyrosine-rich foods include aged cheeses — such as parmesan and blue, mozzarella, Swiss, Gruyere, and feta — red wine, yogurt, sour cream, cured and processed meats and fish, yeast products, eggplant, potatoes, spinach, tomatoes, and milk.

✔ **Eat carbohydrates.** Carbohydrates (sugars and starches) fuel a quick energy high, followed by a crash, after which sleepiness and lethargy set in. For the best sleep-promoting effects, dinner should be a light combination of complex carbohydrates and proteins at least four hours before bedtime. A snack that consists mainly of complex carbohydrates — an English muffin, a bowl of cereal (go light on the milk), wheat crackers — eaten one to two hours before bed has the most sedating effect on you.

✔ **Try herbs that calm.** Herbs such as anise, celery seed, chamomile, clove, cumin, fennel, garlic, ginger, honey, lime peel, marjoram, onion, orange peel, parsley, sage, spearmint, sugar, and decaffeinated tea

(continued)

(continued)

can serve as mild sedatives and tranquilizers to aid sleep. To make an herbal tea, add one teaspoon of dried herb to a cup of boiling water. Let steep for 5 to 10 minutes; strain and drink 45 minutes before bedtime.

✔ **Monitor your sleep environment.** A dark, quiet room, a firm mattress, a soft pillow, cozy sheets, and a comfortable temperature can do wonders to help you get your zzzs.

✔ **Take melatonin.** A controversial treatment for insomnia is the use of melatonin supplements. Melatonin is a natural hormone produced by the pineal gland in the brain, and this hormone is believed to regulate the sleep-wake cycle. When melatonin is being produced, the body assumes that it's dark outside, and tells your internal clock that it's time to sleep. But concerns do exist about melatonin: It is sold in the United States as a dietary supplement, promoted as an aid for insomnia, stress, jet lag, and aging, and it is not regulated as a drug. Questions about proper dosage, interactions with other drugs, and long-term effectiveness and safety remain unanswered. Possible side effects include nausea, headaches, nightmares, and possibly depression.

Chapter 13

Depression and Mood Disorders

• •

In This Chapter
▶ Identifying types of depression
▶ Diagnosing depression
▶ Treating depression

• •

*W*inston Churchill, the famous World War II British prime minister, described depression as a "black bear" that comes around periodically, leaving gloom behind. No matter how you describe depression, it's an energy-draining, joy-blocking, motivation-sapping illness that turns life into hopelessness. Affecting more than 17 million Americans, depression is so prevalent in our society that it's called "the common cold of mental illness."

Depression is a "whole-body" illness, involving the thoughts, mood, and body. It affects the way a person thinks about things, the way he feels about himself, the way he eats and sleeps. Depression is not the same thing as a blue mood and is not a sign of personal weakness or a condition that can be wished or willed away. Without treatment, symptoms can last for weeks, months, or even years.

Some types of depression run in families; however, they can also occur in people who don't have a family history of depression. Either way, depression is usually due to having too little or too much of certain brain neurotransmitters. People with low self-esteem, who see themselves and the world pessimistically, or who are easily overcome by stress are vulnerable to depression.

Types of Depression

Depression comes in different types and can be expressed differently within each type. What follows are the most common types of depression:

✔ **Major depressive disorder (or unipolar disorder):** This is the most common type of depression — which is categorized by at least five of the symptoms listed in the following section — and interferes with the ability to eat, sleep, and work. Types of major depressive disorders include *melancholic depression,* which is characterized by loss of interest or pleasure in everything, and *psychotic depression,* marked by delusions, hallucinations, and a permanent sad mood. Close to 15 percent of those with major depression develop psychotic depression, which has a high risk of suicide.

✔ **Dysthymia:** This is a less severe type of depression and is usually long-term (at least two years' duration). Dysthymia doesn't disable but can keep a person in a low mood and keep him from functioning at his normal "tempo." Dysthymia often leads to major depression.

✔ **Bipolar disorder (or manic-depressive disorder):** Not as common as other forms of depression, bipolar disorder is characterized by periods of depression and elation (mania). Periods of depression generally last six to nine months, whereas periods of mania last one to three months. Other signs are inappropriate irritability and social behavior; poor judgment, excessive energy and talking; flamboyant notions and delusions of grandeur; and racing, disconnected thoughts.

✔ **Atypical depressive disorder:** People with this type of depression tend to oversleep, overeat, and gain weight quickly. They are very sensitive to rejection and may have little or no interest in life.

Diagnosing Depression

The first obstacle a depressed person and his doctor must overcome is recognizing and accurately diagnosing the type of depression. For one thing, men tend ignore the physical effects that are a sign of depression or blame

Down in the dumps

Life is full of changes and not all of them good. People normally react to negative change (such as the loss of a job or some disappointment) with gloom, anger, or a refusal to adjust to the change. Such a response is known as *adjustment disorder with depressed mood* (commonly known in *situational depression*). This type of depression — not to be confused with the normal grieving that occurs after the death of a loved one or other tragic loss — is characterized by prolonged periods of "down in the dumps" feelings.

Adjustment disorder with depressed mood tends to fade when the problem that provoked it no longer exists. However, it's possible for people who are prone to depression to become very depressed. Treatment includes psychotherapy or other type of professional therapy with or without antidepressant drugs.

them on stress. If a man goes to his family doctor, it's likely his doctor may miss the signs of clinical depression. On the contrary, many mental health specialists are likely to attribute mental illness causes to purely physical ills. One way to avoid misdiagnosis is for both the patient and his doctor to be aware of the symptoms that, taken together, almost definitely diagnose depression.

The American Psychiatric Association uses the following criteria to diagnose depression. To be clinically depressed, a person must have at least five of the symptoms listed (including the first two) for the same two-week period. The symptoms can't be the normal reaction to the death of a loved one.

- ✔ Depressed mood most of the day, nearly every day

- ✔ Marked diminished interest or pleasure in all, or almost all, activities most of the day, nearly every day

- ✔ Significant weight loss when not dieting (more than 5 percent of body weight in a month) or decrease/increase in appetite nearly every day

- ✔ Insomnia or hypersomnia (excessive sleep) nearly every day

- ✔ An abnormal speeding up or slowing down of physical activities or mental processes, nearly every day, as observed by others

- ✔ Fatigue or loss of energy nearly every day

- ✔ Feelings of worthlessness or excessive or inappropriate guilt (which may be a delusion) nearly every day (not merely self-reproach or guilt about being sick)

- ✔ Diminished ability to think or concentrate nearly every day

- ✔ Recurrent thoughts of death (not just fear of dying) or suicide with or without a specific plan; or a suicide attempt

In addition to the preceding warning signs, depression may also involve violent outbursts or self-medication, in which you may use drugs or alcohol to cope with difficulties. Withdrawal from family and friends is another sign of depression.

Treating Depression

The worst thing a person can do is handle depression on his own. Unfortunately, that's exactly what many people do: Only around 33 percent of people with depression seek help. The bad news is that people with untreated depression have a suicide rate as high as 15 percent. In fact, suicide is the fifth highest killer of men ages 25 through 44 and has increased 26 percent in men over the past 20 years. The good news is that with proper treatment, close to 85 percent of people with major depression significantly improve and go on to lead productive lives.

Men and depression

Men are more likely to commit suicide as a result of depression. In 1990, three times more men than women chose suicide as a way to end their depression, according to the *Journal of Clinical Psychiatry*. One study found that elderly white men are the group most likely to follow through on a suicide threat as a result of undiagnosed and untreated depression.

Male depression comes in two types: covert and overt. In *overt depression,* men feel fatigue, are sad, and experience changes in sleeping and eating habits. In other words, their depression is apparent.

In *covert depression,* the symptoms are masked by self-medication, isolation, and lashing out. A man self-medicating a covert depression may be drinking, using drugs, womanizing, or living the life of a couch potato. Isolation can be keeping to himself, even if he has a family. Lashing out can mean becoming violent and abusing a spouse or child.

If you are experiencing the symptoms of depression — get help. Depression is very treatable, and many people who seek treatment find that the depression is cured or at least reduced in intensity.

Depression is treated with psychotherapy with or without medication. Each person is different, so the decision to use medication alone or combined with psychotherapy is determined on an individual basis.

If your treatment includes drug therapy, be sure to follow your doctor's orders. Often times, a person may stop taking medication when he starts to feel better, which can result in a relapse of depression. Never stop medication without your doctor's permission or supervision.

Antidepressants are the class of medications most often used in the treatment of depression. These drugs work by stimulating or blocking certain brain chemicals. Types of antidepressants include the following:

- ✔ **Tricyclics (Tofranil, Elavil):** In use since the 1960s, tricyclics affect neurotransmitters. Possible side effects include dry mouth, constipation, bladder problems, weight gain, sexual problems, blurry vision, dizziness, and drowsiness.

- ✔ **Monoamine oxidase inhibitors (Marplan, Nardil, Parnate):** Monoamine oxidase inhibitors (MAOIs) work by limiting the activities of the enzyme monoamine oxidase that breaks down the neurotransmitters serotonin and norepinephrine. MAOIs are generally given to people who don't respond to tricyclics. They were once very popular, but due to their negative interactions (headaches, nausea, seizure, stroke, and possibly coma) with certain foods such as figs, aged cheese, some wines, pickles, salt, and monosodium glutamate, they are used less today. Side effects include those of tricyclics, as well as dizziness, rapid heartbeat, and low libido.

✔ **Lithium:** This drug evens out mood swings. It is used to treat bipolar disorders and some types of depression. Lithium is a salt, so people on lithium should monitor their salt intake. Blood lithium levels are monitored because an effective dose and a toxic dose are not far apart. Possible side effects include drowsiness, weakness, nausea, vomiting, and weight gain.

✔ **Selective serotonin reuptake inhibitors, or SSRIs (Prozac, Zoloft, and Paxil):** They are the preferred drugs for treating depression. SSRIs generally have fewer side effects than other antidepressants. Possible side effects include rash, anxiety, nausea, headache, and diarrhea. Temporary side effects include low libido, difficulty achieving orgasm, and erectile problems.

✔ **Selective serotonin noradrenergic reuptake inhibitors, or SSNRIs (Effexor):** These are some of the newest drugs available for depression. SSNRIs function as SSRIs but have a different chemical composition. Possible side effects include nausea, dry mouth, dizziness, constipation. Less common side effects include abnormal ejaculation and impotence.

Along with antidepressants, other medications may be used. To ease the insomnia and anxiety that often accompany depressive disorders, benzodiazepines may be included in treatment. Hallucinations and extremely disorganized thought patterns may be treated with antipsychotics (Risperdal and Mellaril).

For people with severe melancholic or psychotic depression, or for people who haven't responded to several months of drug therapy, "shock" therapy, or *electroconvulsive therapy,* is used under general anesthesia.

Psychotherapy

Psychotherapy comes in many forms. The most productive for depression seem to be the short-term varieties that last 10 to 12 weeks.

✔ **Talking therapy:** This therapy involves a therapist who helps a patient gain a new, deeper perspective into his problems through two-way conversation.

✔ **Behavioral therapy:** In this treatment, a behavioral therapist helps the patient learn how to gain more satisfaction through action and how to change behaviors that contribute to the depression.

✔ **Interpersonal therapy:** This treatment involves a therapist who focuses on the patient's relationships and how the relationships may cause or aggravate the depression.

✔ **Cognitive/behavioral therapy:** In this treatment, a therapist helps the patient change the negative thoughts and behaviors often associated with depression.

✔ **Psychodynamic therapy:** This treatment involves a therapist who focuses on resolving the patient's emotional conflicts that may have begun in childhood.

Chapter 14

Digestive System Disorders

· ·

In This Chapter

▶ Preventing gallstones

▶ Treating ulcers and hernias

▶ Handling irritable bowel syndrome

· ·

*Y*our digestive system is a complex system of organs responsible for converting the food you eat into the nutrients you need to live. From top to bottom, the digestive system is comprised of the mouth, the tongue, the teeth, the salivary glands, the esophagus, the stomach, the small and large intestines, the rectum, and the anus. As you may already know, perhaps from personal experience, a number of things can go wrong with this important part of your body. In addition to common ailments such as indigestion, heartburn, and hemorrhoids, some of the more troubling digestive system disorders are gallstones, ulcers, hernias, and irritable bowel syndrome. This chapter covers these troublesome problems and tells you what to do about them.

Gallstones

The gallbladder is a small, muscular organ located beneath the liver on the right side of your body. The major function of the pear-shaped sac is to store bile, a digestion-aiding substance, and secrete it into the small intestines and other organs where it's needed to help break down food.

Bile is produced by your liver and contains various substances including fats, cholesterol, pigments, and salts. Bile travels through ducts (tubelike structures) from the liver through the common bile duct to both the small intestine and the *cystic duct,* the duct that leads to your gallbladder. Your liver can make three cups of bile (yummy!) each day, and the gallbladder can store about one cup of concentrated bile.

Are you at risk for gallstones?

It's estimated that about 20 million Americans have gallstones. Women are two to three times more likely to have gallstones than men. In general, obese people have a higher risk of gallstones because they have more cholesterol in their bile. Native American men have a very high risk of developing gallstones; in fact, most have stones by the time they are 60. Extensive fasting, rapid weight loss, and an extremely low-calorie diet also tend to bring about gallstones. It's believed that excessive intake of foods high in starch, fiber, and cholesterol can lead to gallstones.

During digestion, the gallbladder contracts and releases stored bile back through the cystic duct into the common bile duct, where it travels to your intestines to aid digestion. The bile is absorbed in the intestine and returns to your liver through the bloodstream. Sometimes bile can build up in your gallbladder, creating gallstones.

The most common gallbladder problem is gallstones. These solid lumps form when materials in the bile, such as cholesterol and pigments, turn hard and crystallize (see Figure 14-1). Several factors can produce gallstones: buildup of bile in the gallbladder, too much cholesterol in the bile, or proteins in the bile and the liver that encourage crystallization.

Types of stones include *cholesterol stones* and *pigment stones*. Cholesterol stones account for 80 percent of all gallstones. These stones form when the bile is too high in blood cholesterol and not enough salts are present to

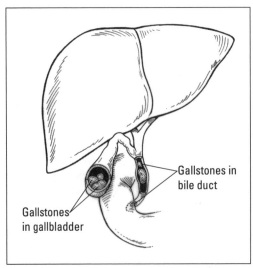

Figure 14-1:
Gallstones.

Gallstones in bile duct

Gallstones in gallbladder

keep the concentration liquid. Pigment stones are made of mostly calcium salts and account for roughly 20 percent of all gallstones. Pigment stones can cause conditions such as the formation of fibrous liver tissue, which results in the loss of functional liver cells (cirrhosis), digestive tract infections, and hereditary blood cell disorders.

Gallstones can be produced in a vast array of sizes, some extremely small and others as large as golf balls. The number of stones can vary from one stone to several thousand.

Recognizing the signs

If you have gallbladder stones, you may never know it. Most gallstones are not harmful and cause no symptoms. However, if a gallstone comes out of your gallbladder and becomes lodged in a duct, you may feel the pain in the right upper abdomen. Typically, the pain begins rather suddenly, builds to a maximum within an hour, and persists for two to four hours until the stone drops back into your gallbladder. This is known as a *gallbladder attack*. You may also feel pain in your shoulders, back, and chest on the right side of your body. For this reason, gallstones can be mistaken for a heart attack. Other symptoms that you may experience include the following:

- ✔ **Vomiting during attacks.**

- ✔ **Periodic attacks.** Gall attacks can occur weeks, months, or even years apart.

- ✔ **Cholecystitis.** This common condition occurs when gallstones get stuck in the cystic duct and block the flow of bile. However, a more uncommon and serious problem occurs when gallstones get stuck in the ducts between the liver and the intestine, preventing bile flow from the gallbladder and the liver. This condition results in pain and jaundice (a bright yellow skin color) or an inflammation of the pancreas. Persistent pain, jaundice, and fever are warning signs of such a blockage. If the blockage remains for an extensive amount of time, it can cause irreversible damage to the gallbladder, liver, and pancreas. This blockage can prove fatal.

Knowing for sure

Stones can be spotted during an abdominal X ray or ultrasound and are often accidentally discovered after an X ray is taken because of another complaint. When your doctor looks specifically for gallstones, he or she will use an ultrasound, which entails sending painless high-frequency sound waves through your abdomen to create an image of the tissues inside. If your gallstones are not causing problems, no treatment is necessary.

Shocking gallstones away

Another option for ridding yourself of gallstones is a procedure called *lithotripsy*. In lithotripsy, gallstones are broken apart into fine pieces by shock waves. The waves are administered by using a machine called a lithotriptor, which is placed against your abdomen, or used while you're seated in a tub of water, which serves to conduct shock waves.

The tiny pieces of bile then pass out of the system. Possible side effects from treatment include some mild bleeding, bruising, or tenderness. Sometimes medications are prescribed to help dissolve the remnants of the stones. Lithotripsy requires general or local anesthesia but no incision.

Treating gallstones

If you have gallstones and have recurrent pain, your doctor may advise you to undergo a surgical procedure called *cholecystectomy*. About 500,000 Americans undergo gallbladder surgery each year, and its risk is considered far lower than the risk of complications from gallstones. Two types of cholecystectomy exist: *standard cholecystectomy* and *laparoscopic cholecystectomy*.

- ✔ A standard cholecystectomy involves removing the stones or the entire gallbladder if necessary, through a 5- to 8-inch incision. A hospital stay may last several days with this treatment.

  If you need your gallbladder removed, don't worry too much — you can function normally without it. Also, gallbladder removal has no known long-term ill effects.

- ✔ The laparoscopic technique involves inserting a small surgical camera through a small incision into your abdomen, giving the surgeon a close-up picture of your insides. The gallbladder is identified, and the cyst formation — not the entire gallbladder — is removed. With this technique, most patients report less postoperative pain, spend only one night in the hospital, and return to their normal activities within two weeks. A potential side effect for both standard and laparoscopic cholecystectomy is infection.

If surgery isn't an option for you, your doctor may treat your gallstones with oral medications such as Actigall and Chenix. These drugs may take months to years of treatment to dissolve the gallstones. A possible side effect of these drugs, although rare, is diarrhea. As your body adjusts to the medication, however, diarrhea normally subsides.

Preventing gallstones

Here are some tips for preventing gallstones:

- **Maintain a healthy weight.** If you're overweight, you're six times more likely to get gallstones than if you're at a healthy weight.

- **Lose weight slowly.** If you need to lose weight, do so slowly because rapid weight loss boosts the levels of cholesterol in the blood, which means more cholesterol ends up in the bile, promoting the formation of gallstones.

- **Don't fast or use crash diets.** If you don't eat, bile is not released to help aid digestion and builds up in the gallbladder instead.

- **Eat *small* meals several times a day.** Doing so results in a regular release of bile from the gallbladder. Spread out your regular calorie intake out over the course of the day.

- **Watch your cholesterol.** High levels of cholesterol in your blood means that bile may become saturated with cholesterol, leading to gallstones.

Ulcers

Ulcers are raw, open sores that form in the lining of your esophagus, stomach, or the *duodenum* (the upper part of the small intestine). Ulcers tend to be named for the area they affect. For example, ulcers of the esophagus are called *esophageal ulcers;* ulcers of the stomach are called *gastric ulcers;* and ulcers of the duodenum are called *duodenal ulcers.* All types of gastrointestinal ulcers are known as *peptic ulcers.*

A variety of factors can cause ulcers. If your stomach, for any reason, isn't able to protect itself from its own digestive fluids (hydrochloric acid and the enzyme pepsin), an ulcer can occur. *Helicobacter pylori (H. pylori)* bacteria — which infect the lining of the stomach, making it more vulnerable to damage from stomach acids and pepsin — often trigger ulcers. Infection usually occurs when contaminated stool comes in contact with hands, water, or food.

Keep a fly swatter handy: Early research points to the common housefly as a carrier of *H. pylori.*

Your lifestyle is also a factor. Consuming too much caffeine and smoking may cause ulcers. Overuse of nonsteroidal anti-inflammatory drugs, such as aspirin and ibuprofen, can make your stomach susceptible to the effects of acid, too.

Painful facts of an untreated ulcer

Left untreated, an ulcer can cause serious complications, such as bleeding, perforation of the walls of the stomach or small intestines, and narrowing and obstruction of digestive tract passages.

Bleeding occurs when an ulcer erodes the muscles of the stomach or the duodenal wall and damages the blood vessels. Blood seeps slowly into the digestive tract if the affected vessels are small. Anemia, weakness, dizziness, and fatigue will result if bleeding continues over time. If a large vessel is damaged, you may feel weak and dizzy when standing and may vomit blood or faint. Stool may look black in color from the blood. These are signs of a serious problem and require immediate medical attention.

Perforation occurs when an ulcer creates a hole in the wall of the stomach or duodenum, and bacteria and partially digested food enter the opening into the abdominal cavity, or *peritoneum.* The result is *peritonitis,* an inflammation of the abdominal cavity and wall. Sudden, sharp, severe pain is the usual symptom of peritonitis, which requires that you receive immediate treatment because this is potentially fatal.

Narrowing and obstructions occur when ulcers located where the duodenum attaches to the stomach cause swelling and scarring. The swelling and scarring may narrow or close the intestinal opening, preventing food from leaving your stomach and entering the small intestine. The main symptom is vomiting.

All these complications can be treated with surgery. Some bleeding ulcers can be treated with *endoscopy,* a procedure that uses a small flexible fiber-optic tube, called an *endoscope,* to see inside the body.

You may have heard that stress causes ulcers. This is no longer thought to be true, though stress can aggravate ulcer symptoms. There's also no proof that drinking alcohol causes ulcers; however, like stress, alcohol is an irritant.

Recognizing the signs

Sometimes an ulcer causes no symptoms, so it's possible you may have an ulcer and not know it. However, when pain occurs, you commonly feel it as a gnawing or burning pain in the abdomen between the breastbone and navel. You're more likely to feel pain between meals and in the early morning that lasts anywhere from a few minutes to a few hours. You may have discovered that taking antacids or eating relieves the pain. Other signs, though less common, include the following:

✔ Nausea.

✔ Vomiting.

✔ Appetite loss.

✔ Weight loss.

✔ Bloating.

✔ Blood in the stool. If an ulcer is bleeding heavily, blood can appear in vomit or in tarlike, black stool.

Knowing for sure

If your doctor suspects that you have an ulcer, he or she may recommend an upper gastrointestinal (GI) series. In this test, you swallow a chalky liquid called barium and then an X ray is taken of your abdomen. The barium coats the digestive tract and makes its structures — as well as any ulcers present — visible on an X ray.

Another option is endoscopy. An endoscope is inserted through your mouth into the esophagus, stomach, and duodenum. The tube lets your doctor view the digestive tract. Samples of the stomach lining or ulcers can also be collected for analysis during this procedure. A local anesthetic and a mild sedative are usually used in endoscopy.

If your doctor discovers that you have an ulcer, he or she will order a blood test or have the sample of tissue that was removed during endoscopy examined for the presence of *H. pylori*.

Treating ulcers

Your ulcer may be treated with medications that block the production of stomach acids or protect the mucosal (thin sheet of tissue cells) stomach lining. Acid-suppressing drugs include H2 blockers, such as cimetidine (Tagamet), ranitidine (Zantac), and famotidine (Pepcid), and acid pump inhibitors such as omeprazole. Protective drugs include sucralfate (Carafate) and misoprostol (Cytotec), as well as antacids. If *H. pylori* are found to exist, antibiotics are prescribed in combination with these drugs. Although most ulcers heal within eight weeks, the chance of recurrence is between 60 and 70 percent without a maintenance dose of ulcer medications.

Medications usually do the trick, but if your ulcer persists, you may need surgery. During surgery, the ulcer is removed, and the lining of the digestive tract is repaired. In some cases, the nerve that controls acid production in your stomach may be severed to decrease the levels of acid.

Hernias

Your body's organs are held in place by a thin wall of muscle. When the muscular wall becomes thin due to an injury or congenital weakness, an organ or tissue can push through it, creating a protrusion. This protrusion of an organ or tissue through an abnormal opening in the body is called a hernia.

Most hernias occur when a piece of intestine slips through a weakness in the abdominal wall, creating a bulge you can see and feel. Hernias can develop around the naval, in the groin, and any place where you may have had an earlier surgical incision.

According to the National Center for Health Statistics, approximately 5 million Americans have hernias. Men suffer hernias at 30 times the rate of women.

Several types of hernia exist:

- **Inguinal hernia** (accounting for about 80 percent of all hernias) occurs when part of the intestine protrudes out of the abdomen (see Figure 14-2). It can push toward the scrotum, creating a bulge in the groin area (a *direct hernia*) or project into the scrotum (an *indirect hernia*), causing pain and swelling. Eighty to 90 percent of inguinal hernias occur in men, primarily because of the unsupported space left in the groin after the testicles descend into the scrotum.

- **Femoral hernia** occurs when the intestine passes through the canal that carries the blood vessels from the abdomen into the top of the thigh. Most femoral hernias occur in women, commonly as a result of pregnancy and childbirth. Only 1 to 5 percent occur in men.

- **Incisional hernia** occurs after surgery if a weakness is present in the abdominal wall along the incision. However, incisional hernias can occur anywhere in the body where an incision has been made.

- **Paraumbilical hernia** is sometimes found in newborns. It is usually caused by a weakness in the abdominal wall surrounding the naval.

- **Hiatal hernia** (not considered to be a true hernia) occurs when the stomach pushes through a small hole in the diaphragm and into the chest cavity, causing heartburn and acid indigestion (see Figure 14-3).

A hernia becomes *strangulated* when an organ or tissues become trapped and the blood supply has been cut off. If this happens, the tissue may die and gangrene (a life-threatening infection requiring emergency care) may set in.

A hernia may result from sudden stress to the abdominal wall (often caused by lifting something heavy), from a weakening of the abdominal wall caused by previous surgery, from a congenital defect, or from a combination of these factors.

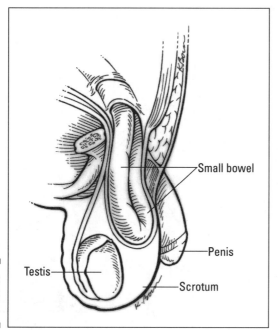

Figure 14-2:
An inguinal
hernia.

Small bowel

Penis

Testis

Scrotum

Recognizing the signs

Here are some of the symptoms of a hernia:

- ✔ Pain or discomfort in the abdominal area while lifting an object or bending
- ✔ Sudden swelling of the affected area
- ✔ Nausea and vomiting if the hernia becomes strangulated (However, in many cases, no symptoms are present.)

Knowing for sure

Your doctor can determine whether a hernia exists either by observation or by a simple digital (manual) examination. In some cases, a visible bulge of tissue in the groin or a mass in the testes may indicate a hernia. To diagnose an inguinal hernia that isn't visible, your doctor will ask you to stand with one leg flexed and with your weight resting on the other. He or she will place a finger against the lower part of your scrotum and push the scrotal skin until the finger enters the inguinal canal. Your doctor then will ask you to cough (not in his or her face!). If he or she feels pressure on the fingertip or on the side of the finger, a hernia exists.

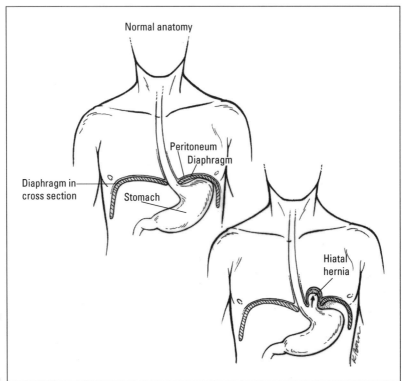

Normal anatomy

Peritoneum
Diaphragm

Diaphragm in
cross section

Stomach

Hiatal
hernia

Figure 14-3:
A hiatal
hernia.

Treating hernias

Except for hiatal hernias — which are usually treated with antacids and diet restrictions — hernias must be repaired surgically. Under no circumstances is a hernia best left untreated. Although you can delay surgery if the hernia is small enough, there's always a chance that the hernia can become strangulated, which is something you want to avoid. At times, a *truss* — a tight-fitting device worn around the abdomen — can help hold a hernia in place until it's repaired. But know this: A truss isn't a permanent solution.

You can have a hernia repaired through outpatient surgery. Possible complications of surgery include *hematoma* (a collection of pooled blood under the skin), infection, or injury to the nerves and vessels of the groin.

About 10 to 15 percent of all hernias recur after corrective surgery.

Preventing hernias

You can't do much to prevent a hernia. You can, however, try to stay fit by keeping your weight at an appropriate level. Also, use a proper technique for lifting heavy objects (see Chapter 9).

If you already have a hiatal hernia, keep yourself more comfortable by wearing loose clothes and avoiding foods and beverages that may trigger heartburn (such as coffee, alcoholic drinks, fatty and fried foods, highly spiced foods, peppermint, and chocolate).

Irritable Bowel Syndrome

Irritable bowel syndrome (IBS), also called spastic colon and irritable colon syndrome, is an involuntary muscle movement in the large intestine. It's considered to be a functional disorder rather than a disease because the colon shows no signs of abnormality, such as a growth or intestinal bleeding. It's estimated that 5 to 19 percent of all men are affected by IBS. Men with IBS are often embarrassed to talk about the problem (and probably are as irritable as their colons). They often don't seek help.

Recognizing the signs

You may have no pain with IBS but may have diarrhea right after you wake up in the morning, during meals, or right after eating. Here are other symptoms you may experience:

- ✔ Abdominal pain
- ✔ Gas (Pain is often relieved by passing gas.)
- ✔ Diarrhea or constipation (or alternating bouts of each)
- ✔ Nausea
- ✔ Feeling full after eating only a small meal
- ✔ Feeling the urge to urinate (and an incomplete emptying)
- ✔ Stress (not everyone who has stress-related bowel problems has the disorder)

Knowing for sure

IBS is diagnosed through a process of elimination. If your symptoms have some semblance of a pattern over time, it may be clear to your doctor that IBS is the cause. But to be cautious, your doctor may order some tests to rule out other causes (such as colitis or inflammatory bowel disease).

After reviewing your medical history and giving you an examination, your doctor will ask you for a small sample of stool. The sample will be tested for blood in the stool. Your doctor may also recommend a *proctosigmoidoscopy* (a procedure that allows the doctor to examine the inside of your rectum and colon through a scope inserted into your anus) and a barium X ray.

Treating irritable bowel syndrome

More than likely, your doctor will recommend some dietary changes. You may find that a change in your diet significantly reduces the effects of IBS. Fat (both vegetable and animal) is often a culprit because it stimulates the colon to contract. Lactose (milk sugar) and gas-producing vegetables such as broccoli and cabbage can also cause IBS symptoms to flare up. Caffeine and alcohol can also affect the colon. Dietary fiber may lessen symptoms by keeping your colon mildly distended, which helps to prevent spasms from developing, and by reducing constipation.

In addition to dietary changes, your doctor may prescribe fiber supplements or an occasional laxative to relieve constipation. Antispasmodic drugs may be prescribed to help reduce abdominal pain and the feeling of urgency for a bowel movement. You may want to try antacid/antigas medications (such as Tums and Mylanta) and antidiarrhea medications (such as Imodium A-D) to treat abdominal pain, cramping, and diarrhea. You can also try smooth muscle relaxants (such as peppermint oil), which help relax the smooth muscles of the gut and relieve cramping.

Don't be surprised if your doctor prescribes antidepressant drugs for you. Studies have shown that these drugs help relieve the symptoms of IBS, independently of their antidepressant qualities.

Sometimes mental health counseling and relaxation training can help relieve IBS symptoms. Emotional stress stimulates colonic spasms in people with IBS, probably because the colon is controlled partly by the nervous system, which is directly affected by stressors in your life. Biofeedback, a relaxation therapy that trains you to control involuntary bodily functions, may be especially helpful in treating IBS.

Chapter 15

Problems with the Plumbing

● ●

In This Chapter

▶ Kicking kidney stones

▶ Treating incontinence

▶ Preventing urinary tract infections

▶ Recognizing penile, urethral, and testicular problems

● ●

*P*lumbing. That's your urinary system — a unit of pipes, connections, and hoses (in a manner of speaking). If you think of your body as being a house, then the urinary system is your body's plumbing system. It's responsible for eliminating liquid waste products from the body. And just like a house with plumbing problems, your body's urinary system may break down, too. Sharing in your body's plumbing are parts of your reproductive organs (namely the penis, testicles, and scrotum). Likewise, these plumbing parts can break down. A house with broken plumbing is inefficient. A body with broken plumbing is annoying, painful, and potentially fatal. But problems with the body's plumbing — such as the kidney stones — are easier to deal with when you know the facts. This chapter covers the most common problems associated with your body's plumbing, including testicular and penile disorders.

Kidney Disease

The kidneys — a pair of bean-shaped organs about the size of your fist and located on both sides of your spine just above the waist — filter liquid waste products (urea, uric acid, and creatinine) out of your body. Each kidney filters about 200 quarts of blood daily.

Blood passes through your kidneys continuously through one million tiny filtering units called *nephrons,* which consist of tufts of small blood vessels called *glomeruli* and some tubules. The kidneys stop blood and protein from passing through the nephrons and return these materials to the bloodstream. The kidneys also clean and filter blood, ridding it of waste that, if left to accumulate, can be fatal.

The average adult produces about two quarts of filtered product, called *urine,* daily. Tiny droplets of urine pass from the tubules in each kidney and collect in the bladder via the *ureters* (tube-like structures). From there, urine is passed from your body through the urethra (a small tube-like structure that drains urine from the bladder). The amount of fluid that passes through the urethra varies daily, depending on how much food and fluid you consume.

Urine can reveal what is happening in your body through a test called urinalysis, which is comprised of any physical, chemical, or microscopic examination of the urine.

Kidney disease is a catchall term for many types of conditions from urinary tract infection (UTI) to serious malformations. If any form of kidney disease goes untreated, further damage can occur, possibly resulting in kidney failure and death.

Figure 15-1 shows a healthy kidney along with a kidney riddled with some of the maladies discussed in this chapter.

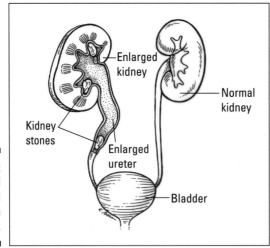

Figure 15-1:
A normal kidney and one with problems.

Kidney failure

The last stage of kidney disease is *end-stage renal disease,* or kidney failure. It means the kidneys have totally shut down. It can result from any kidney condition that has been left untreated. You can live comfortably with half of one normal kidney, but if you suffer total kidney failure, you only have two options: dialysis and kidney transplant.

Forms of kidney disease

Pyelonephritis is an infection of the kidney. Pyelonephritis can affect one or both of your kidneys. Symptoms include fever, nausea, back pain, vomiting, and burning, painful urination. Treatment requires antibiotics, and in severe cases, hospitalization.

Nephritis is an inflammation of the kidney that may affect any of the microscopic structures of the kidney. A drug reaction, an infection, or another form of kidney disease can cause nephritis. Symptoms include retention of fluid and salt, swelling, and protein or blood in the urine.

Glomerulonephritis is an inflammation of the glomeruli, the areas of the kidneys that filter blood. An infection or an inflammatory disease like lupus may cause glomerulonephritis.

Symptoms include discolored urine, high blood pressure, protein in the urine, anemia, severe headaches, and possible convulsions. This condition can lead to kidney failure if not treated. Treatment includes a low-salt diet, blood pressure medication, antibiotics, and sometimes steroids.

Polycystic kidney disease is an inherited, progressive disorder in which cysts form around the kidneys. Symptoms include enlargement of the abdomen, pain, bloody urine, and excessive urination. Patients may also have high blood pressure and kidney stones. Only the symptoms can be treated — high blood pressure can be controlled and kidney stones can be treated. This disease usually leads to kidney failure.

Kidney stones

Perhaps the most painful plumbing problem — and the most common — is the kidney stone.

Men get more kidney stones than women do, and about 12 percent of men can expect a kidney stone by age 70. This problem has a long history — kidney stones have been found in a 7,000-year-old Egyptian mummy.

Also called *nephrolithiasis,* kidney stones form in your kidney, bladder, or ureter (one of a pair of tubes that carry urine from the kidney to the bladder) where there is a buildup of salt or mineral crystals in the urine. They vary in size, shape, and composition, and they can be smooth or jagged.

There are several types of stones. *Calcium stones,* the crystallization of calcium salts, make up 75 to 85 percent of all stones and mostly consist of calcium and oxalate. *Uric acid stones* account for about 8 percent of all cases. *Struvite stones* are large and rough and form as a result of UTIs. They occur mostly in women.

Kidney dialysis

Dialysis involves the use of a machine or mechanism to filter blood and prevent the buildup of toxins in the bloodstream. It must be done frequently (often several times per week) and cannot be stopped unless you receive a kidney transplant.

The type of dialysis you receive depends on your condition and situation. One form of dialysis is *automated peritoneal dialysis*. In this procedure, an incision is made in the abdomen, and a catheter is inserted into the abdominal cavity. During each session of peritoneal dialysis, a special solution is inserted through the catheter and left inside the abdomen for several hours, where it picks up waste products from the body. The fluid then drains from your body. This form of dialysis can be done at night and allows you to be treatment-free during the day. This procedure, done at your home, is performed either manually or by machine.

Hemodialysis involves using a machine to filter your blood. In this process, the blood is diverted to an artificial kidney, called a *dialyzer,* where wastes pass through a membrane. This process takes between two and six hours per session and must be done several times a week.

Continuous ambulatory dialysis requires no machine and cleans the blood continually. A system of tubes and bags flushes your body of toxins. This procedure involves filling the abdomen with cleansing solution and then draining it; it must be done four times daily. Continuous cycling peritoneal dialysis is done by a machine that takes care of the filling, cleansing, and draining process. It is also done at night, usually at your home.

Recognizing the signs

When a kidney stone passes out of your body through the ureter, it produces excruciating pain. Fortunately, most stones pass without causing additional problems or serious damage. Here are the common symptoms of kidney stones:

- ✔ Excruciating pain in the lower back or the abdomen that travels to the groin area
- ✔ Frequent urge to urinate
- ✔ Burning sensation during urination
- ✔ Bloody urine

Knowing for sure

Stones are diagnosed through examination of blood and urine samples. Sometimes an *intravenous pyelogram,* in which a contrast substance (able to be seen on an X ray) is injected into the bloodstream, is done. The contrast substance helps your doctor see the kidney structures, including any kidney stones, on the X ray.

Treating kidney stones

The good news is that about 90 percent of kidney stones don't require surgery. Kidney stones that are small can pass out of your body naturally, and your doctor can prescribe medication to relieve any pain. Also, drinking between six and eight glasses of water daily can help flush out the stones.

If the stones don't pass out of your body, you may be able to undergo a procedure called *lithotripsy,* in which stones are broken apart by shock waves. The waves are created by a machine called a lithotriptor, which is placed against your abdomen or used while you're seated in a tub of water, which helps conduct the shock waves. The small pieces of stones can then be passed out of your body during urination. This procedure requires general or local anesthesia, but no surgery.

Surgical procedures can also remove stones. Open surgery, performed under general anesthesia, is the traditional method. Another option involves the insertion of a fiber-optic scope into the bladder or ureter. Then another instrument is inserted to crush and remove stones.

In addition to removal of stones, your doctor may prescribe medications or dietary restrictions to prevent stones from recurring.

Preventing kidney stones

The best prevention can be found in three simple words: *Drink more fluids*. Drinking lots of fluids can decrease your chances of forming kidney stones by 40 percent. Even beer, wine, and coffee can be beneficial because they increase the flow of urine and decrease the substances responsible for stone formation. But don't overdo them because excessive use of these beverages can lead to other health problems (see Chapter 5).

Conventional wisdom says that too much calcium in your diet causes kidney stones, but this has been proven wrong. One study in which men consumed the highest amount of dietary calcium showed that they were actually less likely than others to get kidney stones. Experts speculate that calcium may reduce the amount of *urinary oxalate* in the body, a substance that may contribute to stone formation.

And recently, a small, three-year study reported in the *Journal of Urology* showed that patients prone to kidney stones who took an experimental compound made of potassium-magnesium citrate daily reduced their risk of recurring kidney stones by 85 percent. Adding the compound increased urinary pH, inhibiting the crystallization of calcium salts.

Incontinence

Of all the male plumbing problems, *urinary incontinence* — or the inability to hold your urine — can be the most embarrassing. Because of this embarrassment, some men fail to seek medical help.

But if you have trouble holding your urine, take heart — you're not alone. An estimated 15 million people have urinary incontinence, including an estimated 3 million men.

The good news is that, in many cases, incontinence is treatable. Millions of Americans are being treated successfully and cured. And because the problem is so widespread, a large number of absorbent products on the market allow people with incontinence to manage their conditions and enjoy normal lives.

Incontinence is not a disease. It's a side effect or symptom of another medical condition such as Parkinson's disease, diabetes, and spinal cord injury. It's not a natural part of aging; in fact, it can happen at any age. Strictly speaking, urinary incontinence means the inability to control urination. It happens when the *urethral sphincter muscles* (muscles that release urine and sperm) — which normally remain tight to keep urine in the bladder — relax and allow urine to leak out.

Incontinence can affect you in many ways — ranging from a little leakage once in a while when you laugh to complete loss of bladder control. The symptoms can change over time.

Incontinence is a common effect of prostate cancer surgery and can persist for up to a year after the surgery. Rarely does incontinence become permanent after prostate surgery. Incontinence may also result from urinary tract infections, constipation, and the effects of some medicine. Or it can be caused by stroke, spinal cord injury, certain birth defects, and chronic conditions such as diabetes. An enlarged prostrate, a condition known as *benign prostatic hyperplasia (BPH),* may also contribute to incontinence (see Chapter 16).

Recognizing the signs

Here are the common symptoms of incontinence:

- Accidental escape of urine from the bladder (either small or large amounts of urine)
- Unable to control urination (either some or all of the time)
- Total loss of bladder control

Several types of incontinence exist: urge, stress, and overflow. You can have more than one type at the same time.

- ✔ **Urge incontinence** is the involuntary escape of urine with little or no warning. With this disorder, you may need to go to the bathroom quite often. You may feel a sudden, severe urge to empty your bladder and lose urine on the way to the bathroom. Some men need to go every two hours, day and night. Others may wet the bed during sleep. This disorder, however, is more common among men with multiple sclerosis, spinal cord lesions, spinal disc problems, and those who have had a stroke and is usually caused by an overactive bladder.

- ✔ **Stress incontinence** is the involuntary loss of small amounts of urine when coughing, sneezing, laughing, walking, or moving in a manner that increases abdominal pressure (such as getting up from a chair or bed). This disorder may occur because the *urethral sphincter,* the part of your urethra that holds the bladder shut, hasn't contracted fully, letting drops of urine escape.

- ✔ **Overflow incontinence** is the involuntary loss of urine from a bladder that doesn't empty completely. It can be caused by an obstruction of the urethra, a stretched or distended bladder, drug side effects, and nerve damage. With this disorder, you may get up often during the night to urinate, you may feel the need to empty your bladder but are unable to do so, and you may produce only a very weak stream of urine despite spending a long time in the bathroom. You may also lose small amounts of urine at various times of the day or night, even though your bladder doesn't feel full.

Knowing for sure

We recommend that you keep a diary to record the exact times and amounts of leakage and to note any problems or anything unusual before you call your doctor. Such a diary can assist your doctor in making a diagnosis.

Be prepared to discuss your complete medical history. Because incontinence is the result of some other medical conditions, your doctor may ask many questions about your health. Don't forget to bring a list of your medications, both prescription and nonprescription.

In addition to reviewing your medical history and any drugs taken, your doctor may perform tests that check your reflexes and muscle tone. Blood and urine tests may also be done to rule out another disease or UTI. Don't be surprised if he or she does a rectal exam to check for internal problems.

If necessary, your doctor may send you to a *urologist,* a specialist who deals with incontinence and diseases of the urinary system and the reproductive organs, such as the prostate.

If simple tests don't prove conclusive, *urodynamic studies* — a series of tests that include *uroflowmetry, cystometry,* and *endoscopic procedures* — may be done. In uroflowmetry, a health practitioner records the volume of the urine you release, how long it takes you to urinate, and whether any dripping occurs after you're finished urinating. In cystometry, a practitioner inserts a catheter (a small, thin tube) through your urethra and into the bladder to measure and monitor your bladder's function. In endoscopic procedures, the practitioner inserts a thin viewing scope into your urethra and bladder to see the internal structures and spot any abnormalities.

Treating incontinence

If a UTI is the cause of incontinence, that condition can be treated with antibiotics to resolve the problem. Here are some things you can do to help if you are incontinent:

- **Teach an old dog new tricks (or retrain your bladder).** Prolong the time between urination gradually, first waiting one to two hours before a trip to the bathroom, then three to four. This training tool stretches the bladder and can improve urge incontinence in up to 75 percent who try it. If you're not sure how to get started, ask your doctor.

- **Avoid *diuretics,* substances that increase urination.** These include alcohol, coffee, and tea. Also, try not to drink anything before going to bed. However, don't cut back severely on liquids, which may contribute to constipation and worsen incontinence.

- **Don't smoke.** Smoking can trigger coughing, which in turn triggers stress incontinence.

- **Empty your bladder before doing exercise.**

- **Try saw palmetto.** This herb has been found to be somewhat successful in treating incontinence associated with BPH. Ask your doctor.

- **Do Kegel exercises.** When experiencing a strong, sudden urge to void, instead of running to the bathroom, take a deep breath, stop what you're doing, and do a series of Kegel exercises (covered in the upcoming sidebar), which not only tighten the urinary sphincter but send signals to your bladder to stop contracting.

Kegel exercises

Kegel exercises can strengthen key muscles, making holding your urine easier. If you tense the muscles around your rectum, while keeping the stomach, thigh, and buttock muscles relaxed, you've done a Kegel. There are two variations: *quick Kegels* (tightening and relaxing the muscles as quickly as possible) and *slow Kegels* (tightening the muscles and holding them for five seconds before releasing them). Start with 10 of each exercise, four times daily. Each week, increase the number of exercise by five, doing four sets daily. Be patient: You may have to do daily exercises for up to two months to notice results.

Treating incontinence with medication

In addition to self-care techniques, your doctor may prescribe medications to help treat incontinence. Oxybutynin (Ditropan) helps to prevent spasms of the bladder muscles. Drugs such as phenylpropanolamine (Propagest) or pseudoephedrine (Sudafed) help to tighten sphincter muscles. If you have BPH, your doctor may prescribe finasteride (Proscar) or terazosin (Hytrin) to reduce the size of an enlarged prostate.

Treating incontinence by other means

When other, less-invasive treatments don't work, your doctor may recommend surgery to treat incontinence. Surgery can remove tissue causing a blockage or strengthen the muscles of your bladder. An artificial sphincter can be surgically implanted. This treatment is 90-percent successful.

A relatively new procedure called the *urethral sling* has been shown to be effective in treating incontinence in women and men. However, its use in males is very experimental and not fully accepted. This surgery involves inserting three small tubes into an incision made under the scrotum. The tubes are pulled tightly against the urethra and sutured into place to help restore urinary control.

Collagen injections may be done to firm up the area around your urethra; however, this treatment is reported to work in about 50 percent of men, and repeated injections are usually necessary to maintain results.

Urinary Tract Infection

Urinary tract infection (UTI), accounting for nearly 8 million doctor visits per year, is one of the most common infections people get. Urinary tract infection is a term that may be used to describe *urethritis* (inflammation of the urethra), *cystitis* (inflammation of the bladder), *pyelonephritis* (inflammation of the kidney), or *prostatitis* (inflammation of the prostate gland).

Here's some good news: UTIs are not common in men and rarely afflict boys. That's in sharp contract to the statistics in women: One woman in five will develop a urinary tract infection sometime during her life (primarily because the urethra in women is shorter than in men, making it easier for bacteria to enter the body and cause infection).

In men, particularly those over age 50, UTIs usually are caused by an obstruction of the urinary tract or an enlarged prostate. They also can result from a medical procedure involving a catheter that unintentionally introduces bacteria.

Urinary tract infections begin when bacteria, usually from the rectum, spread to your urethra and begin to multiply. From there, the bacteria may move into your bladder, causing a bladder infection. Without prompt treatment, the bacteria can then move on to infect your kidneys. Most UTIs are caused by bacteria called *Escherichia coli* (also called *E. coli*), which are found in the colon. Sexually transmitted diseases, such as chlamydia, gonorrhea, and herpes, and nonsexually transmitted infections may cause urethritis in men.

Recognizing the signs

You may have a UTI and not know it. But in most cases, you may have at least one of the following symptoms:

- Frequent urge to urinate (especially at night)
- Pain and discomfort (burning, itching) during urination
- Pain during intercourse and ejaculation
- Cloudy or milky urine
- Blood in the urine
- Urethral discharge (clear fluid or pus from the penis)
- Fullness in the rectum
- Abdominal pain
- Fever
- Fatigue
- Back pain (Lower-back pain is usually associated with prostatitis; high-back pain with kidney infection.)

Knowing for sure

To diagnose a UTI, your doctor reviews your medical history, examines you, and tests a sample of your urine through urinalysis. The test looks for the presence of red and white blood cells, pus, and bacteria. Any bacteria present are grown in a culture medium (a glass dish or bottle containing a jellylike substance in which bacteria grow) to help determine which antibiotic would be most effective in fighting the infection. Your doctor may also include a prostate and rectal exam.

If your infection doesn't clear up with antibiotics, your doctor may order a test that takes an image of the urinary tract, revealing any changes in the structure of the tract. One of these tests is an intravenous pyelogram, which provides X-ray images of the bladder, kidneys, and ureter. Other tests include an ultrasound exam, which produces images from the echo patterns of sound waves from internal organs, and a *cystoscopy,* a procedure in which the urethra and bladder are viewed through a tube inserted into the urethra. These tests can be done at an outpatient setting, in a hospital, or in a clinic.

Treating urinary tract infections

Your doctor will treat your UTI with an antibiotic that fights the particular bacteria responsible for your UTI or with a *broad-spectrum antibiotic* (one that combats a wide range of bacteria). Common drugs to treat UTIs include trimethoprim (Trimpex), trimethoprim/sulfamethoxazole (Bactrim, Septra, and Cotrim), and amoxicillin (Amoxil, Trimox, and Wymox).

Whereas infections of the prostate and kidney require several weeks of antibiotic therapy because they are difficult to cure, most common UTIs often disappear about 24 hours after the drugs are taken. But even if you're feeling better, make sure that you finish taking the full course of antibiotics prescribed or infection may recur.

A warm bath or heating pad can help relieve the pain of UTIs. Drinking plenty of water and cranberry juice is also good to help flush bacteria from the urinary tract. Avoid alcohol, coffee, and spicy foods while you're recovering. If you're a smoker, be kind to your bladder and quit. Smoking has been linked to bladder cancer.

Preventing urinary tract infections

Follow these tips to help prevent UTIs:

- ✔ **Drink plenty of liquids.**
- ✔ **Empty your bladder when you feel the urge to go, and empty it completely.**
- ✔ **Protect yourself against sexually transmitted diseases by using a condom during intercourse.** See Chapter 22 for more information.

Testicular Problems

The testicles are two small, oval organs inside the scrotum, a sac that hangs outside of your body below the abdomen. They produce sperm and secrete testosterone — the hormone that helps you maintain your manly sex characteristics such as a deep voice, facial hair, and muscle mass and strength.

Problems with the testicles can be painful and in some cases may require immediate medical attention.

Epididymitis

This condition is an inflammation of the *epididymis,* the tube that transports sperm from your testicles to the *vas deferens* (another tube that transports sperm to the urethra and out of your body). Symptoms include severe pain in the scrotum that may build over time, fever, and a swollen area that may feel hot to the touch. Epididymitis is diagnosed with a urine sample, a physical exam, and sometimes an ultrasound of the sore tube.

Epididymitis is treated with antibiotics. Your doctor may recommend bed rest, nonprescription pain relievers, and ice packs (applied to the scrotum for 10 minutes three times daily). Fortunately, this condition doesn't cause permanent damage.

Hydrocele

Hydrocele is a buildup of fluid within the sacs that house your testicles (see Figure 15-2). You may notice swelling, but it's usually painless.

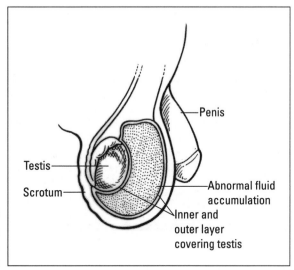

Figure 15-2:
Hydrocele.

Penis

Testis

Scrotum

Abnormal fluid
accumulation

Inner and
outer layer
covering testis

Your doctor can diagnose this condition by manual examination. He or she may also shine a light through your scrotum: If light shines through the swelling, you have hydrocele.

Hydrocele usually goes away on its own. Treatment isn't necessary unless the swelling becomes very large and uncomfortable. Sometimes the buildup of fluid within the sacs must be removed surgically.

Orchitis

Orchitis is an inflammation of the testicle. The condition may be caused by the mumps, but an infection in the prostate or the epididymis can also be a factor. Unfortunately, this condition can cause permanent damage and slight shrinkage to one or both testicles. Infertility may result if both testicles are affected. However, if a man has one normal testicle, he is still fertile. Symptoms include pain in the scrotum, swelling (generally on one side of the scrotum), and a feeling of weight in the scrotum.

Your doctor can diagnose orchitis by manual examination of your scrotum and by the results of a urine sample.

If the infection is bacterial, antibiotics are prescribed. But if the infection is viral, bed rest and pain relievers are prescribed. If the doctor suspects orchitis has interfered with your fertility, he may recommend a sperm analysis (see Chapter 23).

Testicular injury

If you've suffered a blow to a testicle, no doubt you've seen stars from the pain. Fortunately, the painful injury is only temporary and usually causes no permanent harm. That's because the tissues inside your scrotum are spongy and flexible, capable of absorbing a great deal of shock without suffering permanent damage.

The pain is caused by the swelling of the injured testicle within its protective sac. The pressure caused by the swelling inflames the surrounding nerves, causing pain to spread throughout the lower abdomen. An ice pack applied to the scrotum and anti-inflammatory medications can reduce the swelling and pain after an accident. If swelling and pain persist for longer than an hour or if the scrotum is bruised, quickly seek medical care. Too much pressure within the scrotum can damage tissue and could lead to infertility, blood clots, or even the loss of a testicle.

Varicocele

A *varicocele* is a group of varicose veins within the scrotum. The condition is caused by a breakdown of the valves within the veins that causes blood to pool in the testicles. Symptoms include a painless swelling above the testicle that's usually on the left side because the varicose vein travels high into the abdominal region before reaching its area to drain blood. The swelling often goes down when you lie down. Your doctor can make a diagnosis through manual examination of the scrotum.

Although a varicocele isn't harmful in itself, the collection of pooled blood in the testicles may cause infertility. If infertility occurs, surgery can tie off the varicose vein and restore fertility. Otherwise, treatment isn't necessary.

Testicular torsion

Your testicles are suspended within the scrotum by a structure called the *spermatic cord*. Rarely, the cord becomes twisted, cutting off the blood supply to a testicle. This condition is called *torsion*. It may occur after physical activity, but usually there is no known cause. Symptoms include sudden, severe pain in a testicle; one testicle higher within the scrotum; nausea and vomiting; swelling; and fever.

Seek immediate medical attention: If you don't within a few hours, the affected testicle may die from a lack of blood and will have to be removed.

Torsion is diagnosed through manual examination and sometimes ultra-sound of the scrotum. Your doctor may be able to treat testicular torsion by manually untwisting the testicle; however, emergency surgery is generally required.

Undescended testicle

Before you were born, your testicles were housed in your abdomen. About one month before you were born, they descended into the scrotum. Rarely, in 1 percent of men, one or both testicles remain in the abdomen after birth.

Diagnosis is made by manual examination. Usually, the condition corrects itself; however, if the testicle doesn't descend within a year, medications or surgery may bring it into position. The best age for surgery is 12 to 18 months. If a testicle remains undescended in a boy over the age of five, infertility may result. A testicle that was previously undescended is more vulnerable to cancer than a normal testicle and is also more likely to contribute to infertility.

Penile and Urethral Conditions

Along with incontinence, UTIs, and problems with the kidneys, other "plumbing problems" can affect your penis and urethra.

Balanitis

Balanitis is the condition in which the tip of your penis becomes red and sore. It can be caused by UTIs, by irritation from clothing or detergents, or by a yeast infection. Balanitis is more common in uncircumcised men because the foreskin may be so narrow that it can't retract easily. Also, men with diabetes commonly have balanitis; in fact, men with balanitis are often tested for diabetes. Treatment includes antibiotics or antifungal medications when infection is present.

Good hygiene practices — washing the penis thoroughly each day and pulling back the foreskin (if you are uncircumcised) to wash underneath it — are important to your health.

Foreskin and seven years ago . . .

Circumcision — removing the foreskin of the penis — may be controversial, but some studies show it reduces the likelihood of urinary tract infections (UTIs). It's thought that the foreskin tends to trap bacteria, setting the stage for infection of the urethra. Men who are uncircumcised experience a higher rate of UTIs than men who are circumcised. Also, several studies have shown that uncircumcised men are twice as likely as circumcised men to catch sexually transmitted diseases such as human immunodeficiency (HIV), herpes, human papillomavirus, and syphilis. A 1997 study that looked at the data from the National Health and Social Life Survey found *no* preventive benefit to circumcision.

But circumcision may prove beneficial in the case of penile cancer. Almost all cases of this rare type of cancer occur in men who are not circumcised at birth, and areas of the world where circumcision is uncommon have higher rates than countries where boys are routinely circumcised. It is believed that if the penis isn't kept clean, *smegma,* a buildup of mucus and other secretions, can collect under the foreskin and cause irritation and inflammation of the *glans* (the cone-shaped tip of the penis) and can contribute to the development of cancer.

The following illustration shows how a circumcision is performed.

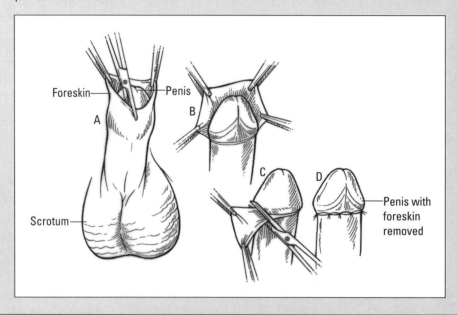

Paraphimosis

Paraphimosis usually develops as the result of a tight foreskin, or *phimosis.* It occurs when the foreskin retracts and becomes constricted, causing pain and swelling. This condition needs to be treated quickly to avoid permanent damage: Seek immediate treatment if the pain and swelling are severe. Often, the foreskin can be gently moved back into its normal position. If not, your doctor may recommend circumcision or partial circumcision.

Peyronie's disease

Peyronie's disease, also known as curvature of the penis, is a progressive condition caused by the formation of scar tissue within the penis. The affected tissue resembles a plaque or a hard lump on the upper or lower side of the penis. It causes your penis to curve when erect and can make sexual intercourse difficult or impossible.

Your doctor can diagnose Peyronie's disease by feeling your penis for the ridge of scar tissue. It is not known why scar tissue forms in some men; however, some studies suggest that it's the result of genetic inheritance or trauma to the penis. There is no specific treatment, although treatment isn't always required in mild cases. Sometimes, Peyronie's disease disappears on its own within 15 months. In extreme cases, surgery can straighten the penis.

Priapism

Priapism is a rare condition marked by prolonged erection. Now that may sound too good to be true, but unfortunately, the prolonged erection is painful and occurs without sexual stimulation. Priapism is caused most commonly as a side effect of drugs such as injection therapy for erection problems or psychiatric drugs like the antidepressant trazadone. It may also be caused by problems within the spinal cord, leukemia, or inflammation of the urethra. Symptoms include an erection in which the tip of the penis is soft and the shaft is hard, and the erection doesn't subside after sexual activity ends. Immediate treatment is necessary to prevent permanent damage to the penis. The erection can be relieved by spinal anesthesia or by drawing blood through a wide needle to help relieve pressure.

Urethral stricture

Urethral stricture is a rare condition in which the urethra — the tube that carries urine through your penis and out of your body — becomes narrowed because of scar tissue from an injury or infection. Symptoms include difficult or painful urination. Treatment involves a local anesthetic and the insertion of a thin instrument to stretch the urethra. This procedure may need to be repeated several times. If the treatment doesn't work, surgery may be required.

Urethritis

Urethritis is inflammation of the urethra. This condition is often caused by sexually transmitted disease, but sometimes the cause remains unknown. Symptoms include pain during urination, an urge to urinate frequently, and discharge from the penis. The condition is diagnosed through examination of the discharge. Antibiotic therapy is the course of treatment, and treatment for a sexual partner may be necessary, too. Urethritis may be *asymptomatic,* or show no symptoms at all, so if your sexual partner is diagnosed with a sexually transmitted disease like chlamydia or gonorrhea, you should be treated for urethritis even if you are asymptomatic.

Chapter 16

Prostate Disease

• •

In This Chapter

▶ Unearthing prostate disease

▶ Recognizing and treating benign prostatic hyperplasia

▶ Identifying and treating prostatitis

• •

The prostate is a gland that plays a key role in reproductive events. It's only as big as a walnut, and it weighs less than an ounce, but along with the *seminal vesicles* (small glands that help sperm to swim), it secretes the seminal fluid in which sperm travel during a man's ejaculation.

The prostate gland, part of the male reproductive system, is located in the neighborhood of the male sex organs, as shown in Figure 16-1. Specifically, you can find it in front of the rectum, at the base of the bladder. The gland surrounds a part of the urethra, the tube carrying urine from the bladder out through the penis. Because of this precarious location inside the body, you can easily see why any enlargement or inflammation of the prostate gland may put the squeeze on the urethra, so to speak, and cause you all kinds of urinary tract complaints. It's also easy to see why many men may sooner or later have some firsthand experience with these complaints. If you are beginning to experience urinary tract difficulties, you can be sure that you are not alone. As this chapter shows, however, we have much good news to share in the treatment — and maybe even the prevention — of serious prostate problems.

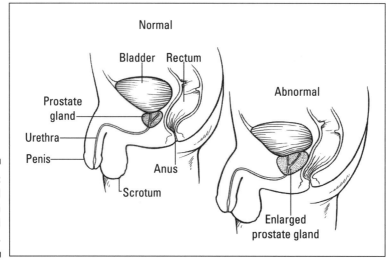

Normal

Bladder Rectum

Abnormal

Prostate
gland

Urethra

Penis

Anus

Scrotum

Enlarged
prostate gland

Figure 16-1:
A normal
and an
enlarged
prostate.

Prostate Disease

The prostate gland can be much more troublesome to men than its small size would suggest. In fact, it causes a range of difficulties that more or less fall into three major categories. Two are common but benign. The third occurs less frequently but is cancerous and, over time, could be life-threatening. Briefly then, here are the three categories:

- **Benign prostatic hyperplasia (BPH):** Otherwise known as *benign enlarged prostate,* BPH is the most common disease of the prostate gland, affecting 6 out of every 10 men between the ages of 40 and 59, according to some surveys. This disease tends to become increasingly problematic for men as they age.

- **Prostatitis:** Prostatitis refers to inflammation or infection of the prostate. This condition affects young to middle-aged men primarily.

- **Prostate cancer:** Prostate cancer is a very serious disease affecting 1 in 8 American men over a lifetime. This cancer usually grows slowly and, with early detection, has an exceptionally good prognosis. We discuss this disease in more detail later in this book (see Chapter 18).

Benign Prostatic Hyperplasia

Benign prostatic hyperplasia (BPH) is more commonly known as a benign, or noncancerous, enlargement of the prostate gland. This form of prostate disease is the most common, and it's the one most likely to cause urinary tract complaints for most men. Fortunately, there is no apparent relationship between BPH and cancer, which occurs far less frequently.

This disease results from the prostate gland's natural growth. When a boy is born, his prostate is about the size of a pea. It grows very slowly until puberty when a period of rapid growth occurs. This first phase of growth ends around age 25 when the prostate reaches its normal size, which is about 20 grams, or less than an ounce.

Sometime around middle age, as if awaking from a long slumber, the gland starts to grow again. It continues to grow steadily during most of a man's life. It's during this second period of growth that the gland has the potential to put pressure on the urethra, which tunnels through the prostate and into the penis. By putting pressure on the urethra, the prostate gland creates an external obstruction on this slender tube. This obstruction — like tightening a too small belt around a too big waist — is the root cause of the symptoms relating to BPH. In addition to creating discomfort, and even pain, urine can back up. This urinary retention can be a serious problem.

Whether or not a growing prostate becomes troublesome has much to do with the direction in which it grows. If the gland grows inward, toward the urethra, then you'll notice it. If, however, the gland grows outward, away from the urethra, then enlargement is not a problem, even if the gland becomes as big as a tennis ball! In other words, although you can expect your prostate to grow as you age, you may never experience the symptoms described next for BPH.

Recognizing the signs

Because the prostate, the urethra, and the bladder are all connected, disorders affecting one or the others often have similar or overlapping symptoms. Symptoms of BPH may include the following:

- ✔ Frequent urination, especially at night
- ✔ Difficulty beginning and stopping the flow of urine
- ✔ Dribbling, hesitant, and thin stream of urine

✔ Sensation of urgent need to urinate

✔ Sensation that the bladder hasn't emptied completely

✔ Blood in the urine

✔ Inability to urinate, which can cause possible infection and increasing pain

✔ Involuntary loss of urine (incontinence)

Knowing for sure

Your doctor can diagnose BPH through a series of tests, your medical history, a physical examination, and a review of your urinary habits. Expect a urinalysis and a urine culture to be done (tests that show any abnormalities in urine, including bacterial infections). Your doctor may also do a few "hands-on" types of examinations, such as palpitating your bladder to tell whether it's distended and a *digital rectal exam* — a manual exam in which the doctor inserts a gloved, lubricated finger into the rectum and, through the wall of the rectum, checks the prostate for hard or lumpy areas (see Chapter 2). Your doctor may also do a series of tests known as a *urodynamic evaluation* to measure urine flow and *residual urine,* or urine that is left in the bladder after urination. Sometimes a catheter (a thin tube that drains the bladder) is inserted through the penis to measure residual urine.

Other tests include blood tests to rule out kidney disease. A blood test that checks for prostate cancer — *prostate-specific antigen (PSA)* — may also be done. In addition, imaging tests, such as X rays and ultrasound scans, can provide an image of the prostate. A *cystoscopy,* a procedure in which a lighted viewing tube is passed through the urethra into the bladder, may also be done to allow visual examination of the bladder.

Treating BPH

Many treatment options exist for men with BPH. You can determine which treatment is right for you only by discussing your particular situation with a *urologist,* a doctor who specializes in diseases of the urinary and reproductive systems in men. Many physicians believe that men whose symptoms are mild (do not interfere with their quality of life) and who are at low risk of urine retention may benefit from a period of "watchful waiting." Interestingly, it has been observed that as many as one-third of all mild cases of BPH clear up without any treatment at all.

Measure your symptoms

The following questions, based on the American Urological Association questionnaire, can help you and your practitioner measure the severity of BPH. Give yourself a 0 for never; 1 for less than one time in five; 2 for less than half the time; 3 for half the time, 4 for more than half the time; and 5 for almost always. The time frame is over the past month.

✔ How often have I had a sensation of not emptying my bladder completely after I have finished urinating?

✔ How often have I had to urinate again less than two hours after I finished urinating?

✔ How often have I found I stopped and started again several times when I urinated?

✔ How often have I had a weak stream of urine?

✔ How often have I found it difficult to postpone urination?

✔ How often have I had to strain to begin urination?

✔ How often have I typically had to get up to urinate from the time I went to bed at night until the time I got up in the morning?

A score of 7 or less may indicate a mild problem; 8 to 19 may indicate a moderate problem; and 20 to 35 may indicate a severe problem. Talk with your doctor about your symptoms and your score.

If symptoms become more progressive — and often they do not — medication may be appropriate. Other men with severe symptoms may need to consider surgery or another medical procedure.

Treating BPH with medication

If your doctor suggests medication, he or she may prescribe one of two major kinds of medications used to treat an enlarged prostate: alpha blockers (brand names, Hytrin, Cardura, Flomax) or finasteride (Proscar).

Alpha blockers were first marketed about a decade ago to treat hypertension. When it was noticed that these drugs indirectly relieved urinary symptoms, doctors began prescribing them to treat BPH. These drugs relax muscles in the prostate and neck of the bladder, increasing urinary flow rates and decreasing outflow obstruction and symptoms of irritation associated with BPH. They are believed to benefit men with smaller prostate glands who, nevertheless, are thought to require medication. An example is terazosin (Hytrin). Possible side effects include low blood pressure, dizziness, fainting, and headache. Reduced fertility has been observed in animal studies. A newer alpha blocker, tamsulosin (Flomax), has a more selective ability to relax the muscles in the prostate and neck of the bladder without lowering blood pressure.

Finasteride, belonging to the chemical family 5-alpha-reductase inhibitors, blocks the enzyme 5-alpha reductase, which converts testosterone to DHT. DHT is one of the hormones that prompts the prostate gland to grow. Finasteride relieves the symptoms of BPH by reducing the size of the prostate. Results occur after three to six months of use, and although this may seem rather slow, the results show that the prostate reduces in size by up to 30 percent. Sixty percent of the men who use finasteride show some improvement; however, the improvement may not be substantial. In some cases, sexual problems such as a lowered libido and erection problems may result from taking the drug. Also, evidence shows that finasteride reduces PSA, the marker to detect early-stage cancer of the prostate, in the bloodstream by almost 50 percent. This, in turn, must be taken into account when screening for prostate cancer.

Along with sexual problems, another possible side effect includes a condition called *gynecomastia,* or enlarged and tender breasts. Rarer still, gynecomastia has been associated with breast cancer in men. This uncommon side effect from finasteride is not yet understood.

Treating BPH with surgery

Sometimes medication alone is enough to reduce an enlarged prostate and relieve the symptoms associated with BPH. At other times, surgery is necessary. Although a number of studies suggest that surgical procedures to relieve prostate symptoms can safely be put off for years, thousands of men a month undergo surgical treatment to relieve their symptoms of BPH.

Surgical procedures called *prostatectomy* or *partial prostatectomy* center around removing or reducing prostate tissue. In an open prostatectomy, the gland is removed through an incision in the abdomen. Closed prostatectomy involves surgery performed through the urethra. Open prostatectomy has been largely replaced by closed prostatectomy, though it's still used if the prostate is very large, if other procedures need to be done simultaneously, or if an open procedure is preferred to the more technically difficult closed procedure.

Transurethral resection of the prostate (TURP) is a closed method and is commonly performed, accounting for 90 percent of all prostate surgeries done for BPH. This procedure — which typically lasts about 90 minutes — involves inserting a narrow instrument, called a *resectoscope,* into the urethra to remove obstructing tissue in the prostate gland one piece at a time. This procedure is fairly successful: Ninety percent who opt for this surgery show improvement, although an estimated 10 percent report erection problems, and 3 percent report incontinence. However, men who have erection problems after TURP often had poor erections to start with. Also, about 10 percent of men who have TURPs need a second prostatectomy at some time in their lives because the glandular tissue continues to grow.

Another closed procedure is *transurethral incision of the prostate (TUIP)*. This surgery differs from TURP in that it requires the surgeon to make slices in the prostate to lessen the stranglehold the gland has on the urethra. This method reduces the risk of erection problems and other sexual problems. Again, a repeat procedure is sometimes required.

Newer surgical methods have been developed and include *transurethral microwave thermotherapy, intraurethral stents,* and *transurethral needle ablation (TUNA)*. Microwave thermotherapy (also known as hyperthermia) uses heat to eliminate some of the prostate tissue. Intraurethral stents are small, tubelike structures inserted into the urethra that enlarge it to give relief from urinary problems. TUNA uses a needle and heat to eliminate excess prostate tissue. To date, long-term effects of these procedures are unknown.

Risks of benign prostatic hyperplasia surgery

For some men surgery for BPH isn't necessary, or it can be safely delayed for years — perhaps indefinitely — with watchful waiting if they can handle the symptoms and if no dangerous complications develop. If after discussing your options with your doctor you decide to forgo surgery, expect regular checkups and monitoring to keep track of the progress of the condition. And remember: If surgery is recommended, seek a second opinion before agreeing to the procedure (see Chapter 2).

As with any surgery, there can be side effects. Here, then, are the potential ones:

✔ **Incontinence:** This problem may occur after surgery for BPH. But it's not usually a permanent problem unless muscles of the external urethral sphincter have been damaged somehow during surgery, or unless there was a prolonged problem with an enlarged prostate for months or years prior to surgery.

✔ **Sterility:** Sterility is not uncommon after certain forms of prostate surgery, such as a radical prostatectomy.

✔ **Erectile dysfunction (impotence):** Most prostate problems do not lead to erectile dysfunction. Although all surgical approaches to BPH involve some risk, these risks are small, and they are usually temporary. Recovering sexual function sometimes takes up to a year after surgery. Ultimately, most men who are able to have an erection before the procedure recover that ability afterwards and report no difference in the sensation of sexual climax after surgery.

✔ **Retrograde ejaculation:** Sometimes ejaculate leaks backward into the bladder instead of moving forward out of the penis after surgery. This does not alter the ability to achieve orgasm.

✔ **Stricture:** A scar may form in the urethra that leads to a narrowing that may cause recurrent symptoms of obstruction.

✔ **Bleeding:** This problem is more common with TURP. Usually this bleeding does not require transfusion and typically stops on its own.

✔ **Infection:** Placing any instrument from outside to inside the urinary tract risks introducing infection. Surgeons prescribe antibiotics after prostate procedures to minimize this risk.

Treating BPH through self-care

For all men, a low-fat, low-cholesterol diet plays a key role in helping to reduce and prevent the symptoms of BPH. Here are other steps you can take to make you more comfortable and slow the progress of BPH (and other prostate problems):

- ✔ **Reduce your intake of fluids in the evening.**

- ✔ **Limit your intake of coffee and other caffeinated drinks.**

- ✔ **Urinate frequently.** If you overtax your bladder, you only aggravate the symptoms.

- ✔ **Take your time while urinating.** Allow several minutes to empty your bladder as completely as possible.

- ✔ **Avoid spicy foods, citrus juice, and other acidic drinks to make your urine less acidic and less irritating.**

- ✔ **Exercise regularly to increase the flow of blood and oxygen to the prostate area.** Walking and swimming are especially good exercises for men with BPH.

- ✔ **Take a warm bath to soften the prostate and relax the pelvic muscles.**

- ✔ **Avoid constipation, which worsens the symptoms of BPH.**

- ✔ **Watch your blood sugar level if you are diabetic.** Poorly controlled diabetes weakens the bladder, which then cannot push the urine past the enlarging prostate.

- ✔ **Watch out for certain over-the-counter and prescription drugs that may trigger the bladder neck to suddenly tighten like a clamp, blocking urine flow.** Talk with your doctor and pharmacist about possible side effects of drugs that can worsen BPH symptoms. Medications that could be troublesome include oral bronchodilators (drugs that relax airways, making it easier to breathe), diuretics, tranquilizers, cold and allergy preparations that contain decongestants, and antidepressants.

Prostatitis

Prostatitis is an inflammation of the prostate and can affect a man at any age. This condition is common, and most men at least once in their life visit the doctor for this problem. There are two types of prostatitis: nonbacterial and bacterial.

Nonbacterial prostatitis

Nonbacterial prostatitis is the most common form of prostatitis diagnosed and occurs eight times more frequently than bacterial prostatitis. Nonbacterial prostatitis is somewhat puzzling because no microorganisms have yet been discovered that might cause the condition; yet infection-fighting cells are sometimes found in the seminal fluid from the prostate of men with prostatitis. Shrouded thus in mystery, the condition is often treated with antibiotics and with drugs that relax the muscles of the prostate gland. These treatments are not always effective; nonetheless, the symptoms often disappear eventually, only to return again at a later date. Nonbacterial prostatitis describes two separate conditions: congestive prostatitis and prostatodynia.

Congestive prostatitis occurs when *prostatic fluid* — a rather creamy, souplike fluid — is stored in the gland instead of being ejaculated out of the body. It's normal for the prostate to routinely produce prostatic fluid because this fluid accompanies sperm. Some practitioners believe that chronic, unrelenting stress is responsible for most cases of prostatic disease, particularly when no sign of bacteria is present. And some scientists are still searching for a mystery microorganism. But in the absence of other evidence, some urologists have concluded that sex — too much or too little — is to blame. That's the hunch of Stephen N. Rous, M.D., author of *The Prostate Book*, and the late Monroe E. Greenberger, M.D., author of *What Every Man Should Know About His Prostate*.

Every day, a healthy prostate secretes between one-tenth and two-fifths teaspoon of prostatic fluid. When you're sexually aroused, however, you produce between 4 to 10 times that amount. Normally, you release it through ejaculation. But if you don't ejaculate, the fluid builds up and the prostate becomes congested.

Prostatodynia (which means "painful prostate") indicates a condition in which pain seems to be coming from the prostate gland, though usually it's coming from surrounding muscles. In most cases of prostatodynia, the prostate is normal. This is another somewhat mysterious form of prostate disease because no one is sure what causes it. Some physicians suspect that prostatodynia, and maybe even other prostate disorders, are stress related.

Bacterial prostatitis

Bacterial prostatitis is clearly caused by a bacterial infection. The disease can be either acute or chronic.

Acute bacterial prostatitis is a rare and serious disease caused by bacteria in the prostate gland. *Neisseria gonorrhoeae,* responsible for gonorrhea, and the *Trichomonas* protozoan may cause bacterial prostatitis. Other suspected organisms include *Chlamydia trachomatis* and *Ureaplasma urealyticum.* Bacterial infections of the prostate can also occur as an indirect consequence of BPH. If urine retention were to become a problem, for example, the urine lingering in your bladder might serve as a breeding ground for bacteria, putting you at high risk for an infection. Similarly, you are at higher risk for bacterial prostatitis if you've recently had a urinary catheter, which can introduce bacteria into your body.

Chronic bacterial prostatitis is a recurring prostate infection that usually results when invading bacteria are not eradicated for various reasons. For example, bacteria can take hold because of some defect in the prostate. In this case, correcting the problem in the gland is necessary before treatment with antibiotics. Because of the complicated nature of this problem, these infections are not treated easily.

Recognizing the signs

The symptoms for nonbacterial and bacterial prostatitis are similar and also include many of the symptoms described for BPH. They include the following:

- Pain or tenderness in the prostate area that can radiate toward the genitals, the lower back, and even the upper thighs
- Discharge of fluid from the penis, especially after a bowel movement
- Pain or itching deep within the penis
- Discomfort and burning during urination
- Pain following ejaculation
- Fever, aches and pains, and lower-back pain (for acute bacterial prostatitis)

Many of these symptoms are also symptoms of sexually transmitted diseases (see Chapter 22).

Knowing for sure

Along with physically examining you and reviewing your medical history, your doctor relies on several diagnostic tests to determine whether you have prostatitis. One such test is a urinalysis and urine culture to check for signs of infection. If bacteria are found, further tests may be unnecessary. To check for nonbacterial prostatitis, your doctor may use a digital rectal exam to measure the size of your prostate. If the prostate is enlarged and spongy, you may have nonbacterial prostatitis.

If symptoms of acute bacterial prostatitis are present, a digital rectal exam should be done very gently (if at all) because the prostate is highly inflamed or irritated during this disease. Too much probing may force the infection into other parts of the reproductive system. Therefore, ask your doctor whether this examination under these conditions is necessary.

To diagnose chronic bacterial prostatitis, a *segmented urine culture* may be done. In this test, your practitioner takes one routine urine sample and one from the midstream of the urine. Afterword, he performs a digital rectal exam and massages the prostate to release prostatic fluid. Then another urine sample, which contains the released prostatic fluid, is taken. All these urine samples may leave you feeling as dry as the Mojave Desert, but they're necessary to determine if the infection lies in the prostate or in the urethra.

Treating prostatitis

Bacterial prostatitis is treated with a regimen of antibiotics, which must be thorough and complete to rid yourself of bacteria responsible for the disease. Treatment often lasts up to a month because the bacteria often remain hidden within the prostate. If your symptoms are severe, your doctor may prescribe painkillers. Hospitalization is sometimes necessary if the urethra becomes blocked, if fever leads to dehydration, or if there is a risk that the bacteria may spread throughout your body (for example, when your health is compromised by another condition such as cancer).

Prostatectomy is a last resort for men with chronic bacterial prostatitis. If the condition is causing complications such as urinary retention or kidney problems, prostatectomy may be considered. Increasing evidence, however, shows that recurring prostate infections may be related to diet. Interestingly, more zinc is found in a healthy prostate than anywhere else in the body, and it appears that when zinc moves out, bacteria move in. Unfortunately, eating a diet high in zinc has not translated to greater zinc in the prostate.

Antibiotics are not effective for nonbacterial prostatitis. Prostatodynia can be treated with over-the-counter drugs such as ibuprofen or aspirin. Sometimes muscle relaxants are prescribed for prostatitis if a doctor suspects that the condition may be stress related. Other measures may include alpha blockers (such as those discussed under treatment of BPH) and warm baths to relax the pelvic muscles.

Sexy ways to treat congestive prostatitis

You don't need pills to treat this type of non-bacterial prostatitis. And fortunately, the therapy is quite enjoyable: regular ejaculation, whether through intercourse or masturbation. As you may recall, congestive prostatitis occurs when prostatic fluid builds up in the prostate gland instead of being ejaculated from the body. In this case, ejaculation may be just what the doctor ordered — but beware: Too much sex can make you uncomfortable, irritating your prostate, especially if you've been celibate for a while. So gradually increase how often you engage in sexual behavior, and keep it a regular part of your life.

Chapter 17

Heart Disease

. . . .

In This Chapter

▶ Exploring coronary heart disease

▶ Decreasing your risk of heart disease

▶ Exposing the "hidden killer" — hypertension

▶ Lowering blood pressure

▶ Recognizing the signs of stroke

▶ Keeping tabs on your cholesterol and triglyceride levels

. . . .

*H*eart attack. The words alone can send a chill down even the strongest man's spine, and with good reason.

American Heart Association data show that heart disease is the leading cause of death for Americans. Men have a greater risk of heart attack at a younger age than women. But the risk increases for women as they near menopause and, eventually, surpasses that of men.

For all that we have romanticized it in song and fable, the heart is just a muscle about the size of your fist, but a most vital muscle it is. Your heart pumps about 2,000 gallons of life-sustaining blood through your body in the average day. When it stops working right, so do you.

If the nicest thing we can say about someone is that he has a good heart, the most important thing we can say is that he has a healthy heart.

Your heart will beat 2.8 billion times by the time you're 70. But you shouldn't take any of its beats for granted. This chapter gives a broad overview on heart disease and what you can do to keep your heart beating strong.

Coronary Heart Disease

Unlike the more easily understood ailments such as appendicitis or kidney stones, heart disease is not a readily defined condition. Health practitioners use the term to cover a wide range of cardiac and circulatory problems. Unfortunately, what this means, among other things, is that pinpointing a single, identifiable cause for heart disease is not possible. There are many causes for many conditions or a lot of causes for a single condition.

The type of heart disease you are probably most concerned about is coronary heart disease, or coronary artery disease — those conditions in which the arteries (large blood vessels) that nourish your heart with blood become blocked, cutting off the blood and oxygen supply to your heart muscle. The heart muscle starves, causing *angina pectoris* — chest pain brought on by exertion (a warning sign of coronary heart disease) — and *myocardial infarction (MI),* also known as heart attack.

It's fair to say that coronary heart disease is in large part a by-product of who we are, what we do, and how we live. Some heart problems are hereditary or congenital (existing from birth) and can be treated or managed but not eliminated. The American Heart Association has identified the following other risk factors:

- **Smoking and passive smoking:** You're taking a big risk if you smoke. The record shows that smokers have twice the risk of heart attack compared with nonsmokers, and that cigarette smoking is the greatest single risk factor for sudden cardiac death (death that occurs unexpectedly and suddenly). If you're a smoker who suffers a heart attack, you're more likely to die within the hour than a nonsmoker is. Evidence shows that if you smoke or are chronically exposed to secondhand smoke, you may irreversibly damage your blood vessels, which can lead to heart attack and stroke (discussed later in this chapter). *Peripheral vascular disease* (an abnormal condition affecting blood vessels outside of the heart), which can cause gangrene and requires leg amputation, is almost exclusively confined to smokers. The good news is that if you quit, your rate of risk declines rapidly. Within three years of stopping, if you smoked a pack a day or less, your risk of coronary heart disease is almost the same as someone who never smoked at all.

- **High cholesterol levels:** Cholesterol is a fatlike substance found naturally in animal sources such as meat, fish, poultry, whole-milk dairy products, and egg yolks. Too much cholesterol, above the accepted norms, can dramatically increase your risk of heart attack, especially when combined with other factors such as cigarette smoking. Excess cholesterol causes fatty deposits to form along the walls of your arteries. We discuss cholesterol in more detail later in this chapter.

- ✔ **High blood pressure:** High blood pressure makes your heart work and pump harder, which can lead to heart failure. High blood pressure in particular presents no obvious symptoms or early warning signs and thus requires close attention. We talk about high blood pressure later in this chapter.

- ✔ **Inactivity:** You may want to abandon your couch potato ways for regular exercise. Exercise controls cholesterol and obesity and also lowers blood pressure.

- ✔ **Diabetes:** If you're a diabetic, carefully monitor your blood glucose levels. More than 80 percent of people with diabetes die from some form of blood vessel disease or coronary heart disease.

- ✔ **Obesity:** Being obese puts a strain on your heart and may lead to high blood pressure and high cholesterol levels.

- ✔ **Stress:** Stress can cause your blood pressure to rise.

Arteriosclerosis and atherosclerosis

The origins of coronary heart disease often lie with arteriosclerosis and atherosclerosis. *Arteriosclerosis,* or "hardening of the arteries," describes a number of conditions in which fatty deposits and minerals collect in your arteries, causing the vessels to become rigid and inflexible, as shown in Figure 17-1. In *atherosclerosis,* the most common form of arteriosclerosis, the walls of your arteries become thick and irregular due to the accumulation of cholesterol, fats, and other substances, called *plaque.* Arteriosclerosis sets the stage for heart attack by narrowing your arteries and reducing blood flow to your heart. Also, your rigid blood vessels can't expand to allow greater blood flow when needed. Because you can't feel the buildup of plaque, the only signs of atherosclerosis may be angina pectoris or heart attack.

Angina pectoris

Atherosclerosis leads to angina pectoris (often abbreviated as *angina*). During stress, exercise, or an emotional situation — even after a large meal — your heart beats faster and works harder, which means that your heart muscle must get more oxygen-rich blood to maintain the pace. But if you have arteriosclerosis, the arteries leading to your heart become rigid and narrow, and they don't allow enough oxygen-rich blood, filled with nutrients, to reach your heart muscle during these situations. The pain felt during this oxygen deficiency is angina. Nearly 3 million American men have angina.

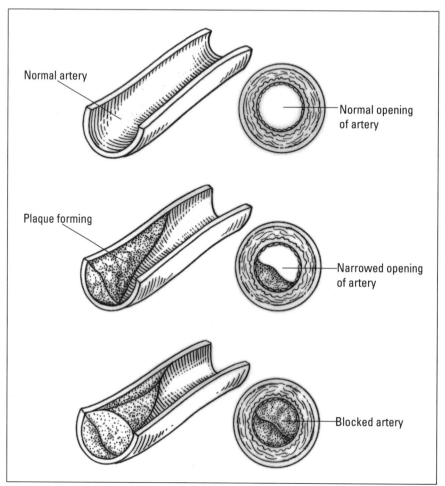

Normal artery

Normal opening
of artery

Plaque forming

Narrowed opening
of artery

Blocked artery

Figure 17-1:
Arteriosclerosis.

Angina is a warning sign of coronary heart disease. Some doctors call angina
"God's gift to humans" because many heart problems are silent, without
symptoms, and go unnoticed until they cause sudden death.

Recognizing the signs

Here are the common signs of angina:

- A heavy, strangulating, suffocating pain
- Pain that seems to begin under the breastbone, on the left side of
  the chest

✓ Pain that radiates to other parts of the body, including the throat, neck, jaw, and left shoulder and arm

✓ Pain that reaches the right side of the body. A heavy meal, stress, emotional excitement, cold weather, and physical exertion, such as climbing the stairs, can trigger an episode of angina. It commonly occurs at night

An episode of angina usually lasts longer than 5 minutes and less than 30 minutes. Anything longer than this may be a heart attack.

Knowing for sure

Angina is usually unmistakable, but at times it mimics noncardiac conditions, such as heartburn, indigestion, and gas. Diagnosis can be done through a physical exam and an *electrocardiogram (EKG),* a test in which electrodes, attached to your chest, measure your heart's electrical activity. A stress test — an EKG in combination with exercise, such as running on a treadmill — may also be done. If your stress test is abnormal, an angiography — an invasive test in which dye is injected in your blood vessels and viewed with an X ray — is done.

Treating angina through self-care

Angina must be treated under your doctor's care. However, along with doctor's orders, here are some self-care techniques:

✓ Don't smoke.

✓ Eat a balanced, very low-sodium diet.

✓ Lose weight if necessary.

✓ Have your blood pressure monitored.

✓ Remain calm in stressful or emotional situations.

Treating angina through medication

Along with self-care, medication is necessary and, in some cases, invasive and noninvasive surgery. Medications don't resolve the problem of buildup in your arteries, but instead get around it by reducing blood pressure, slowing your heart rate, and enlarging your blood vessels. These are the more commonly used medications:

✓ **Beta blockers** slow your heartbeat and reduce the contraction strength of your heart muscle, reducing your heart's need for oxygen. Beta blockers include propranolol (Inderal), nadolol (Corgard), and metoprolol (Lopressor).

✔ **Vasodilators** relax your arteries and increase your blood flow. The most common one prescribed is nitroglycerin (Minitran and Nitrol). Other vasodilators include minoxidil (Loniten), hydralazine (Apresoline), and prazosin (Minipress).

✔ **Calcium channel blockers** are prescribed to ease the load on your heart. They work by blocking the passage of calcium, which your muscle cells use to control the size of your blood vessels. When the muscles of your arteries are prevented from constricting, your blood vessels open up, allowing blood to flow more easily through them. Calcium channel blockers include nifedipine (Procardia) and diltiazem (Cardizem).

✔ **Thiazides** (types of blood-pressure-lowering medications) and **digitalis** (a drug that increases the strength of your heart's contraction, while slowing and regulating your heartbeat), when heart failure is a factor, are two other drug regimens to combat angina.

Treating angina with surgery

In addition to lifestyle changes and medication, your surgeon may perform bypass surgery (surgery that restores blood flow to the heart), angioplasty, or stenting (a flexible tube placed in the artery). However, most experts agree that they are not necessary for those with mild angina.

Heart Attack

A heart attack, or myocardial infarction (MI), takes place when a blockage (clot) — perhaps caused by a buildup of plaque — occurs in your heart artery. As a result, blood-containing oxygen is cut off from your heart and your oxygen-deprived heart muscle is damaged. The area of dead or damaged tissue is known as an *infarct*.

You have close to a 90 percent chance of survival after a heart attack if no complications arise. Alarmingly, 23 percent of previous heart attack victims will have another attack within six years of their first attack.

Recognizing the signs

Unfortunately, denial is often the first reaction to outward signs of an occurring or impending heart attack. People tend to explain away warning signals by attributing them to other, less lethal causes. Quite frankly, a heart attack is scary, and no one is eager to deal with its implications. But the fact is that certain symptoms — although they do not definitely prove the presence of heart disease — clearly indicate that you should consult your doctor as soon as possible.

A heart attack is not necessarily the giant and immobilizing blow that literally strikes you down. An attack isn't always that severe, at least not the first time around. Some heart attacks (known as "silent heart attacks") are either so minor that they are almost unnoticed or the outward symptoms pass and are dismissed as just another angina attack or heartburn. A massive heart attack, on the other hand, can be compared with being tackled by an entire football team; an episode of angina can be compared with being tackled by one football player. Many victims pass out due to pain and panic.

Here are some common signs associated with painful heart attacks:

✔ Crushing, breathtaking pain that starts in the chest and radiates into the left arm, back, or shoulder

✔ Cold, clammy sweat

✔ Vomiting

✔ Pain that lasts longer than 15 minutes or is not affected by nitroglycerin medication

---

Symptoms of heart trouble

Excluding obvious symptoms, such as angina and heart attack, other common signs of coronary heart disease include:

✔ **Shortness of breath:** Sure, we all run out of breath now and then after exertion, especially as we age or put on weight (perhaps just a wee bit too much weight). However, when things that you used to do as a matter of routine begin to leave you breathless and gasping for air, you need to think about having some tests done. This is especially important if you tend to awaken during the night with the feeling that you are choking or suffocating. Also, breathing difficulties, especially during exercise or while lying flat, may be additional signs. Shortness of breath can sometimes be nothing more than a reaction to nervous tension or stress, but it never hurts to be sure.

✔ **Dizziness and fainting spells:** Thankfully, these conditions may motivate you to see your doctor and head off a potential heart attack. Although other conditions — such as low blood pressure or a middle-ear infection — can cause dizziness and fainting, these signs have been associated with heart disease.

✔ **Extreme fatigue:** Finding yourself extremely tired, especially if paired with either chest pain or shortness of breath (or both) may be a sign of heart disease.

✔ **A dry, hacking cough:** This is a rare sign.

✔ **Swelling of your legs, feet, ankles, or abdominal area**

Aspirin: Can it increase your chances of surviving a heart attack?

Taking aspirin at the first sign of a heart attack may increase your chances of surviving a heart attack. In the Second International Study of Infarct Survival, 17,000 men and women were randomly given either 162 mg of aspirin or a placebo daily over a 30-day period within 24 hours of the onset of suspected heart attack symptoms. The study ended after five weeks and showed a decrease in complications only in people taking aspirin. Experts estimate that aspirin taken at the beginning of a heart attack could save between 5,000 and 10,000 lives annually. However, aspirin is not safe for everyone and can increase the risk of stroke for some. Discuss whether aspirin is a safe alternative with your doctor.

Knowing for sure

Your doctor may check you for a heart attack through an EKG and a series of blood tests that measure enzymes in your blood. Silent heart attacks are usually diagnosed by a stress test.

Getting treatment

A heart attack is a medical emergency! Call for help. When you arrive at the hospital, the staff will treat you as if you definitely had a heart attack until it is proven otherwise. This is a good thing, no matter how frustrating it may become if you're suddenly feeling better.

If you encounter someone having a heart attack, call for help immediately. Help the person into a comfortable, lying down position. Unloosen his or her collar, belt, cuffs, and shoes. If the heart and breathing have stopped, perform cardiopulmonary resuscitation (CPR) if you are qualified to do so, or keep the person as comfortable as possible until someone properly trained in CPR arrives.

At the hospital, clot-busting (thrombolytic) drugs are given to dissolve the clot responsible for the attack and restore blood flow to your heart, preventing further damage. Thrombolytic drugs are most effective when administered within two hours of a heart attack. Thrombolytic drugs include streptokinase, urokinase, tissue-type plasminogen activator, and recombinant plasminogen activator. Depending upon the circumstances, you may also receive injections of painkillers, blood pressure medications, or other drugs.

After your condition stabilizes, the long process of determining exactly what happened and what to do next about it has just begun. The main treatment is rest to relieve any stress or anxiety that may have brought on the attack. You may leave the hospital within a matter of days after an attack if your physical condition warrants it, but expect various tests, procedures, and possibly surgery in days and weeks following a heart attack.

Knowing for sure

Following a heart attack — or, better yet, before an attack occurs — diagnostic tests may be done to diagnose coronary heart disease and determine its extent.

If your doctor suspects that your heart vessels are blocked, an angiography is performed. A form of angiography called a *cardiac catheterization* is also helpful in diagnosing heart disease. In this procedure, your doctor inserts a small plastic tube (catheter) through a blood vessel in your groin and into your heart. Dye is then injected, and an X ray shows detailed images of your heart's blood vessels. In addition to showing blockages and clot formations, heart chamber pressure and blood samples may be taken during the procedure.

EKGs and stress tests are another way of diagnosing heart problems. In addition, a number of imaging techniques can be used. Computer axial tomography (CT or CAT) scans, a computerized, three-dimensional X-ray process, and magnetic resonance imaging (MRI) scans (which create the heart's image by using a magnetic field) are also procedures that your doctor may order to diagnose heart disease. Your doctor may also order X rays to examine your heart's structure or an echocardiogram, which sends ultrasonic waves through your heart to create its image.

Treating with surgery

A number of procedures can help restore blood flow to your heart, whether or not you have experienced angina or heart attack. Angioplasty is a procedure to open blockages. Two main types are *percutaneous transluminal coronary angioplasty (PTCA),* or balloon angioplasty, and *direct angioplasty.* Laser angioplasty is an additional type of angioplasty currently under development. *Coronary bypass* and *coronary-stent placement* are two other surgical procedures.

In PTCA, a catheter with a balloon on the tip is inserted into a narrowed artery where the balloon is inflated to push aside any blockages. Direct angioplasty involves the same procedure, but the balloon catheter is inserted into a totally blocked artery rather than one that is simply narrowed. Laser angioplasty may be an option in the future. With this technique, a laser catheter would be inserted into an artery and used to burn away the blockage. The procedure is still experimental and has not been perfected, but is expected to be easier to perform, is less expensive, and is less painful than balloon angioplasty.

When your doctor knows that certain arteries are blocked and normal blood flow to your heart must be restored, he or she may recommend coronary bypass surgery. In this procedure, the surgeon takes a vessel — usually from your leg or thigh — and transplants it to the aorta and coronary artery to replace, or bypass, the clogged artery. About 75 percent of all bypasses are done on men. Bypass surgery is usually recommended over angioplasty for high-risk patients (who suffer severe conditions with more than two blocked arteries).

In coronary-stent placement, done with the aid of ultrasound (an imaging technique that creates an image using sound waves), a small, stainless-steel mesh tube — called a stent — is placed on the end of a balloon catheter and threaded into your blocked artery. The doctor then inflates the balloon, which expands the tube and lodges it firmly in place. The stent pushes the blockage out of the way and props open your artery to increase blood flow. Stents are not appropriate for difficult-to-reach blockages because they need to be positioned carefully without puncturing the vessel.

Treating with medication

Drug therapy is best if you're at low risk for heart attack — that is, you have mild angina or have had a heart attack with no subsequent angina. However, bypass surgery relieves angina pain and other symptoms of coronary heart disease better than medication therapy. Nonsurgical alternatives to treat your clogged heart arteries include calcium channel blockers, aspirin, beta blockers, and nitroglycerin. If heart failure is also a factor, you may be given *angiotensin converting enzyme (ACE) inhibitors,* diuretics, and digitalis.

ACE inhibitors work by breaking apart the fatty deposits that form along the walls of your arteries. They are successful in preventing heart failure and have been credited with preventing heart attacks in those who take them. Diuretics remove water and salt from your body by causing you to urinate frequently, which results in lower blood pressure. Digitalis helps keep your heart pumping more effectively by relaxing your heart vessels and helping blood flow to your heart. It also strengthens your heartbeat and reduces the size of your heart.

A low, daily dose of aspirin may also be prescribed after heart attack to prevent repeat attacks. According to a 1996 report in the *Journal of the American College of Cardiology* that monitored close to 1,000 patients, 2 percent of the aspirin users died from cardiac causes, compared with 5 percent who didn't use aspirin. The benefits were greater for those who had been treated with clot-dissolving drugs, the study said.

Cholesterol-lowering drugs such as lovastatin may be used if you've had bypass surgery. The drugs help reduce the progression of atherosclerosis, the artery-clogging disease that initially causes the need for surgery.

Preventing heart attack

Granted, you can do little about your age, gender, or family history. However, you probably can decrease your risk of heart attack by changing your lifestyle in the following areas:

- ✔ **Keep tabs on your cholesterol levels.** The Framingham Heart Study found that heart attack rates rise 2 percent for each 1 percent increase in blood cholesterol over 200 milligrams per deciliter (mg/dl). To control your cholesterol, avoid saturated fat, eat fewer calories, and try to eat foods rich in fiber, such as vegetables and fruits. If your cholesterol is very high, drugs to lower it may be an option for you. We talk about cholesterol later in this chapter.

- ✔ **Ask your doctor about aspirin.** Daily intake of aspirin may reduce your risk of heart attack by thinning your blood and preventing clots from forming. However, you should talk with your doctor before doing so because aspirin is not safe for everyone.

- ✔ **Drink moderately.** Studies show that one drink a day (12 ounces of beer, 5 ounces of wine, or $1^1/_2$ ounces of liquor) may have a protective effect on the heart. However, the effects are more beneficial if you are middle-aged or older and have suffered a heart attack or stroke or already have cardiovascular disease, according to a study reported in the January 8, 1998, issue of *Medical Tribune*.

- ✔ **Exercise.** Regular exercise is good for you because it helps reduce stress, cholesterol levels, high blood pressure, and excess weight, and it can make your heart stronger, leading to a lower pulse rate. But overdoing exercise isn't a good thing, especially weight-lifting exercises that can trigger heart attacks. Talk with your doctor before beginning an exercise program.

- ✔ **Relax.** Because stress is such a factor in heart disease, eliminating or decreasing it can do wonders for your cardiovascular health (see Chapter 6 for stress-reducing tips).

✔ **Control your blood pressure.** Your heart has to work harder to push blood through your body when your blood pressure is high. This causes your heart to enlarge and can speed up atherosclerosis. Fortunately, by reducing your diastolic blood pressure by only 2 mm Hg (millimeters per mercury), you can decrease your risk for cardiovascular disease and stroke. The average healthy blood pressure is 120/80 mm Hg. We talk more about blood pressure later in this chapter.

✔ **Stop smoking.** We've already told you that smoking is hurtful to your cardiovascular health. If you need additional convincing, see Chapter 5.

Other Forms of Heart Disease

As if coronary heart disease isn't enough, other types of cardiovascular disease exist, too. These include valve disorders, congestive heart failure, congenital heart defects, heartbeat irregularities, heart muscle diseases, and pericardial disease.

Valvular heart disease

Your heart's valves — thin, tough, membranous "door flap" tissues — keep watch over which way blood flows through your heart. They guide blood through your heart in the right direction by opening or shutting flaps. Diseases, such as rheumatic fever, can damage the valves and lead to endocarditis (inflammation of the heart's inner lining). When the valves heal, the valves' flaps develop scar tissue, preventing them from closing properly. Blood can leak back through the opening. The scarring can narrow valve openings, too. Over time, the narrowing worsens and usually needs surgery to repair or replace the valve. Another way the valve flaps degenerate is through thickening or calcification (calcium deposits). And if the previously mentioned isn't enough to make your heart flutter, there are a number of additional, nonrheumatic valve disorders: floppy valve syndrome (which is pretty much what it sounds like), syphilitic heart disease, tumors, and drug-induced valvular difficulties, among others.

When the valves are damaged, your heart's chambers — where nutrient-rich blood passes through — need to work overtime to maintain the proper pumping pressure despite the narrowing and the leaks. The extra work can lead to serious complications affecting the size of the chambers and the thickness of the chamber walls (not to mention exhausting your heart's ticker — the pumping mechanism).

Knowing for sure

Usually, cardiac catheterization and angiography are used to determine the type and extent of the valve disorder.

Getting treatment

Valve disorders can be corrected by surgically separating the valves that are stuck together with scar tissue, by cutting valves to fit more snugly (valvuloplasty), or by reconstructing the valve tissue through plastic surgery (annulopasty).

Congestive heart failure

Congestive heart failure, commonly referred to as "water on the heart," involves problems with your heart's pump, usually caused by muscle failure. When your heart doesn't pump efficiently, blood backs up into the vessels of your lungs, draining into the lung tissue itself. As a result, your body becomes overloaded with water and sodium, often leading to death by total heart failure.

Don't confuse congestive heart failure with heart attack. A heart attack means the heart no longer pumps blood, but with congestive heart failure, your heart keeps on ticking, but not as efficiently.

Recognizing the signs

Symptoms include breathing difficulty, coughing, fluid retention, chest and liver pain, and diminished urination. The heart often enlarges to compensate for its inefficiency.

Getting treatment

Treatments include a pacemaker to regulate your heartbeat, dietary restrictions, and medications such as digitalis, diuretics, and vasodilators. Sometimes beta blockers and calcium channel blockers are also used.

Congenital heart defects

Congenital defects are abnormalities that occur at birth, perhaps because of a developmental problem in the womb. About 925,000 Americans live with heart defects today. Heart defects may be caused by disease in the mother during pregnancy, by drugs or alcohol taken by the mother, or by genetic or environmental factors.

Knowing for sure

Congenital defects can usually be detected through a stethoscope as an unusual sound, or murmur. However, not all murmurs mean a heart defect. Murmurs that are not dangerous occur naturally in many people. Imaging techniques such as CAT scans, MRI, and ultrasound are used to see heart defects.

Getting treatment

Treatment depends on the type of defect. Congenital heart defects are usually corrected with surgery. Drugs may also be used to treat the conditions.

Heartbeat irregularities

Perhaps you've felt your heart speed up, slow down, or flutter and become out of control. Although everyone's heart skips a beat occasionally (you see a pretty woman, come within two numbers of winning the lottery, or get pulled over by a police officer for "creative driving"), conditions of abnormal heartbeat and rhythm, known as *arrhythmias,* may warn of heart disease. In themselves, they're usually not life-threatening.

A blockage in an artery, a lack of oxygen to your heart muscle, a slow heartbeat, changes in the electrical activity of your heart, or certain drugs can trigger arrhythmias. The most serious form of arrhythmia is *ventricular fibrillation,* in which the heart contracts wildly and blood stops being pumped. Death usually occurs unless immediate treatment is given.

Medications such as lidocaine, propranolol, procainamide, and quinidine are used. The type of drug used depends on the type of arrhythmia present. In emergencies, CPR can keep the heart beating during an attack. A *defibrillator* — a piece of equipment that provides a jolt of electricity — can also be used in emergencies.

Heart pacemakers are available to control irregularities in the heart's rhythm. These are tiny devices (the size of a silver dollar) that weigh only two ounces. They are placed in the chest to help regulate the heartbeat by emitting an electrical charge. This charge is generated by batteries within the device and carried to the heart by an electrode-containing wire. Pacemakers are implanted when a complete heart vessel blockage is present.

Heart muscle diseases

Several types of heart muscle disease, or *cardiomyopathy,* exist with a number of causes — some of them unknown. In this condition, the heart muscle may thicken or shrink, causing problems that include congestive heart failure, lazy pumping action, or valve problems. Cardiomyopathy can be caused by infection, illness, degenerative disease (such as muscular dystrophy), high blood pressure, chemicals, alcohol, drugs, and chemotherapy drugs.

Treating cardiomyopathy depends on the type of disease and its cause and often includes surgery or medications.

Pericardial disease

The *pericardium* is the fluid-filled sac that protects your heart, and it may be affected by various types of infection.

- ✔ **Pericarditis.** This condition is the inflammation of the pericardium due to infection. In *acute pericarditis,* a general infection affects the sac, causing chest pain and fever. It can be treated with antibiotics. *Acute nonspecific pericarditis* is a condition in which the pericardium is attacked directly by a virus.

- ✔ **Pericardial effusion.** This condition occurs when the sac becomes flooded with liquid. It can be caused by infection or injury to your heart or by drugs, including radiation therapy used to treat cancer. It isn't dangerous unless the fluid causes your heart to fill with blood, a condition called *cardiac tamponade.* In this case, a surgical procedure called *pericardiocentesis* is done to drain the fluid from the sac.

- ✔ **Constrictive pericarditis.** The sac becomes hard with calcium deposits and interferes with the functioning of your heart. Treatment includes surgical removal of the pericardium.

Hypertension

Hypertension, or high blood pressure, is a serious and insidious health issue that affects 50 million Americans. Not only does it greatly increase your chance of heart attack, but it also increases your risk of stroke, arteriosclerosis, and kidney failure. Recent research shows that high blood pressure can reduce memory and mental sharpness.

High blood pressure makes your heart work harder, straining both it and the arteries as they try to push more blood through your vascular system. The heart compensates for high blood pressure by enlarging itself. In reality, a large heart is less efficient than a normal-size one. In the end, your overworked vessels can become scarred and more susceptible to atherosclerosis. Hypertension is sneaky, usually giving no outward sign that it exists or is steadily doing damage to your heart and circulatory system. This is why hypertension is often called "the silent killer." You can have high blood pressure for years without knowing it (like that moldy mass of Chinese food leftovers hiding in the dark corner of your refrigerator). Most people only discover they have hypertension when they have their blood pressure checked (like when you finally decide to clean out your refrigerator) or when life-threatening conditions occur.

One in four American adults suffers from hypertension. Some 90 percent of people with hypertension have no obvious causes. For about 10 percent of people with hypertension, a definite cause — or combination of causes — may trigger the disease, including a genetic predisposition, kidney diseases, sleep apnea (sudden stoppage of breathing during the night), and environmental conditions. According to the American Heart Association, those most at risk are people with low educational and income levels, men up until the age of 55 (women age 55 and over are at a greater risk than men), and African Americans and white Americans who live in the Southeast.

Blood pressure

Blood pressure is the force your blood exerts on the walls of your blood vessels while it travels throughout your body. It's measured using two numbers, the *systolic* and the *diastolic*. The systolic, the higher number in the blood pressure fracture, represents the force of your blood at its strongest as the heart contracts. The diastolic, the lower number, represents the force of your blood between heartbeats, when your heart is resting.

There is no such thing as a "normal" blood pressure level, and you're unlikely to actually have a measurement of exactly 120/80 mm Hg, for example. Yet guidelines have been devised to give health practitioners a tool to help diagnose the stage of the disease.

Though it was once taken for granted that older people had higher blood pressure, we now know that hypertension is not a natural effect of aging, and, if anything, older people should watch their blood pressure levels more carefully than younger people.

Following is a listing of the standards that most practitioners use to diagnose hypertension:

	Systolic (mm Hg)	Diastolic (mm Hg)
Optimal	<120	<80
Normal	120 - 129	80 - 84
High normal	130 - 139	85 - 89
Stage 1 hypertension	140 - 159	90 - 99
Stage 2 hypertension	160 - 179	100 - 109
Stage 3 hypertension	180 - 209	110 - 119
Stage 4 hypertension	>210	>120

Recognizing the signs

Because hypertension usually shows no symptoms in the majority of people, it is difficult to recognize. However, you may experience the following, common indicators of hypertension:

- ✔ Headaches
- ✔ Heart palpitations
- ✔ Flushed face
- ✔ Blurry vision
- ✔ Nosebleeds
- ✔ Labored breathing after moderate exertion
- ✔ Fatigue
- ✔ Strong and frequent need to urinate
- ✔ Ringing or buzzing in the ears
- ✔ Dizziness and spinning (vertigo)

Knowing for sure

Blood pressure is measured by using a *sphygmomanometer,* or blood pressure cuff, which is inflated around your upper arm to get a reading. This inflation compresses the *brachial artery,* a large artery in your arm, which momentarily stops the flow of blood. As the pressure is released, a stethoscope is used to listen to the sound your blood makes as it again starts to pulse through the artery. The systolic pressure is measured when the first sound is heard, the diastolic pressure is measured just after the last sound is heard.

An examination for changes to your retina, the membrane at the back of your eye, can also help to diagnose hypertension. The retina is the only place in your body where arteries can be seen directly.

If your systolic pressure is greater than 140 mm Hg and/or your distolic pressure greater than 90 mm Hg over an extended period of time (blood pressure readings are taken several times at varying intervals because they do change), your blood pressure is considered to be borderline high. As these numbers increase, indicating that blood is having a harder time flowing, the danger of complications from high blood pressure becomes greater. Such complications include heart disease, stroke, and kidney and eye damage.

You can also take your blood pressure at home with a traditional sphygmo-manometer or an automatic device. Home monitoring is helpful in distin-guishing true hypertension from *"white-coat" hypertension,* high blood pressure that occurs only in the doctor's office, probably because of nervousness.

Using self-care and prevention

By taking measures to control or eliminate the known factors of hyperten-sion, you can often reduce high blood pressure or, if you don't have hyper-tension, prevent it from occurring. Most medical experts recommend the following:

- ✔ **Begin a moderate aerobic exercise program, such as running, walk-ing, swimming, or biking, with your doctor's okay.** Most experts advise against weight-lifting exercises, which can raise blood pressure. If you're elderly, you may want to try T'ai chi, which has been shown to lower systolic blood pressure in elderly people.

- ✔ **Quit smoking.** The nasty habit increases your heart rate and narrows your blood vessels, directly causing a rise in blood pressure.

- ✔ **Avoid alcohol.** Studies show that as few as two drinks daily can raise your blood pressure.

- ✔ **Reduce personal stress and anger.** As a man, you're especially prone to high blood pressure levels.

- ✔ **Lose excess weight.** Obesity and high blood pressure go hand-in-hand.

- ✔ **Toss your salt shaker out if you have high blood pressure.** Reducing sodium in your diet can lower your blood pressure between 4 and 5 mm Hg of systolic pressure and between 1 and 3 mm Hg of diastolic pres-sure. The National Heart, Lung, and Blood Institute advises those with hypertension to limit their intake of sodium to 2,400 mg or less daily. In addition to table salt, watch out for processed foods, which supply three-fourths of the sodium in the average diet. Reduce or cut out canned meals and soups, certain frozen foods, lunch meats, catsup, salad dressings, and other condiments, cereals, cheeses, and snack foods, such as pretzels, salted nuts, and potato chips, from your diet. Hypertension is a very rare disease in cultures where salt intake is minimal.

- ✔ **Eat foods high in potassium and calcium.** According to a National Institutes of Health study, a diet rich in fruits, vegetables, and low-fat dairy products provides enough potassium and calcium to help reduce blood pressure. The study, called DASH (Dietary Approaches to Stop Hypertension), found that this type of diet reduced systolic pressure by an average of 11.4 mm Hg and diastolic pressure by 5.5 mm Hg in people with hypertension.

✔ **Lighten up on NSAIDs because they can increase blood pressure, particularly if you are old.** They can also interfere with certain antihypertensive drugs, such as beta blockers. Popular nonprescription NSAIDs include ibuprofen (Motrin IB and Advil) and naproxen (Aleve).

✔ **Watch your caffeine intake.** Although some studies have shown no risks from caffeine, others have seen a correlation between hypertension and higher intake of the stimulant. To see whether caffeine affects your blood pressure levels, try going without coffee and other caffeinated foods and drinks.

Treating hypertension with medication

If lifestyle changes don't do the job, your doctor may prescribe an antihypertensive medication. A wide range of medications is available, all designed to relieve hypertension by allowing blood to flow through the body more easily. Because people react quite differently to various antihypertensives, a trial period is often necessary to determine which is the most effective and causes the fewest side effects. Common medications for treating high blood pressure include the following:

✔ **Angiotensin converting enzyme (ACE) inhibitors:** These medications block the production of angiotensin, a chemical your body produces to raise blood pressure. Angiotensin's normal role is to maintain equilibrium when your blood pressure drops by tightening your arteries. Examples of these drugs include enalapril (Vasotec), lisinopril (Prinivil and Zestril), and captopril (Capoten).

✔ **Calcium channel blockers:** Calcium channel blockers work by blocking the passage of calcium, which your muscles' cells use to control the size of your blood vessels. When the drugs prevent the muscles of your arteries from constricting, your blood vessels open up, letting blood flow more easily through them. Calcium channel blockers include nifedipine (Procardia), diltiazem (Cardizem), isradipine (DynaCirc), and verapamil (Calan).

✔ **Diuretics:** These drugs cause your body to excrete excess salt and water, reducing blood volume. Consequently, your heart doesn't have to work as hard (hey, we all need a break now and then). Examples of these drugs include chlorothiazide (Diuril) and hydrochlorothiazide (Hydro-DIURIL).

✔ **Beta-blocking drugs:** Beta blockers lower high blood pressure by reducing the force and rate of your heartbeat. Examples of these drugs include atenolol (Tenormin), metoprolol (Lopressor), and propranolol (Inderal).

✔ **Vasodilators:** Vasodilators relax your arteries and increase your blood flow by working directly on the muscles that comprise the walls of your arteries, causing them to dilate. An example of these drugs includes hydralazine (Apresoline).

Antihypertensive drugs may cause such minor side effects as dizziness, fainting, and stomach upset. More serious possible side effects are specific to each drug and range from disorientation, depression, and anxiety to a decrease in libido, sexual dysfunction, impaired circulation, and congestive heart failure. Discuss the possibilities with your doctor before beginning treatment. Once you begin treatment, tell your doctor immediately about any side effects.

Your doctor will work with you to find the best medication or combination of medications to bring your blood pressure to normal and keep it there with minimal or no undesirable side effects. After you agree on an approach, following your doctor's guidelines is important in terms of both the amount taken and the schedule followed.

Don't stop taking an antihypertensive suddenly because doing so may cause a dramatic rise in blood pressure with serious consequences.

Finally, if you tend to have high blood pressure, regular physical checkups become even more important (see Chapter 2).

Stroke

A stroke, or *cerebrovascular accident,* is often called a *brain attack.* The brain, which consists of more than 10 billion cells, uses 25 percent of the oxygen you breathe in order to function. Oxygen gets into your brain through your bloodstream. When the blood supply is interrupted and the oxygen can no longer be delivered, its cells, which run the various functions of your brain, begin to die. This injury, which can affect any part of your brain, is called a stroke.

Stroke is the third largest cause of death (behind heart disease and cancer) and the leading cause of serious disability in the United States. According to the American Heart Association, about 600,000 Americans suffer new or recurrent stroke every year. Young African-Americans have a two to three times greater risk of ischemic stroke (covered in the next section) compared with white Americans. Fortunately, the risk of dying from a stroke is less than half of what it was 20 years ago.

According to the American Heart Association, hypertension is the most important risk factor associated with stroke. Even a high-normal systolic blood pressure (130-139 mm Hg according to the Joint National Committee on Detection, Evaluation, and Treatment of High Blood Pressure) is linked to stroke. Other factors associated with stroke include high cholesterol levels, coronary heart disease, high red blood cell count (a high red blood cell count encourages the development of blood clots, increasing risk of stroke), cigarette smoking, lack of exercise, and excess weight combined with too much sodium in the diet.

If you've been described as hot-tempered, you may want to cool down your anger. A study of Finnish men found that men who act out their angry feelings have a two times greater risk of stroke compared with men who control their anger before it reaches an extreme level.

No two strokes are exactly alike. For one thing, the effect of stroke is determined by which part of your brain it attacks and the severity of that attack. A stroke may be mild, with few permanent or serious effects. However, a stroke may be severely debilitating, leaving you weak or paralyzed, uncoordinated, off-balance, and unable to use language.

Types of strokes

Your oxygen supply can be interrupted in two ways: through a blockage or through bleeding. A blockage of a blood vessel in your neck or in your brain is called an *ischemic stroke*. A rupture of a blood vessel in or near your brain causes the second type of stroke, called *hemorrhagic stroke*.

Ischemic stroke is more common, accounting for 80 percent of all strokes. In ischemic stroke, one of your blood vessels may become blocked by thrombosis, an embolism, or stenosis, cutting off the oxygen supply to your brain. *Thrombosis* is a blood clot that forms within a blood vessel of your brain or neck. *Embolism* is a clot that forms in another part of your body and then moves through your bloodstream to lodge in a vessel of your brain or neck. *Stenosis* indicates severe narrowing of an artery in or leading to the brain.

Hemorrhagic stroke can be caused by a head injury, by the rupture of an *aneurysm* (a bulge in the wall of one of your blood vessels), or by a weak or abnormal blood vessel. A hemorrhage causes a hematoma (pooled blood) in your brain and can increase pressure on your brain. This rise in pressure decreases the circulation to the damaged parts of your brain.

Ministroke

Perhaps you've heard of someone who had a "ministroke." *Ministroke,* or *transient ischemic attack (TIA),* occurs when a narrowed artery, blood clot, or some other foreign material temporarily blocks blood flow to the brain (see the following figure). The result is stroke-like symptoms that last from a few minutes to several hours (no longer than 24 hours).

TIAs can occur days, weeks, or months prior to major stroke, and those who suffer a TIA usually make a full recovery within a day or so. About 36 percent of those who have more than one TIA will later have a stroke. Half of those subsequent strokes occur within a year of the mini-attack, and 20 percent of them happen within a month.

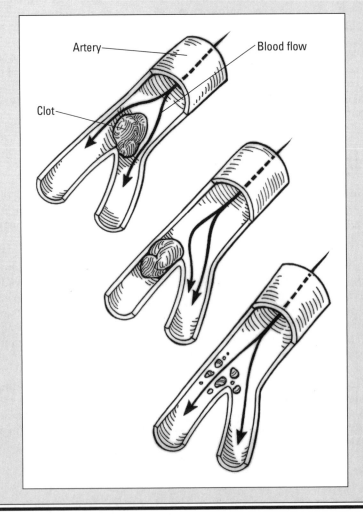

Artery — — Blood flow

Clot —

Recognizing the signs

If you observe one or more of these signs of a stroke or a TIA, seek emergency help:

✔ Sudden weakness or numbness of your face, arm, or leg

✔ Sudden dimness or loss of vision, particularly in one eye

✔ Sudden difficulty understanding speech or speaking

✔ Sudden severe headache with no known cause

✔ Unexplained dizziness, unsteadiness, or sudden falls, especially accompanying the other signs

These are some of the effects of a stroke:

✔ **A stroke may weaken or paralyze one side of the body.** The affected side of your body is opposite the side of your brain that has been injured. Your whole side may be affected or just your arm or leg.

✔ **A stroke may affect your balance and coordination.** You may find it hard to coordinate movements in order to sit, stand, or walk — even if your muscles are strong enough.

✔ **A stroke may cause you to ignore or be unaware of things on one side of your body.** You may not even look toward the injured side of your body.

✔ **A stroke can create pain, numbness, or odd sensations.** These symptoms can make relaxing and getting comfortable hard for you.

✔ **A stroke may affect your memory, thinking, attention, and learning abilities.** You may have problems with mental activities, such as following directions or keeping track of the date or time.

✔ **A stroke may cause problems using language.** Depending on what areas of the brain have been damaged, you may have difficulty understanding speech or writing, or you may be able to understand but cannot think of the words to speak or write. Also, you may have difficulty saying words clearly.

✔ **A stroke may make swallowing difficult.**

✔ **A stroke may impair your bowel or bladder control.**

✔ **A stroke may cause sudden bursts of emotions.** You could find yourself laughing, crying, or feeling angry easily. A stroke can also bring on depression.

Knowing for sure

Your doctor will diagnose your condition by evaluating your symptoms and medical history and by peforming a physical exam, a series of neurological tests (entailing simple questions to check communication and memory skills and motor skill tests, such as standing up and walking), and a series of blood tests. In addition, several imaging tests can be done to determine what type of stroke you suffered and the level of damage. CAT scans, X rays, and MRIs can assess the severity of your stroke, its location in your brain, and cause. Other tests detect blockages and narrowing in your arteries and check the blood flow through them. These include *carotid ultrasound, ocular pneumoplethysmography (OPG),* and *arteriography.*

- ✔ Carotid ultrasound is a painless, noninvasive test. A gel is applied to the skin of your neck over your carotid artery (the blood vessel that starts at the large artery of your heart and runs along through your neck), and a probe runs along your artery to send an ultrasound signal. This signal shows how fast your blood is flowing and the degree of narrowing in your carotid artery.

- ✔ OPG is another painless, noninvasive test. Drops are placed into your eyes to numb them, and then a small eyecup (similar to a contact lens) is placed in the corner of your eyes. The test takes only a few minutes and evaluates whether your carotid artery is letting in enough blood to your eyes and brain.

- ✔ Arteriography, or cerebral angiography, provides detailed images of your blood vessels with the aid of an X ray. You will be awake during this test but will be given a medication to relax you. A dye is injected into one of your blood vessels through a catheter that allows your doctor to see your blood vessels. You may experience minor discomfort during this test, such as feeling pressure when the catheter is inserted and a momentary feeling of warmth when the dye is injected. The test lasts between one and two hours and detects impaired blood flow and blockages in arteries that supply blood to your brain. This test can also check for an aneurysm.

Getting immediate treatment

Immediate, prompt treatment may help to reduce the effects of stroke and prevent permanent damage. Emergency treatment after the onset of a stroke involves stabilizing you and preventing any additional damage to your brain. For either ischemic or hemorrhagic stroke, your blood pressure must be lowered slowly with medication. A quick drop in blood pressure can lead to further damage.

With ischemic stroke, treatment focuses on improving blood and oxygen flow to your brain by using *anticoagulants,* or blood-thinning drugs. Anticoagulants help prevent the formation of clots in arteries that have narrowed. *Carotid endarterectomy surgery* may be done to open your carotid artery by removing plaque deposits and to restore blood flow to your brain.

With hemorrhagic stroke, treatment focuses on stopping the bleeding, correcting the cause of the hemorrhage, and protecting your brain from further damage. Treatment is complicated and must be individualized. You will probably be given medications to decrease the swelling of your brain tissue. Your intake of liquids may be limited as well. If necessary, evacuation surgery may be done to drain blood clots within the injured area of your brain.

As part of your medical treatment, rehabilitation may be necessary. Rehabilitation is an important aspect of treating stroke because physical disability and dependence are serious psychological factors that can inhibit your recovery. The goal is to make you as independent and productive as possible within whatever limitations may result from a stroke. You may have to develop new skills to replace ones that you no longer can perform. Also, don't be afraid to ask the help of your family and friends who can be significant factors in your rehabilitation.

Rehabilitation may take place at your home, hospital, nursing facility, or outpatient clinic. If the damage caused by the stroke is extensive, expect to be treated at a hospital or nursing facility. If you're able to move and your daily routine is not greatly affected, you can have therapy in your home. The total recovery time depends on the severity of your stroke. You may recover in as few as six to nine months, or your recovery may take longer.

Preventing stroke

To help prevent a stroke, you must take steps to reduce your risk. Many risk factors can be controlled, and although the risk of stroke is never zero at any age, by starting early and controlling your risk factors, you can lower your risk of death or disability by stroke.

✓ **Eat a low-salt, low-fat, high-fiber diet.** A balanced diet with less than 30 percent of calories from fat reduces your risk of coronary heart disease, high cholesterol, and hypertension.

✓ **Eat at least five servings of fruits and vegetables daily.** Research shows that for every three servings of fruits and vegetables daily, middle-aged men may be able to reduce their risk of stroke by 22 percent.

✔ **Control your blood pressure.** We mention earlier that hypertension is the most important risk factor in stroke.

✔ **Don't smoke.** Smoking increases your risk of stroke, heart disease, and numerous types of cancer (see Chapter 5 on how to quit).

✔ **Exercise.** A regular program of aerobic exercise helps to reduce your blood pressure and your risk of heart disease. It also can help keep off excess pounds that may contribute to stroke risk.

✔ **Maintain a healthy weight.** Obesity increases the risk of stroke by contributing to risk factors such as heart disease and hypertension.

✔ **Lower your homocysteine levels.** Several studies have found that people with low amounts of B6 and folate in their blood have higher levels of homocysteine, an amino acid (see Chapter 1), putting them at an increased risk of atherosclerosis. Recent research from the department of neurology and geriatrics at the University of Maryland in Baltimore found that the triple therapy of vitamins B6, B12, and folate also reduced *homocysteine* and *thrombomodulin* (a marker for injury in the blood vessels) levels in stroke survivors. However, evidence of whether these vitamins can prevent a stroke in people who have never had a stroke is lacking.

✔ **Stay calm.** Angry outbursts increase your risk of stroke two-fold. Don't suppress your anger, but learn to manage it so that it doesn't reach explosive levels. When very angry, try to distract yourself momentarily with constructive, gentle, physical activity, such as walking or raking leaves, until you cool down.

✔ **Control diabetes.** If you have diabetes, treating this disease can delay complications that increase your risk of stroke. Monitoring your blood pressure, too, is especially important to you.

✔ **Monitor your cholesterol levels.** High cholesterol levels can contribute to atherosclerosis, which in turn can lead to hypertension.

✔ **Ask your doctor whether you have *atrial fibrillation*, a heart condition that encourages the formation of blood clots.**

Cholesterol

Cholesterol is a confusing subject. You hear that it's bad for you — then you hear that certain types are good for you. You're told to stay away from foods high in cholesterol, but then you find out that the cholesterol you eat may have little bearing on your blood levels of it. The confusion of what's what about cholesterol is enough to make the burliest of men sink in a tub of Calgon bath bubbles to escape.

What exactly is cholesterol anyway, you may ask?

Cholesterol is a soft, fatlike, waxy substance found in your body's cells. Although cholesterol is often described as a *lipid,* or blood fat, it is not truly a fat. Rather, it's a closely related substance that belongs to the class of compounds called *sterols.* Like wax or fat, cholesterol does not dissolve in water and needs to be carried around in your bloodstream by a protein shell of sorts; this combination is called a *lipoprotein.*

The primary lipoproteins are high-density lipoprotein (HDL) and low-density lipoprotein (LDL). Your small intestine and liver make and release HDL into your bloodstream. HDL then carries cholesterol back to your liver to be processed and disposed. Because this lipoprotein removes excess cholesterol from your body and helps excrete it, HDL is called *good* cholesterol. Therefore, you want a high level of HDL.

LDL carries cholesterol to cells in your body where it is used to form your cells' membranes. However, if you have more cholesterol than your cells can use, LDL recirculates cholesterol in your bloodstream until, eventually, the cholesterol sticks and builds up on the inside of your arteries forming plaque (the accumulation of cholesterol, fats, and other substances). For this reason, LDL is called *bad* cholesterol. Therefore, you want a low level of LDL.

You can remember the difference between which cholesterol is good and bad by associating the "H" in HDL with "healthy" and the first "L" in LDL with "lousy."

Knowing your cholesterol level

In the past, cholesterol guidelines focused on total cholesterol levels. However, recent research suggests that the ratio of high-density lipoprotein (HDL) and low-density lipoprotein (LDL) to total cholesterol provides a more accurate indication of risk. In other words, the problem is not how much cholesterol you have in your bloodstream but how it circulates and whether it is in the form of HDL or LDL. Most experts favor tests that give the ratios of *good* and *bad* cholesterol to total cholesterol. The real danger is having low HDL levels and high LDL levels. However, if your total cholesterol is high because of high HDL, then you usually have no need for concern.

Table 17-1 lists the current recommendations for cholesterol levels from the National Cholesterol Education Program.

Table 17-1	What Should Your Cholesterol Level Be?	
Risk	*LDL Cholesterol (mg/dl)*	*Total Cholesterol (mg/dl)*
Men with heart disease	100 or less	160 or less
Men with no heart disease, but with two or more risk factors	129 or less	199 or less
Men with no heart disease and fewer than two risk factors	159 or less	239 or less

Source: National Cholesterol Education Program, 1993.

Lowering cholesterol through self-care

When you reduce your cholesterol levels, you lower your risk of coronary heart disease. An important way to lower your cholesterol level is through diet (see Chapter 1). Most doctors believe that too much fat, especially saturated fat, plays a major role in raising cholesterol levels. However, some controversy does exist over whether eating cholesterol affects the levels of cholesterol in the blood. Food sources of cholesterol are animal products, such as meat, eggs, milk, yogurt, and cheese. The American Heart Association recommends less than 300 mg of cholesterol from food daily (the equivalent of three to four large eggs weekly) and no more than 200 mg if you have heart disease. The average man gets about 450 mg of cholesterol in his diet daily.

Here are more tips to help lower your cholesterol level:

✔ Eat fewer calories because losing excess weight helps.

✔ Limit your dietary fat intake to 30 percent of your daily calories.

✔ Eat foods rich in fiber.

✔ Eat more fruits and vegetables and replace saturated fats with monounsaturated fats.

✔ Limit your dietary cholesterol level to less than 300 mg daily. Use a food chart that lists dietary cholesterol in food sources.

✔ Include aerobic exercise. Research shows that regular aerobic exercise raises HDL. The more intense the exercise, the higher the level of HDL. (Please check with your doctor before beginning any exercise program.)

Lowering cholesterol with medication

You may not be able to lower your cholesterol level even with diet. For you — along with diet and exercise changes — cholesterol-lowering drugs are necessary.

The drugs commonly used to lower cholesterol are *bile acid sequestrants* because of their few side effects (constipation and hard stools). Bile acid sequestrants reduce the amount of fat absorbed from the foods you eat and help lower your cholesterol levels. These are synthetic resins, called cholestyramine (Questran), and come in powder form to be mixed with a liquid, or as a bar, called colestipol (Cholybar), that you must chew thoroughly.

The next potent class of drugs are HMG CoA reductase inhibitors (sometimes referred to as *statins*). They work by inhibiting the enzyme HMG CoA and interfere with the natural process of cholesterol-making in the body to produce a harmless by-product. In the Scandinavian Simvastatin Survival Study, simvastatin (Zocor) performed impressively. It reduced the risk of death from heart attack by 42 percent and overall risk of death by 30 percent. It also cut the risk of having to undergo bypass surgery.

Another statin, pravastatin (Pravachol), has been found to rapidly reduce the risk of first-time heart attack in people with high cholesterol. Other examples of statins include fluvastatin (Lescol) and lovastatin (Mevacor). Don't take statins if you have liver disease. Possible side effects are skin rashes and gastrointestinal upset. Further studies are needed to determine the effects of long-term usage.

Triglycerides

Triglycerides are often discussed along with cholesterol. Although they're not related to cholesterol — triglycerides are also fats but have a different chemical structure — they can affect your cholesterol levels and increase your risk of heart disease.

Triglycerides, found in animal fats and plant oils, provide fats that your body uses for energy or places in your body's fat stores for later use. Triglycerides from food sources travel through your bloodstream via large lipid carriers, or *chylomicrons*. Triglycerides also come from your liver, which makes them from leftover carbohydrates and alcohol for use as energy stores. These triglycerides travel through your bloodstream through carriers called *very low-density lipoproteins (VLDLs)*. Unlike cholesterol, triglycerides do not stick to artery walls.

Researchers have known for some time that high triglyceride levels are a risk factor for heart disease, but it's not clear whether the risk comes directly from high triglyceride levels or the combination of high triglyceride and low HDL levels.

Although the combination of high triglyceride and low HDL levels is a factor in coronary heart disease, two recent studies also show that triglycerides may have an impact on coronary heart disease all by themselves. Triglycerides may slow blood down and make it harder to transport oxygen through the bloodstream, and triglycerides are dangerous at half the level once thought safe.

The first study, at Rush-Presbyterian-St. Luke's Medical Center in Chicago, found that triglyceride levels of 190 mg/dl and above may contribute to thickening of the blood. This in turn may contribute to coronary artery disease (narrowing of the coronary arteries) and heart attack.

The second study, at the University of Maryland Medical Center in Baltimore, concluded that people with triglyceride levels as low as 100 mg/dl had twice the risk of suffering from future coronary artery disease than those with lower levels. The researchers concluded that triglyceride levels previously considered normal may be predictive for future coronary artery disease. They advise that recommended triglyceride levels be revised.

Table 17-2 presents a list of triglyceride levels from the American Heart Association.

Table 17-2	Current Triglyceride Levels
Category	*Levels (mg/dl)*
Very high	Above 1,000
High	1,000 - 400
Borderline high	400 - 200
Normal	200 and lower

Lowering your triglyceride levels

As with lowering your cholesterol level, dietary factors play an important role in reducing triglyceride levels. People with high triglyceride levels tend to be inactive, overweight, diabetic, and heavy alcohol drinkers. Here are some tips for lowering your triglyceride levels:

✔ **Lose excess weight.** Doing so can lower your triglyceride level.

✔ **Eat a balanced diet including five servings of fruits and vegetables daily.**

✔ **Avoid simple sugars because they are notorious for increasing triglyceride levels.** Instead, replace them with complex carbohydrates, but keep your carbohydrate level around 60 percent of your daily calories. Anything over this amount can increase your triglyceride levels.

✔ **Replace saturated fats with monounsaturated fats (see Chapter 1).** Fish oil and omega-3 fatty acids in supplement form can also help reduce triglyceride levels. However, talk with your doctor before taking them as they can interfere with blood clotting and diabetic control and increase your risk of stroke.

✔ **Avoid alcohol.** It encourages triglyceride production.

✔ **Exercise.** Aerobic exercise for 30 to 40 minutes, three times weekly, can reduce triglyceride levels 30 to 40 percent, according to research.

✔ **Try medication.** If dietary and lifestyle changes alone don't lower your triglyceride level, you may have to use lipid-lowering drugs. HMG CoA reductase inhibitors that lower cholesterol, such as simvastatin and pravastatin, are often prescribed. Other types of lipid-lowering drugs used to lower triglyceride levels include fibric acid derivatives, such as gemfibrozil. A micronized fenofibrate (Tricor) is a new drug that lowers triglyceride levels and also increases the good cholesterol, HDL. You shouldn't use fenofibrate if you have liver, gallbladder, or severe kidney disease.

Finding out your cholesterol and triglyceride levels

For cholesterol levels, a basic test done at your doctor's office uses a few drops of blood taken from your fingertip (see Chapter 7 for home testing). It can measure total cholesterol and sometimes HDL. However, this form of testing may not be as accurate as a complete lipid profile. To find out your cholesterol and triglyceride levels, a tube of blood needs to be drawn from your arm. A complete lipid profile shows your total cholesterol, HDL, LDL, and triglyceride levels. For accurate readings, you have to fast for 12 hours. (Even having as little as a cup of coffee with milk can throw off your results.)

Chapter 18

Cancer

In This Chapter

▶ Recognizing the warning signs

▶ Treating cancer

▶ Preventing cancer

*J*ust the thought of cancer may give you a shiver, like a penetrating chill on a winter day. However, all is not bleak. On the positive side, the search for a cure for various types of cancer is racing ahead. Knowledge is power, and this chapter tells you what you need to know to help gain control of your medical options and quality of life. And you can do many things to reduce your risk of getting cancer and improve your chances of survival should you require treatment.

How Cancer Occurs

Cancer occurs when cells in the body divide abnormally without control or order. Many kinds of cells make up all your body's organs. Under normal conditions, these cells divide in an orderly way and produce more cells only when your body needs them. Think about your skin, for example. When you fall down and scrape your elbow, your body acts to fight infection by generating new skin to help you heal.

But when cells start to divide even though new cells are not required, the resulting mass of extra tissue is called a tumor. Three different types of tumors exist:

✔ **Benign (noncancerous) tumors:** These tumors don't spread to other parts of the body and are rarely life-threatening. They can be removed and often do not grow back.

✔ **Malignant (cancerous) tumors:** Unlike their benign counterparts, these tumors' cells can invade other organs throughout the body and affect their proper function. They can spread by invading neighboring tissues or by entering the bloodstream through the *lymph nodes* (glands that are part of the immune system), traveling to various parts of the body. The spread of cancer is called *metastasis*.

Lymph nodes are found in strategic parts of our bodies. After the skin, they are an important defense barrier when your body is invaded by harmful substances such as bacteria.

✔ **Precancerous lesions:** These are limited areas of the body that show abnormal, but not necessarily cancerous, changes. For example, a lesion may consist of rapidly growing normal cells. Lesions can result from an injury or disease. If left untreated, lesions have the potential of becoming malignant.

Recognizing the signs

The American Cancer Society lists seven basic warning signals. If you have any of these symptoms, talk with a doctor as soon as possible. Early detection and proper treatment greatly increase your chances of being cured.

✔ A change in bowel or bladder habits

✔ A sore that does not heal

✔ Unusual bleeding or discharge

✔ Thickening or a lump in any part of the body (for example, in the testicles)

✔ Indigestion or difficulty swallowing

✔ An obvious change in a wart or mole

✔ Nagging cough or hoarseness

Don't wait until you experience pain. Pain is not an early indication of cancer; on the contrary, pain is usually a late symptom. Remember, too, that pain can also be related to other conditions that are not cancerous — a trip to your doctor can put your mind to rest.

Cancer: Are you at risk?

Our current understanding of what causes cancer is not complete, but it's clear that you can't get cancer from an injury such as a bump or a bruise. Although being infected with certain viruses may increase the risk for contracting certain types of cancer (for example,

contracting HIV may increase the risk for lymphoma), cancer is not contagious.

Doctors know that specific factors can increase your risk of contracting cancer. Some of these risk factors are hereditary, so you cannot avoid them. Others, roughly 80 percent, are environmental or lifestyle factors over which you do have some control. Just because you have a particular risk factor doesn't mean you get cancer. In fact, according to the National Cancer Institute, most people at risk don't get the disease. However, you can lower your risk by avoiding certain risk factors whenever you can. You can further improve your chances by getting regular checkups. That way, if cancer develops, it's likely to be detected and treated while it's still in an early stage, thereby greatly increasing your chances for survival!.

Here are some of the factors known to increase the risk for cancer:

- **Tobacco use:** The National Cancer Institute reports that tobacco use causes cancer. In fact, one-third of all cancer deaths in the United States each year are attributed to smoking tobacco, using "smokeless" (chewing) tobacco, and being regularly exposed to secondhand, or environmental, tobacco smoke.

- **Diet:** The 60s pop culture proclaimed, "You are what you eat!" The same holds true today. What you eat can increase or decrease your chances of contracting cancer. Researchers believe that a link exists between a high-fat diet and cancer of the breast, colon, and prostate. Also, weighing 20 percent more than your ideal weight can increase your risk for cancer of the prostate, pancreas, and colon. More important, some believe that certain foods may help protect against some forms of cancer (such as foods high in fiber, fruits and vegetables, whole-grain breads, and cereals, peas, beans, and rice).

- **Sunlight:** If you're a sun worshipper, you ought to find something else to worship. The American Cancer Society predicted that nearly 90 percent of the estimated 1 million skin cancers reported in 1998 could have been prevented by protection from the sun's rays, more specifically, ultraviolet (UV) radiation. Keep in mind that UV radiation doesn't just damage the skin once with a sunburn. All damage is permanent and cumulative. And don't be fooled into thinking that sun lamps or tanning booths are safe — they emit concentrated UV radiation, increasing your risk of skin cancer.

- **Alcohol:** Like anything in life, moderation is the key, which is certainly true of alcohol consumption. Drinking large amounts of alcohol increases the risk for cancer of the mouth, throat, esophagus, and larynx. Alcohol can also damage the liver and lead to liver cancer.

- **Radiation, chemicals, and other substances:** An occasional X ray taken for medical purposes provides very little exposure to radiation and far outweighs the risk. But repeated, regular exposure to radiation can be harmful. Ask your practitioner or dentist about using shields to protect the areas of your body not pictured in the X ray. The risk for cancer also increases with exposure to various substances commonly found in the workplace. According to the National Cancer Institute, asbestos, nickel, cadmium, uranium, radon, vinyl chloride, benzidine, and benzene are well-known *carcinogens* (substances known to cause cancer) in the workplace. Be sure to follow work and safety rules to avoid contact with dangerous materials.

- **Family history of cancer:** A small number of cancers, such as melanoma (a type of skin cancer) and cancers of the prostate and colon, tend to occur more often in some families than in the rest of the population. If a close relative of yours had cancer, talk to your practitioner and follow his or her recommendations for close monitoring, prevention strategies, and early detection.

Knowing for sure

Many cases of cancer are accidentally discovered during a routine physical, an important reason to see your practitioner regularly. The tools and techniques used to diagnose cancer may include imaging tests (such as X rays and CT scans), endoscopy, and laboratory tests. If these diagnostic tests show a tumor or other abnormality, a sample of tissue is removed to determine if it's cancerous or benign. This procedure, called a *biopsy,* is the only sure way to determine whether cancer is present. The following list takes a closer look at some of these tests:

- **X rays:** X rays involve the use of radiation to create an image of a particular part of the body.

- **Radionuclide scanning:** In this procedure, you swallow a radioactive substance, and then a scanner measures the radioactivity in certain organs and provides a picture of any abnormal areas on paper or film.

- **Ultrasound:** Sound waves are used to create an image of internal structures.

- **Magnetic resonance imaging (MRI):** A magnet and a computer are used to create a picture that can show size, shape, and location of a tumor and whether the cancer has spread to other areas of the body.

- **Computerized tomography (CT):** A beam that rotates around the body is used to create a three-dimensional X ray. CT scans (also known as CAT scans) can show the relationship of a tumor to other structures, the size of the tumor, and whether the cancer has spread to other organs.

- **Endoscopy:** In this procedure, an endoscope (a flexible, fiber-optic tube) is inserted through an incision or opening in your body. The scope provides a view of your body's interior.

- **Lab tests:** Lab tests, such as blood and urine tests, are also performed and may show whether cancer has affected the body in any way.

- **Biopsy:** If an image technique or a lab test reveals that cancer may be present, a biopsy is done. This procedure involves removing a small amount of tissue from a suspicious area or growth for microscopic examination. In most cases, a biopsy is the only sure way to determine whether a problem may be cancer.

Treating cancer

Several basic methods are available for treating cancer. They can be used individually or in combination. The type of cancer, its stage, and the age and overall health of the patient determine the method used.

Stages of cancer

Cancer is classified according to stages that indicate how far the cancer has spread from its original site or how large a tumor has grown. The stages vary slightly, according to type of cancer, but generally range from stage 0 (the earliest stage, known as *in-situ cancer*) to stage 5 (cancer that has spread, or metastasized, throughout the body). Another stage, recurrent cancer, indicates cancer that has reappeared even though there was no evidence of it after previous treatment was completed. The stages of cancer are used to determine the course of treatment. The earlier a cancer is diagnosed, the easier it is to cure.

✔ **Surgery:** This technique is used to remove cancerous tissue and any affected lymph nodes. For most forms of cancer, surgery is the primary treatment, although other treatments may be used along with, or instead of, surgery. One possible side effect is infection at the incision site.

✔ **Radiation therapy (also called radiotherapy):** This treatment involves the use of high-energy rays to destroy the reproductive material of cancerous cells and prevent them from multiplying. Depending upon the type of cancer and primary site, radiation therapy may be used after surgery as a supplemental therapy to destroy any cancer cells that may remain. Some possible side effects include red, sunburned skin in the treated area, nausea and vomiting, hair loss, and loss of appetite.

✔ **Chemotherapy:** This treatment uses anticancer drugs to kill cancer cells. The drugs are administered orally or through an injection and travel through the bloodstream and throughout the body. Although the prescribed dose is chosen to damage cancer cells only, chemotherapy affects normal cells as well. Chemotherapy is given in cycles of a treatment period that is followed by a recovery period, then another treatment period, and so on. Side effects depend on the type of drug used and the dose. Generally, anticancer drugs affect cells that divide rapidly, such as blood cells and the cells that line the digestive tract. As a result, those who have chemotherapy are vulnerable to infections, bruise easily, and feel tired. Other temporary side effects include loss of appetite, nausea and vomiting, infertility, hair loss, and mouth sores.

✔ **Hormone therapy:** This treatment fights certain types of cancer that depend on hormones to grow — for example, prostate cancer and breast cancer. This therapy is designed to prevent cancer cells from getting the hormones they need by surgically removing the hormone-producing organs (such as the testicles) or by using drugs that stop hormone production or change how the hormones work. Temporary side effects include nausea and vomiting, swelling, weight gain, erection problems, tender breasts, infertility, and lowered libido.

✔ **Biological therapy (also called immunotherapy):** This treatment involves the injection of a substance into the body — for example, the protein interferon — to enhance the body's natural defenses against cancer. This relatively new form of treatment is still considered experimental. Biological therapy can also help to protect the body from some other cancer treatments' side effects, such as infections that occur during chemotherapy. Possible side effects include flulike symptoms — chills, fever, muscle aches, weakness, loss of appetite, nausea and vomiting, and diarrhea.

✔ **Bone marrow transplants:** These may be used for particularly aggressive or recurrent forms of cancer such as lymphoma, lung cancer, and leukemia. Bone marrow is the tissue that produces new cells and helps to maintain the immune system, and it can be damaged by high doses of chemotherapy and radiation needed to treat some forms of cancer. In a bone marrow transplant, the marrow is removed, stored, and then replaced after the high-dose treatment is completed. In this way, the cell-producing bone marrow is preserved rather than destroyed by the cancer treatment.

✔ **Cryosurgery (also called cryoablation):** This relatively new form of treatment — still considered experimental by most doctors — involves using liquid nitrogen to freeze cancer cells when cancer is localized (hasn't spread to other areas of the body).

Overview of Types of Cancers

This section looks at the specific cancers that either most often affect men or have the greatest impact on men's lifestyles.

Colorectal cancer

Colorectal cancer (cancer of the colon or rectum) is the growth of abnormal cells in the large intestine. Each year, more than 150,000 people in the United States learn that they have colorectal cancer. The American Cancer Society estimated 131,600 new cases in 1998, consisting of 95,600 cases of colon cancer and 36,000 of rectal cancer. Colorectal cancers account for about 11 percent of new cancer diagnoses. That's the bad news. The good news is that colorectal cancer is highly treatable if it's caught early.

Recognizing the signs

Early colorectal cancer and *polyps* (small protrusions on the colon lining) usually have no symptoms. But if they do occur, symptoms include bloody or black stools, rectal bleeding, pain in the lower abdomen, cramping and gas, bloating or a full feeling ever after a bowel movement, weight loss, and tiredness. Diarrhea, constipation, or unusually narrow stools lasting for more than 10 days are also symptoms.

Keep in mind that other problems can cause these symptom, such as ulcers, an inflammation of the colon, and hemorrhoids. Visit your practitioner if the symptoms persist for more than 10 days.

Knowing for sure

To detect colorectal cancer, a doctor may use any or all of the following tests:

- ✔ **Digital rectal examination (DRE):** The practitioner inserts a lubricated, gloved finger into the lowest four inches of the rectum to check for abnormalities.

- ✔ **Occult stool blood test:** This laboratory test checks for blood in the stool and may also be done during the DRE.

- ✔ **Lower gastrointestinal (GI):** This test (also called a *barium enema*) examines the colon by X ray after a contrast dye, known as barium, is administered. The barium outlines the lower gastrointestinal tract on the X rays.

- ✔ **Sigmoidoscopy or colonoscopy:** In sigmoidoscopy, an endoscope (see Chapter 26) is inserted into the rectum to inspect the lower portion of the colon. A colonoscopy inspects the upper portion of the colon. During either of these procedures, photographs may be taken, or a biopsy may be done to remove tissue for microscopic examination.

Colorectal cancer: Are you at risk?

Factors that increase your risk for colorectal cancer include the following:

- ✔ **Personal or family history of this cancer.**

- ✔ **Polyps.** These develop in the lining of the colon. Polyps are not cancerous, but they may develop into colon cancer.

- ✔ **Inflammatory bowel disease.** This includes *Crohn's disease,* an inflammation of the intestines, and/or *ulcerative colitis,* a condition in which sores occur in the colon.

- ✔ **High-fat, low-fiber diet.**

- ✔ **Sedentary lifestyle.** Exercise helps to speed digestion and quickly move along any possible harmful chemicals in the digestive tract.

- ✔ **Obesity.**

- ✔ **Heavy alcohol consumption (three or more drinks daily).**

Other tests include CT and MRI scans, blood tests (such as CEA assay, which measures the blood level of *carcinoembryonic antigen,* a substance sometimes found in higher-than-normal amounts when colorectal cancer is present, especially when the disease has spread), and staging tests to determine whether the cancer has spread to other parts of the body.

Treating colorectal cancer

The most effective method for treating colorectal cancer is surgery to remove the tumor and nearby lymph nodes. If the cancer is more extensive, a section of the colon containing the tumor and surrounding tissue can be surgically removed in a procedure called a *wedge resection.* If the lymph nodes are also removed, the procedure is known as a *bowel resection.* Radiation therapy or chemotherapy most often accompanies surgery to destroy any remaining cancer cells.

In most cases where a section of the colon is removed, the remaining segments are reattached. When necessary, a colostomy is done — this procedure involves the creation of a hole in the abdominal wall through which waste passes into a bag outside of the body. A colostomy is permanent in about 15 percent of cases when the cancer is extensive and part of the colon must be completely removed. Otherwise, the temporary colostomy bag is removed after the colon heals from the surgery.

Preventing colorectal cancer

Here are tips to prevent colorectal cancer:

- ✔ Eat high-fiber, low-fat foods such as whole-grain cereals and breads, pasta, fruit, and fibrous vegetables (such as broccoli, cauliflower, and cabbage). Also, reduce your total fat intake to 30 percent or less of your total calories.
- ✔ Get 30 minutes of regular exercise at least three to four days weekly.
- ✔ Avoid smoking, and if you must drink alcohol, do so moderately.
- ✔ Have regular checkups, especially if you have a family history of the disease.

Lung cancer

Lung cancer, the uncontrolled growth of abnormal cells in the lung, is the number one cause of death from cancer among men. Approximately 93,000 men die of lung cancer every year, according to the American Cancer Society. However, the incidence of lung cancer in men is declining. It reached a high of 87 per 100,000 in 1984 and declined to 74 per 100,000 in 1994.

Lung cancer: Are you at risk?

Factors that increase your risk of lung cancer include the following:

✔ **Smoking:** Unless you've been asleep for many years like Rip Van Winkle or just returned to Earth from another planet, you've probably heard the message that smoking causes lung cancer. And the message is a simple one: The longer you smoke, the more likely you are to die of lung cancer. The National Cancer Institute strongly encourages smokers to quit. The risk for lung cancer begins to slowly decrease as soon as you quit smoking (see Chapter 5).

✔ **Exposure to industrial substances and chemicals:** Avoid things such as asbestos, radon gas, arsenic, nickel, chromates, coal gas, mustard gas, and vinyl chloride.

✔ **Exposure to excessive air pollution and heavy doses of radiation:** Researchers believe that these substances may cause lung cancer.

Lung cancer has a high mortality rate because it's usually discovered after the cancer has spread from the lungs to other parts of the body. According to the American Cancer Society, 49 percent of patients with localized lung cancer live an average of five or more years after diagnosis. Unfortunately, only 14 percent of patients with lung cancer that has spread live an average of five or more years after diagnosis.

Recognizing the signs

Lung cancer can be present for years and you may not even know it. Typically, lung cancer is discovered after a person has a chest X ray for another medical reason. Early symptoms of lung cancer — coughing, wheezing, and shortness of breath — are often mistaken for a cold or bronchitis or ignored. Other symptoms include coughing up blood, ongoing chest aches and pains, fever, weakness, weight loss, and repeated bouts of pneumonia. Advanced symptoms include hoarseness; shortness of breath; swollen lymph nodes in the neck; difficulty swallowing; shoulder, back, or arm pain; and drooping of the upper eyelids. Other symptoms may include headaches, blurred vision, dizziness, and bone pain.

Knowing for sure

The practitioner first begins with a medical history by asking the patient whether he smokes and, if so, how frequently. A physical examination tells the doctor how well the heart and lungs are functioning. In addition to the medical history and physical examination, a number of diagnostic techniques are used to check for lung cancer. These include chest X rays and radionuclide, MRI, and CT scans. If an abnormal area is located, a biopsy is done. Other diagnostic tests include the following:

✔ **Lab tests:** Examination of *sputum,* a thick fluid coughed up from the airways, can determine whether the cells in the sputum are cancerous and, if so, the type of lung cancer present.

✔ **Bronchoscopy:** A tube with lighting and a magnifying device is inserted through the nostril or mouth into the bronchial tubes. While viewing abnormal areas through bronchoscopy, the doctor takes samples of tissues, and tumors are viewed for location and size.

✔ **Thoracotomy:** This exploratory surgery is done if other tests are negative but the physician still has a concern that cancer is present.

As part of the diagnosis, staging is an important factor to find out whether the cancer has spread to other areas of the body.

Treating lung cancer

Surgery, radiation therapy, and chemotherapy are the standard treatments for lung cancer. Depending on the size and location of the tumor, part or all of the lung is removed during surgery. An operation to remove only a small part of the lung is called a *segmental* or *wedge resection.* When a surgeon removes a lobe (semi-detached portion) of the lung, the procedure is called a *lobectomy. Pneumonectomy* is the removal of an entire lung. Following surgery, radiation is used to damage cancer cells and stop them from growing and dividing. Chemotherapy also may be used. A patient may have just one form of treatment, or a combination, depending on his needs.

Another method of treatment under study is *photodynamic therapy.* In this treatment, cancer cells are destroyed with a combination of laser light and light-sensitive drugs.

Preventing lung cancer

Here are tips to prevent lung cancer:

✔ **Don't smoke.** For tips on quitting, see Chapter 5.

✔ **Avoid secondhand smoke.** Encourage a smoke-free environment at home and at work.

✔ **Avoid pollution.** Exercise in the early morning or evening, after the sun has set, when pollution levels are lowest. Also, covering your nose and mouth with a mask helps to filter out pollution.

✔ **Avoid industrial chemicals on the job.** If you work around chemicals or fumes, protect yourself with a face mask or other protective equipment.

✔ **Have your home checked for radon gas (a radioactive gas) if you live in an area known for such problems.**

✔ **Maintain your daily recommended dose of vitamins and minerals.** Studies show vitamins C and E may help protect against lung cancer.

Radon gas, the second leading cause of lung cancer (after smoking), contributes to as many as 21,800 lung cancer deaths in the United States each year. Exposure to radon gas markedly increases lung cancer risk among smokers, according to a report by a committee of the National Research Council.

Oral cancer

Cancer can appear in any part of the *oral cavity,* the area that includes your lips, tongue, mouth, and throat. Oral cancer is more than twice as common in men as in women, and it occurs more often after the age of 45, although it can develop at any age.

The American Cancer Society estimated 30,300 new cases of oral cancer in 1998, with 8,000 deaths. Fortunately, the mortality rates have been decreasing since the early 1980s.

Recognizing the signs

Once a month, examine your mouth (cheeks, gums, lips, tongue, and mouth lining) by looking in a mirror. Symptoms include sores that bleed easily and don't heal, lumps or thickenings, white or red patches that persist, soreness or feeling that something is stuck in your throat, difficulty chewing or swallowing, difficulty moving your tongue or jaw, numbness of your tongue or other area of your mouth, swelling of your jaw that causes dentures to fit poorly or uncomfortably, pain in your ear, and change in your voice.

A less serious problem may cause these symptoms, but you still need to see a doctor or dentist if any symptom lasts longer than two weeks.

Knowing for sure

Diagnosis usually begins with an examination and X rays of the mouth. If an abnormal area is found, a biopsy is done (the only definitive test for oral cancer). If cancer is diagnosed, staging tests — such as dental X rays, X rays of the head and chest, ultrasound, and CT and MRI scans — are done to see whether the cancer has spread to other areas of the body.

Treating oral cancer

As with other cancers, treatment depends on the location, size, type, extent of the tumor, and stage of the disease. Treatment typically involves surgical removal of the affected areas, followed by radiation therapy to destroy any remaining cells. Chemotherapy is also used. Hyperthermia, which uses a special machine to heat the body for a period of time to kill heat-sensitive cancer cells, is now being tested as a treatment for oral cancer.

Oral cancer: Are you at risk?

Factors that increase your risk for oral cancer include the following:

- **Tobacco use:** According to the National Cancer Institute, tobacco use (whether smoking, chewing, or dipping snuff — keeping fine, powered tobacco tucked under the lip or tongue) accounts for 80 to 90 percent of oral cancers. Smokers are four to 15 times more likely to develop oral cancers than nonsmokers. The risk for smokeless tobacco users increases significantly for long-time dippers or chewers.

- **Heavy alcohol consumption:** Excessive alcohol use has also been linked to oral cancer. Those who drink heavily but do not smoke may have a higher risk than people who do smoke. The chances for oral cancer increase for people who use both alcohol and tobacco.

- **Ultraviolet (UV) radiation:** Exposure to UV radiation can cause lip cancer.

- **Certain nutritional deficiencies:** A lack of vitamins B and A have been linked to oral cancer.

- **Poorly fitting dentures and bridges or sharp and broken teeth that irritate or infect the gums:** These may contribute to oral cancer.

- **White or red patches inside the mouth:** Studies indicate that oral cancer sometimes develops in people who have white patches (leukoplakia) or red, velvety patches (erythroplakia) inside their mouths.

As with other cancers, treatment for oral cancer can cause unpleasant side effects. These depend on the type and extent of the treatment, the specific area being treated, and the reaction to the treatment. Some side effects are temporary; others are permanent. Surgery to remove a large tumor inside the mouth may require partial removal of the palate, tongue, or jaw, changes that can affect the person's ability to chew, swallow, or talk, and that may change appearance. Radiation therapy can make the mouth sore and dry, causing chewing and swallowing difficulty, which can contribute to weight loss. Many patients cannot wear dentures during radiation therapy and up to a year after treatments.

You must have a complete dental examination before oral cancer treatment begins. Because the treatments may make your mouth more sensitive and more easily infected, doctors often advise patients to have any needed dental work done before treatment begins.

Preventing oral cancer

Here are tips to help prevent oral cancer:

- Stop smoking and using tobacco products.
- Drink moderately.

✔ Protect your lips by using a lip balm that contains sunscreen.

✔ Have regular checkups of the oral cavity (your doctor or dentist can check your mouth).

Prostate cancer

Other than skin cancer, prostate cancer — the rapid growth of abnormal cells in the prostate gland — is the most common type of cancer in American men. The American Cancer Society estimated nearly 185,000 new cases of prostate cancer in 1998, with incidence rates nearly two times higher for African-American men compared with white men. Nearly 40,000 deaths were estimated in 1998, making prostate cancer the second leading cause of cancer-related deaths among men.

As you may recall from Chapter 16, the prostate gland — about the size of a walnut and located near the rectum just below the bladder — is part of the male reproductive system. Its job is the production of prostatic fluid, which becomes part of semen.

Talk of prostate cancer — or any type of cancer, for that matter — is often surrounded by an aura of fear, bolstered by daunting statistics and concerns about complications such as impotence and incontinence. You can't deny that prostate cancer is serious. However, you need to understand that cancer, and especially prostate cancer, is not an automatic death sentence. In fact, the reality of prostate cancer is quite the contrary: Prostatic cancers grow so slowly that the vast majority of these cancers never become life-threatening — hence the common statement that "most men die *with* prostate cancer, not *of* it." The good news is that this slow-growing cancer may grow so slowly that treatment isn't needed (a man may die of old age rather than from the cancer). Fifty-eight percent of all prostate cancers are discovered while still localized. Consequently, the five-year survival rate during the early stages is 100 percent, according to the American Cancer Society. And over the past 20 years, the survival rate for all stages has increased from 67 percent to 89 percent.

Rehabilitation and oral cancer

If you've ever sustained a sports injury, such as a badly sprained ankle, then you know the importance of physical therapy in rehabilitating weakened muscles. Similarly, rehabilitation is a very important part of treatment for patients with oral cancer. Depending on the extent of the disease, this treatment may include dietary counseling, surgery, a dental prosthesis, and speech therapy.

Prostate cancer: Are you at risk?

Factors that can increase your risk of prostate cancer include the following:

✔ **Age:** Studies in the United States show that prostate cancer is found mainly in men over age 55 (the average age of patients at diagnosis is 72).

✔ **Being African-American:** The disease is more common in men of color than in white men.

✔ **Father or brother with prostate cancer:** Some studies show that a man has a higher risk for prostate cancer if his father or brother had the disease. However, researchers are uncertain why some families have a higher incidence of prostate cancer than others.

✔ **High-fat diet:** Some evidence suggests that a diet high in fat increases the risk for prostate cancer, whereas a diet high in fruits, grains, and vegetables decreases the risks. These links have not been proven.

Recognizing the signs

In the early stages there are no obvious symptoms. As the disease progresses, the major symptoms include problems with urination such as needing to urinate frequently (especially at night), difficulty starting and stopping the flow of urine, inability to urinate, weak or interrupted flow of urine, blood in urine or semen, and painful or burning urination. As you can see, these symptoms are similar to those of benign prostatic hyperplasia (see Chapter 16). However, in benign prostatic hyperplasia, these symptoms develop gradually, but the onset is usually rapid if the cause is cancer. Other symptoms of prostate cancer include painful ejaculation and pain or stiffness in the lower back, hips, and upper thighs.

Knowing for sure

Because of its initially slow progression, prostate cancer often goes undetected for a long time before it's found and diagnosed, usually discovered accidentally while screening for another condition. The practitioner may use several diagnostic tools to determine prostate cancer, including the following:

✔ **Digital rectal examination (DRE):** A doctor inserts a gloved, lubricated finger into the rectum and feels the prostate through the rectal wall to check for hard or lumpy areas. This procedure is illustrated in Chapter 2. DRE doesn't diagnose cancer; rather it's used only to locate abnormalities that may be cancerous. Even though DRE is used to check for prostate cancer, studies show that it may not be effective in catching cancer before it spreads. Also, tumors in their early stages are too small to be felt or are located in an area where the doctor may not feel them. Regardless, the American Cancer Society recommends that all men over the age of 40 have a DRE as part of their yearly physical.

✔ **Prostate-specific antigen (PSA) test:** This blood test measures levels of an enzyme called prostate-specific antigen, produced by the prostate gland. This enzyme is produced by both normal cells and cancerous cells. However, cancerous cells produce larger amounts of PSA than normal cells and may indicate cancer. Similarly, an enlarged prostate gland also produces more PSA. Although the PSA test is not specific for cancer, it is a highly sensitive test that may be able to indicate cancer before a obvious lump is present in the prostate. However, the test is so sensitive that it's highly controversial.

✔ **Prostatic acid phosphatase (PAP) test:** This test — done when a biopsy is positive — checks for the presence of PAP in the blood, urine, or prostatic secretions. PAP levels are generally elevated in men with prostate cancer that has spread beyond the capsule of the prostate gland.

✔ **Transrectal ultrasound:** This procedure involves the insertion of a probe into the rectum. Ultrasound waves bounce off the rectum, and a computer uses the waves to create a picture called a *sonogram*. Ultrasound is used to help diagnose and determine the stage of cancer.

Other tests used to diagnose or determine the stage of prostate cancer include MRI and CT scans, bone scans, and *lymphadenectomy,* a biopsy of the lymph nodes surrounding the prostatic area.

Treating prostate cancer

Treatment depends on the stage of the disease, the man's age and general health, and his feelings about the treatments and possible side effects. *Radical prostatectomy* (removal of the prostate gland and seminal vesicles) is done when the cancer is confined to the prostate gland. Possible side effects include risk of infection, urinary incontinence, and erection problems. Radical prostatectomy is usually not recommended for men over age 70 because it's not proven to add any years to life and because of the risk for side effects. Radiation therapy may follow surgery or be used as a treatment tool by itself to treat small tumors or cancer that has spread beyond the gland. Possible side effects include rectal, urinary, and erection problems. For men with advanced cancer who can't have surgery or radiation, hormone therapy may be an option. Side effects include erection problems, tender breasts, and hot flashes. Other treatments may include cryosurgery (in which cancer cells are frozen and removed) and biological therapy (in which the body's immune system is triggered to attack cancer cells).

You should consider both the benefits and possible side effects of each option, especially the effects on sexual activity, urination, and other concerns that can affect your quality of life. Many older men whose prostate cancer is slow growing and is found at an early stage may not need treatment. Instead the doctor may suggest *watchful waiting,* following the patient closely and treating the patient later for symptoms that may arise.

Prostate-specific antigen (PSA) — a controversial blood test

The PSA test, a highly sensitive blood test to detect prostate cancer, has two major problems. The first is that PSA may give the wrong answer. PSA test results are often false negatives — that is, they're normal even if cancer is present. A number of factors can result in false positives, such as prostatitis, major trauma or injury to the prostate (such as an operation or biopsy), ejaculation one or two days before the test is taken, and age. More than any other reason, age can elevate PSA levels, simply because the prostate grows larger in men as they age. And because benign prostatic hyperplasia is so common in the same age-group that's at risk for prostate cancer, many in the medical community consider the PSA test unreliable for diagnosing prostate cancer.

To resolve the problem surrounding PSA levels and age, age-adjusted PSA reference ranges have been created. These ranges allow for higher PSA levels in older men, with a lower cutoff point for younger men. Age-specific reference ranges have also been designed for African-American men.

Age-Adjusted PSA Levels

Age	Acceptable PSA Level (nanogram/milliliter)
40-49	2.5
50-59	3.5
60-69	4.5
70-79	6.5

Age-Adjusted PSA Levels for African-American Men

Age	Acceptable PSA Level (nanogram/milliliter)
40-49	2.0
50-59	4.0
60-69	4.5
70-79	5.5

The second problem with the PSA test is that it may tell you more than you need to know. No evidence to date shows that screening with a PSA test improves the health or extends the life of a man with prostate cancer. A critical issue is whether an early finding of cancer increases a man's life span or just his anxiety level. For older men with prostate cancer, many doctors believe that ignorance may be bliss. Men with small, slow-growing cancer may opt for treatment that could actually prove to be more dangerous than the cancer itself.

Other doctors argue, however, that men should be informed about the PSA test and then decide what they want to do. Not every older man who learns he has prostate cancer elects treatment.

Preventing prostate cancer

Here are tips to help prevent prostate cancer:

- ✔ **Maintain a healthy weight:** Your rate for prostate cancer increases if you are overweight.

- ✔ **Eat less fat:** Studies have linked a high intake of saturated fat with an increased risk of prostate cancer.

- ✔ **Eat green leafy vegetables rich in beta-carotene (such as spinach and broccoli):** Beta-carotene has been noted as a possible factor in lowering cancer risk.

- ✔ **Eat a lot of tomatoes:** Recent research indicates the risk for prostate cancer is dramatically reduced in men who eat 10 or more servings of tomato products (such as tomatoes, tomato sauce, and pizza) a week. Experts believe that *lycopene,* the substance that gives tomatoes their red color, has positive effects on the prevention of prostate cancer. Strawberries and guava also contain lycopene.

Skin cancer

Cancer of the skin is the most common of all cancers, even though it can be prevented in most cases. The American Cancer Society estimated nearly 42,000 new cases of malignant melanoma, the most serious form of skin cancer, in 1998, with 9,200 deaths. Each year, about a million people in the United States learn that they have basal cell or squamous cell skin cancer — highly curable cancers.

Recognizing the signs

The most common warning sign is a change in the skin, especially a new growth or a sore that doesn't heal, and changes in the size or color of a mole or other darkly pigmented growth or spot. Skin cancers don't look the same. For example, the cancer may start as a small, smooth, shiny, pale, or waxy lump. Or it can appear as a firm red lump. Sometimes the lump bleeds or develops a crust. Skin cancer can also start as a flat, red spot that is rough, dry, or scaly. Both basal and squamous cell cancers are found mainly on areas of the skin exposed to the sun. Changes in the skin are not sure signs of cancer; however, seeing a doctor is important if any symptom lasts longer than two weeks. Don't wait for the area to hurt because skin cancers seldom cause pain.

Types of skin cancer

The three types of skin cancer are basal cell cancer, squamous cell cancer, and malignant melanoma:

✔ **Basal cell cancer:** This common cancer forms in the deepest layer of the skin. It is the most easily cured form of skin cancer, though it can still cause death if not treated early. About 75 percent of all skin cancers are basal cell cancers. Ninety-five percent of these cancers are caused by prolonged sun exposure. It typically develops on the face and ears, taking the form of a white or gray, raised, pearly nodule (a small, irregular mass), which may become an open sore.

✔ **Squamous cell cancer**: Also caused by sun exposure, this cancer makes up 20 percent of all skin cancers. It grows in the topmost layer of skin. This cancer grows quickly and is hard to treat. It generally begins as small, round, painless lumps or as flat, crusty, red areas, which may grow to resemble warts. It can also develop into lesions such as scars or open sores.

✔ **Malignant melanoma:** This deadly form of skin cancer accounts for only 5 percent of all cases but 75 percent of all deaths. It begins in the melanocytes, the cells that produce the pigment melanin. When caught early, it is highly curable. Unfortunately, this cancer grows quickly and often spreads throughout the body before it can be treated. Melanoma usually occurs where there is a mole, though it can appear anywhere on the body. The tumors most frequently appear on the chest, back, and abdomen and are common in white men. Though this cancer is rare in African-Americans, it can occur on the palms, the skin under the nails, and the soles of the feet.

Skin cancer: Are you at risk?

Factors that increase your risk of skin cancer include the following:

✔ **Fair skin:** Fair-skinned people, especially with blond or red hair, are at a higher risk for skin cancer because their cells have less melanin (meaning they sunburn more easily).

✔ **Freckles**

✔ **Burning rather than tanning**

✔ **Frequent vacations in sunny places, especially near the equator**

✔ **Exposure to UV radiation:** Exposure counts whether through sun lamps, tanning beds, or sunlight.

✔ **Exposure to occupational hazards:** These include such things as coal tar, pitch, creosote, arsenic compounds, radium, or ionized radiation from X rays.

✔ **Family history of skin cancer**

✔ **Being male:** Men are slightly more likely than women to develop skin cancer, possibly because they tend to hold more outdoor jobs and industrial jobs than women.

The American Cancer Society suggests the "ABCD Rule" for identifying melanoma:

✔ **A** is for **asymmetry.** One-half of the mole does not match the other half.

✔ **B** is for **border irregularity.** The edges are ragged, notched, or blurred.

✔ **C** is for **color.** The pigmentation is not uniform.

✔ **D** is for **diameter** greater than 6 millimeters.

Knowing for sure

Diagnosis begins with an examination by a practitioner. If he or she suspects cancer, a biopsy is performed. If cancer cells are detected, a pathologist (an expert in the examination of tissues) determines what type of cancer cells they are and how far the cancer has progressed.

How to do a skin examination

The National Cancer Institute recommends regular self-examination of the skin.

The best time to do this examination is after a shower or a bath. Check your skin in a well-lighted room by using full-length and hand-held mirrors. Begin by learning where your birthmarks, moles, and blemishes are and what they usually look like. Check for anything new such as a change in the size, texture, or color of a mole, or a sore that doesn't heal. Then take the following steps:

1. **Look at the front and back of your body in the mirror; then raise your arms and look at the left and right sides.**

2. **Bend your elbows and look carefully at your palms, forearms (including the undersides), and upper arms.**

3. **Examine the front and back of your legs.**

   Also look between your buttocks and around your genital area.

4. **Sit down and closely examine your feet, including the soles and the spaces between the toes.**

5. **Look at your face, neck, and scalp.**

   You may want to use a comb or a blow dryer (on the cool setting) to move your hair so that you can see better.

By checking your skin regularly, you become familiar with what is normal. If you find anything unusual, see your doctor right away. Remember, the earlier skin cancer is found, the better the chance for cure.

Treating skin cancer

Ninety percent of all skin cancer cases are treated with some form of surgery. Small lumps or abnormal areas may be removed in a practitioner's office. Common surgeries include the following:

- ✔ **Curettage:** After a local anesthetic numbs the affected area, the cancer is scooped out with a sharp, spoon-shaped instrument. Electric current from a special machine is used to control bleeding and kill any cancer cells remaining around the edge of the wound. Most patients develop a flat, white scar after the treatment.

- ✔ **Mohs' surgery:** The patient is given a local anesthetic, and the cancer is shaved off one thin layer at a time. Each layer is checked under a microscope until the entire tumor is removed. This surgery is especially helpful when the doctor is not sure of the shape and depth of the tumor. In addition, this method is used to remove large tumors, those in hard-to-treat places, and cancers that have recurred. Some scarring may occur with this surgery.

- ✔ **Laser therapy:** A narrow, concentrated beam of light is used to remove or destroy cancer cells.

Other types of treatment include cryosurgery, *electrodessication* (tissue destruction by heat), radiation therapy, biological therapy, and chemotherapy. When a large tumor is removed, a skin graft is needed. For this procedure, the doctor takes a piece of healthy skin from another part of the body to replace the skin that was removed.

Preventing skin cancer

Here are some tips to prevent skin cancer:

- ✔ **Try to avoid the sun when its rays are at their strongest — between 10 a.m. and 3 p.m.:** The National Cancer Institute's "shadow method" states that if your shadow is shorter than you are, which indicates the UV rays are at their strongest, stay indoors. Keep in mind that UV rays are still present even on cloudy days.

- ✔ **Wear protective clothing to block the sun's harmful rays:** Wear a hat to protect your face and head. Wear sunglasses with UV protection.

- ✔ **Use sunscreens rated with a sun protection factor (SPF) of at least 15:** The higher the SPF number, the longer it takes to sunburn.

- ✔ **Don't use sun lamps or visit tanning salons:** Sun lamps and the equipment in tanning salons intensify UV rays.

- ✔ **Avoid the sun when you are using medications containing Retin-A, sulfa drugs, tetracycline, thiazide diuretics, or indomethacin:** These substances make the skin more sensitive to sunlight, increasing the chance of burning.

Testicular cancer: Are you at risk?

Factors that increase your risk for testicular cancer include the following:

✔ **Cryptorchidism:** This is a congenital condition, characterized by undescended testicles, which occurs in infants. The risk for testicular cancer is 3 to 17 times higher than average for boys born with undescended testicles. The risk increases if the condition is not surgically corrected in early childhood.

✔ **Klinefelter's syndrome:** This rare, chromosomal disorder is characterized by small testicles, enlarged breasts, and a lack of secondary sex characteristics such as beard growth and voice change.

✔ **Gonadal aplasia:** With this condition, the testicles don't develop.

✔ **Hermaphroditism:** This condition is the development of both male and female sex characteristics.

✔ **Conduct a monthly skin examination.**

✔ **Protect your children from skin cancer by using these tips, especially the use of sunscreen:** Using sunscreen correctly for the first 18 years of your child's life can lower his or her risk of skin cancer by 80 percent.

Testicular cancer

Cancer that develops in a testicle is called testicular cancer. The American Cancer Society estimated 7,600 new cases of testicular cancer in 1998, with 400 deaths. Testicular cancer can affect men at any age, but it's more common among men between the ages of 15 and 34.

The two most common types of testicular cancer are seminoma and nonseminoma. *Seminomas,* which account for almost 40 percent of all testicular cancer, are comprised of immature germ cells. *Nonseminomas* make up about 55 percent of testicular cancer. Both cancers are fast growing and can often be felt before they spread beyond the testicle. Fortunately, testicular cancer is almost always curable if it is diagnosed and treated early. The key to early detection is regular testicular self-examination.

Recognizing the signs

Most cases are discovered by the man himself, either unintentionally or by self-examination (which is covered in Chapter 7). Symptoms of testicular cancer include a lump in either testicle, enlargement of a testicle, a feeling of heaviness in the scrotum, a dull ache in the lower abdomen or the groin (where the thigh joins the abdomen), a sudden collection of fluid in the scrotum, pain or discomfort in a testicle or in the scrotum, and enlargement or tenderness of the breasts.

These symptoms are not sure signs of cancer, so you should see your doctor if any of these symptoms lasts as long as two weeks.

Knowing for sure

When symptoms suggest that a problem may exist, the doctor reviews the patient's history and does a physical examination, including careful inspection of the scrotum. Tests include a chest X ray, ultrasound, as well as blood and urine tests. If no sign of an infection is present, the doctor may suspect cancer.

At present, a biopsy is the only one sure way to know whether cancer is present. To obtain the tissue, a surgeon does an *inguinal orchiectomy* (removal of the affected testicle through the groin). The surgeon does not cut through the scrotum and does not remove just a part of the testicle because if it is cancer, cutting through the outer layer of the testicle may cause the cancer to spread to the surrounding tissue and lymph nodes. Although this treatment may seem drastic, removing the affected testicle can halt further growth if the cancer is present. Removing one testicle doesn't interfere with fertility or the ability to have an erection. Also, an artificial testicle (a prosthesis), can be implanted into the scrotum for cosmetic purposes.

Treating testicular cancer

Treatment of testicular cancer depends on the stage and cell type (seminoma or nonseminoma) of the disease. Treatments for testicular cancer include surgery, radiation therapy, and chemotherapy.

Seminoma cells grow slowly and are usually diagnosed before they have spread. They are sensitive and responsive to radiation therapy. Chemotherapy is also another treatment option.

Nonseminoma cells grow rapidly and are not usually caught before they spread. Fortunately, the cure rate is still quite high. Surgical removal of the lymph nodes is often necessary after the cancer has spread beyond the testicle, because nonseminomas do not respond well to radiation therapy. Chemotherapy also may be used. Regular follow-up examinations are necessary in both types of testicular cancer to ensure that the cancer is completely gone. Testicular cancer seldom recurs after a patient has been cancer-free for three years. Men who have been treated for cancer in one testicle have about a 1 percent chance of developing cancer in the other testicle.

Chapter 19
Chronic Conditions

• •

• •

Some 100 million Americans suffer from one or more *chronic conditions* — diseases and conditions that recur frequently and have no medical cure. Like infomercials that keep cropping up on late-night TV, chronic conditions are always with you. But unlike those annoying infomericals that you can eliminate with a zap of the TV remote control, chronic conditions are persistent, physically debilitating, and emotionally exhausting. Fortunately, many chronic conditions are manageable, and with some persistence and diligence, you can lead a productive life.

In this chapter, we provide basic understanding of chronic conditions, present up-to-date treatments, and outline preventive measures whenever possible.

Allergies

Think of your body as a castle protected against harmful invaders by an army within you. This army is your immune system, which consists of cells, glands, tissues, and organs. Your immune system is normally ready to attack harmful invaders such as viruses, bacteria, and parasites.

At times, however, the immune system makes a mistake and sees some substances as invaders. Allergy attacks occur when your immune system overreacts and produces antibodies to fight irritants like food, drugs, house mites, pollen, mold, and pet dander (minute particles of skin that come from hair or feathers). Any substance that triggers the immune system to cause an allergic reaction is called an *allergen*.

Antibodies are proteins designed to eliminate foreign substances from the body. Antibodies attach themselves to cells in the respiratory and gastrointestinal tracts, skin, and blood. These cells then release powerful chemicals — histamines, prostaglandins, and leukotrienes — that cause common allergic symptoms.

Recognizing the signs

Table 19-1 lists the common signs of allergies:

Table 19-1	Common Allergies and Their Symptoms
Allergy Type	*Symptoms*
Allergic rhinitis (including seasonal allergic rhinitis)	Clear and watery nasal discharge, nasal congestion and sneezing, itchy nose and eyes
Allergic contact dermatitis (see Chapter 11 for more information)	Rash, skin irritation, redness, itching
Allergic reaction to foods	Hives (skin eruptions of varying shapes and sizes with clear borders and pale centers), swelling, abdominal pain, nausea, vomiting, diarrhea
Allergic reaction to drugs	Breathing difficulty, wheezing, hives, itchy skin, rash
Allergic reaction to insect bites and stings	Hives, itching, constriction or swelling in the throat and chest

With many types of allergies, symptoms can quickly escalate to a rare, potentially life-threatening reaction known as *anaphylaxis* or *anaphylactic shock.* Signs include sudden drop in blood pressure, constricted airways, swollen throat, and hives. This reaction occurs in seconds to minutes after the person has come in contact with an allergen. Death can occur if not treated immediately. For those who have severe reactions to bee stings or foods, emergency kits, which usually contain an injection of epinephrine, are available.

Knowing for sure

You eat a bowl of strawberries and, within an hour, you're covered with hives. Some darling sends you cologne for your birthday, and at the first whiff, you sneeze. Many times you can diagnose an apparent allergy and avoid it. At other times when the allergen is unknown, you may need to consult an *allergist,* a medical specialist who deals with allergies.

Types of allergies

Allergies may be temporary or chronic. Temporary allergies are often seasonal, whereas chronic allergies can annoy year-round if you don't get treatment. Several types of allergies exist: allergic rhinitis, allergic contact dermatitis, and allergic reaction to foods, drugs, and insect bites and stings.

✔ Allergic rhinitis, a swelling of the nasal passages, has symptoms similar to the common cold. This type of allergy may be chronic or may occur seasonally. Seasonal allergic rhinitis (commonly occurring in spring and fall) is also called hay fever, though it has nothing to do with hay or fever. With this type of allergy your immune system may react to spores, molds, and the pollens of trees, weeds, and grass.

✔ Allergic contact dermatitis may result when you come into contact with a particular allergen. Think of poison ivy and you have the general idea. Other potential allergens include sunlight, dyes, cosmetics, and metal compounds.

✔ Allergies from foods, drugs, and insect bites and stings result from eating various foods (for example, chocolate, milk, wheat products, eggs, soybeans, nuts, and shellfish), from ingesting or receiving injections of certain drugs (penicillin and related antibiotics, sulfonamides, anticonvulsants, insulin, anesthetics, and barbiturates), and from being bitten or stung by venomous insects (such as spiders, ants, bees, and wasps).

After your doctor has examined you and has concluded that you do indeed have an allergy, he or she may order specific tests to determine the one or more allergens that plague you. Such tests include blood tests (for example, *radioimmunosorbent* test and *radioallergosorbent* test) that check for the presence of antibodies. Several skin tests are available:

✔ **Scratch test:** In this test, the doctor makes a series of short, superficial scratches on the skin — usually the forearm — and then rubs different extracts of suspected allergens into them. This test is rarely used today.

✔ **Skin-prick test:** This test involves placing a drop of allergen extract on the back or arm and then pricking the skin with a small needle under the drop.

✔ **Intradermal test:** In this test, the allergen-containing extract is injected directly into the skin.

✔ **Patch test:** This test involves placing a small amount of an allergen on the skin and covering it with an adhesive patch. This type of test is usually done to confirm contact dermatitis.

Foiling food allergies

Determining specific food allergies is difficult. After skin and blood tests suggest certain foods are allergens, you have two choices to confirm a suspected food allergy. The simpler is food avoidance. The suspicious food is removed from your diet, and you are observed to see whether allergic symptoms disappear. If they do, the food is reintroduced into the diet to see whether symptoms recur. If they do, the food is then assumed to be the culprit.

Another method is blind testing. In this test, you're given a dose of a suspected food allergen or a placebo, an inactive substance. This test allows the doctor to determine whether the food really triggers a reaction.

Treating allergies

After your doctor diagnoses allergies, he or she may prescribe an antihistamine, decongestant, or corticosteroid for you.

- ✔ **Antihistamines:** As the name implies, these drugs counteract the effects of histamines, such as a runny nose, nasal congestion, hives, itchy and watery eyes. They work best when taken before you come in contact with an allergen because the antihistamine's job is to bind to tissue sites such as the cells lining the breathing tubes before the histamines do. Antihistamines are available over the counter and through a prescription. Common brands include Benadryl, Chlor-Trimeton, Tacaryl, and Tavist. These types of antihistamines can cause drowsiness, so some manufacturers counteract this effect by adding a decongestant to give an "upper" effect. Antihistamines sometimes are also combined with pain relievers to reduce headaches and pain associated with allergies. Newer antihistamines that are nonsedating include Allegra, Claritin, Hismanal, and Zytec.

- ✔ **Decongestants:** These drugs reduce the swelling of the nasal passages and stop nasal congestion. And unlike antihistamines, decongestants are effective when an allergy attack is underway. Decongestants are available as pills, drops, and sprays. Popular over-the-counter decongestants include Afrin, Neosynephrine, and Sudafed. Decongestants have a stimulating effect, and possible side effects include high blood pressure, rapid heart rate, headaches, and jitteriness. Also, decongestant nasal sprays may become addictive and shouldn't be used continuously for longer than five days.

✔ **Corticosteriods:** These hormonelike anti-inflammatory drugs treat respiratory and skin allergies. They come in spray or inhalant form for respiratory tract problems; in injectable or topical form for skin rashes; and in injectable or oral form for systemic (whole body) therapy. Systemic forms should be used only in short-term allergy treatments. Corticosteroids have few side effects when used in low doses for short periods of time. Possible side effects include stomach ulcers, high blood pressure, psychological disorders, and weight gain.

Treating allergies through self-care

The best way to control an allergy is to minimize your exposure to the allergens. Here are some tips on how to do that:

✔ **Check the weather.** A dry, sunny, and windy day (in spring, summer, and fall) may inspire you to fly a kite, but you're better off inside with a good book instead. That's because the picture-perfect day is actually the perfect time for plants to release their pollen into the air. Humid or rainy days are better times for venturing outdoors because offending plants don't pollinate under these conditions. But rainy days may worsen a person's allergy to mold.

✔ **Keep windows and doors closed when the pollen count is highest.** Generally between 4 p.m. and 10 a.m.

Immunotherapy

Immunotherapy — an allergy-desensitizing therapy — may help bring relief to allergy sufferers who don't respond to medications. It's also used in conjunction with medications. The process involves desensitizing an allergic person through a series of gradually potent injections of whatever he is allergic to — for example, ragweed and mold. The shots allow the allergy sufferer to build a tolerance to the allergen and reduce or eliminate allergic reactions. If successful, the course of treatment can continue five years or more. Potential side effects include a reaction to the injection such as swelling at the site or, rarely, more serious reactions such as breathing and swallowing difficulty, hives, stomach pain, and fainting. Plus, injections are not available to treat every type of allergy.

A new version of this treatment is under study — nasal immunotherapy in which the allergen is absorbed into the body through a nasal spray. The advantage of the spray is that the user has fewer side effects.

✔ **Use an air conditioner or an air purifier, particularly in the bedroom.** Be sure to clean the filter regularly.

✔ **Use a dehumidifer to help reduce the growth of fungi, dust mites, and molds during summer humidity.** Again, keep the machine clean to avoid mold.

✔ **Skip the yard work.** Avoid mowing the lawn or raking the leaves if you can. But if the neighbors begin to complain about the herds of sheep flocking to your lawn, then don a mask or filter to keep pollen and molds out of your system while you do yard work.

✔ **Clean your home as often as possible to remove allergens.** Avoid dust-gathering knickknacks and draperies, bedspreads, and carpeting, especially in the sleeping area.

✔ **Wash your bedding, synthetic pillows, and mattress pads often in hot water.**

✔ **Encase your mattress and pillows in plastic to reduce dust mite waste in the air.**

✔ **Avoid hanging clothes, sheets, and blankets outside to dry.**

Asthma

Asthma is a chronic respiratory disease in which airways in the lungs periodically become narrowed, obstructed, or even blocked. An estimated 15 million Americans suffer from asthma, and the number of new asthma cases increases yearly. Figure 19-1 shows a healthy respiratory system.

Asthma generally develops in childhood but may develop in adults with no previous history of asthma. Males develop this disorder twice as often as females.

Asthma attacks, periods of breathing difficulty, occur in reaction to certain stimuli, usually something inhaled. Allergens responsible for allergies often trigger asthma attacks. Other triggers include strenuous exercise, cold air, upper respiratory infections, and emotional stress.

Recognizing the signs

Asthma attacks may be so mild that you may barely notice it, or an attack can be life-threatening and require emergency medical treatment. Here are the most common symptoms of asthma:

✔ Shortness of breath (gasping or panting)

✔ Pressure in the front of the chest, in the area of the breastbone

✔ Wheezing (whistling or rasping sound)

✔ Excessive mucus

✔ Coughing

✔ Anxiety

Knowing for sure

Because other conditions can mimic asthma (such as chronic bronchitis, an inflammation in the lungs, and emphysema, a respiratory disorder that leads to permanent damage to the alveoli, or tiny air sacs, in the lungs), getting a proper diagnosis is important. Your health-care practitioner determines whether you have asthma by a physical examination, medical history, chest X rays, ultrasound scans, allergy testing, and diagnostic tools such as a spirometer, which measures the breathing capacity of your lungs.

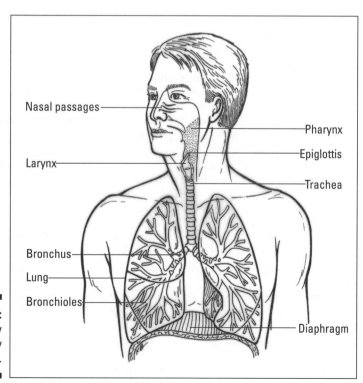

Figure 19-1:
A healthy
respiratory
system.

A *bronchodilator,* an asthma drug that opens the airways, is also used in testing. If airflow improves after using the drug, then a diagnosis of asthma may be made. If airflow doesn't improve immediately and your health-care practitioner suspects asthma, he or she may put you on bronchodilators and anti-inflammatory drugs for several weeks. The test is then repeated, and if readings improve, asthma is the likely diagnosis.

Other possible tests include *bronchoprovocation,* which involves exposure to a suspected or known allergen to provoke a mild asthma attack. Another is an *exercise-challenge test,* which involves jogging on a treadmill or riding an exercise bike to trigger an asthma attack. This test is also used to measure the airway's sensitivity or to gauge the effectiveness of medication or self-care treatment.

Treating asthma

The bad news is that asthma can't be cured. The good news is that it can be controlled through medication and self-care methods. Asthma drugs come in pill, syrup, solution, aerosol, and powdered form. Those in solution form require a machine called a *nebulizer,* which converts the solution into a fine, medicated mist that is inhaled over a four- to five-minute period. Inhalers are small aerosol canisters that deliver measured doses of medication as small "puffs."

Asthma drugs are generally grouped into two categories: quick-relief medications used to treat acute symptoms and attacks (bronchodilators) and long-term control medications (anti-inflammatories and leukotriene modifiers). As we already said, bronchodilators help relax airways and improve airflow. Examples include albuterol (brand names Proventil and Ventolin), bitolterol (Tornalate), ipratropium bromide (Atrovent), and theophylline (Bronkodyl and Elixophyllin). Possible side effects include increased blood pressure, tremors, irregular heart-beat, nervousness, throat irritation, and cough.

Special precautions are necessary with theophylline, which has a narrow therapeutic range (meaning that the body can handle only a specific amount of theophylline in the bloodstream for positive effects). If below the range, the drug doesn't work. If above the range, adverse reactions can occur, such as irritability, restlessness, sleeping difficulties, and mild headaches.

Theophylline's side effects can be serious and include the following toxic reactions: nausea, vomiting, stomachache, loss of appetite, irregular heart-beat, severe headache, confusion or disorientation, and seizure. You should call your doctor immediately if you experience any of these reactions.

Anti-inflammatory drugs are used to prevent inflammation in the airways or, if inflammation is already present, stop it from worsening. Examples of these drugs include beclomethasone (Beconase and Vancenase), cromolyn sodium (Intal), and nedocromil sodium (Tilade). Possible side effects include fungal infection of the mouth and throat, changes in the lining of the nose, increased cataract risk, spasm of bronchial tubes, and increased wheezing.

Leukotriene modifiers are a relatively new class of drugs used in long-term asthma treatment as substitutes for anti-inflammatories. They attack leukotrienes, substances that constrict the airway, increase mucus secretions, and activate inflammatory cells. Although these drugs' usefulness and safety are still being studied, they are primarily used to prevent asthma attacks. Examples of these drugs include zileuton (Zyflo Filmtab), zafirlukast (Accolate), and pranlukast (Ultair). Possible side effects include headache, upset stomach, nausea, and diarrhea.

Other drugs used to treat asthma are mucokinetics. These drugs help clear thick mucus from the lungs. One such mucokinetic drug is guaifenesin, an expectorant (found in many cough and cold syrups) that helps a person with asthma cough up more mucus. Possible side effects include nausea, vomiting, and drowsiness.

Antihistamines are sometimes helpful for people whose asthma is triggered by allergens. These drugs help to relieve nasal congestion, sneezing, and the hives that often accompany allergic reactions.

Treating asthma through self-care

Asthma is a complicated disease, but the control of this disease rests in your hands and your family's. Along with medication, self-care is essential. Your overall goal should be to control asthma so that you can live a full, productive life. One important step is the use of a *peak flow meter*. With this portable device, you can measure the maximum speed at which air leaves your lungs. As you exhale forcefully into the mouthpiece of this tube-shaped device, an indicator scale measures the greatest speed of air exiting the lungs. Doing several measurements over time and recording the results on a chart help you compare your readings with an established normal range. Levels that begin to drop can predict an asthma attack. In that case, you can take preventive medications or notify a doctor.

Here are some other helpful tips:

✔ **Avoid or control your exposure to allergens, food allergies, and irritants such as cigarette smoking.** During pollen and mold season, keep your windows closed, especially in the bedroom. Seal central heating and cooling system ducts to keep allergens from other rooms entering your bedroom. For other ways to avoid allergens, refer to the allergy section of this chapter.

✔ **Keep active.** A sedentary lifestyle is associated with long periods of shallow breathing. Routine aerobic exercise conditions your body's muscles and builds lung strength. Moderate activity, and the deep breathing that accompanies it, protects your lungs by acting as a clearing agent so that inhaled allergens spend less time in your body. Check with your health-care practitioner before beginning a new exercise program (see Chapters 1 and 4).

✔ **Try postural drainage:** This technique uses gravity and gentle rapping on the chest to loosen and eliminate thick mucus. Nurses and physical or respiratory therapists trained in this technique can show family members how to perform postural drainage on you.

✔ **Use stress management:** Everyone experiences stress in life, but stress plays an even more complex role in your life if you have asthma. To help deal with tension and reduce the fear you experience during an asthma attack, learn a stress management technique such as the ones we discuss in Chapters 2 and 6.

Diabetes

Diabetes is a chronic disease that affects the way your body turns food into energy. A healthy body changes carbohydrates, such as starches and sugars (for example, breads, fruits, and vegetables), into a form of sugar called *glucose.* Glucose is to your body what gasoline is to a car — fuel and energy. The bloodstream carries glucose to cells, and *insulin* (a hormone made in the pancreas) helps glucose enter the cells. When a man has diabetes, either his pancreas doesn't make enough insulin or his body can't use the insulin correctly.

When glucose begins to build up in the bloodstream, the result can be serious. Untreated diabetes can cause damage to the eyes, heart, kidneys, legs, feet, nerves, and blood vessels. Diabetes-related health conditions include blindness, heart disease, kidney disease, amputations, strokes, and birth defects.

About 16 million Americans have diabetes, and it's the fourth leading cause of death by disease in the United States.

Diabetes is generally classified simply as type 1 or type 2. In type 1 diabetes, the body's immune system attacks the insulin-producing cells in the pancreas and destroys them. As a result of this "cannibalizing" action, glucose in the bloodstream increases and upsets the blood-sugar level. The results are either hyperglycemia (too much glucose) or hypoglycemia (too little glucose). Also, people with type 1 diabetes can develop *ketoacidosis,* which is a poisoning of the body with ketones (toxic acids caused by the disintegration of fats for fuel). In extreme cases, ketoacidosis can result in unconsciousness, diabetic coma, or death.

Type 1 diabetes is typically first diagnosed in children and young adults, but it can appear at any age. There may be a genetic link. Symptoms normally develop over a short period of time, but cell damage can occur years before the symptoms begin to appear.

Type 2 diabetes is much more common, accounting for about 90 percent of all cases of diabetes. It's also very sneaky because symptoms of the disease sometimes don't show up until damage to the body has already occurred. You can have this disease for years before you know it.

People diagnosed with type 2 diabetes are typically over 30 and are obese. Four out of five people with this condition are overweight. In type 2 diabetes, the pancreas produces insulin, but the body is unable to use it successfully. Some speculate that excess weight and a high carbohydrate intake cause the body's cells to become resistant to insulin. In addition, the cells that produce insulin work overtime and eventually become exhausted, resulting in inadequate insulin production. Type 2 diabetes may also have a genetic link, but it generally is thought that the disease must be triggered by age or excess weight.

Recognizing the signs

Here are the most common signs of diabetes:

- Sudden weight loss
- Frequent urination
- Frequent thirst and/or hunger
- Vision problems
- Weakness, fatigue, and irritability
- Circulation problems such as tingling or numbness in legs, feet, or fingers
- Slow healing of cuts (especially on the feet)
- Frequent infections
- Itchy skin

Knowing for sure

You should expect a routine blood test first to check for diabetes. In healthy, fasting adults (anyone who has not eaten in three or more hours), a normal blood-sugar level is between 60 and 100 milligrams per deciliter (mg/dl). If your fasting blood sugar is between 115 and 140 mg/dl, periodic testing may be necessary to monitor blood-sugar levels. If your fasting blood sugar is over 140 mg/dl, two additional tests are necessary to diagnose diabetes: fasting plasma glucose test and oral glucose-tolerance test.

✔ The fasting plasma glucose test is performed after you haven't eaten for 8 to 12 hours. This test is repeated on different days, and diabetes is diagnosed if glucose levels are higher than 140 mg/dl on two successive tests.

✔ The oral glucose-tolerance test is a fasting blood sample taken after you eat a high-carbohydrate diet for three days. After that sample is taken, you must drink a glucose solution and then blood samples are taken every 30 minutes for two hours, with another sample taken an hour later. You may feel like you were run over by a porcupine after this test, but all the blood samples are necessary to show how your body is handling glucose. Blood-sugar levels normally rise after glucose is consumed, but the levels should return to normal rather quickly. Blood-sugar levels higher than 200 mg/dl one to two hours after a meal confirm a diagnosis of diabetes. And if your blood sugar is more than 200 mg/dl after the fasting segment of this test, there's no doubt that you have diabetes.

Treating diabetes

We won't kid you — diabetes has no cure. But the disease is controllable, and you can expect a normal life span as well as an active lifestyle if you follow a prescribed treatment plan. Each type of diabetes has a different treatment plan. Those with type 1 diabetes must take injections of prescription insulin to regulate their sugar metabolism, whereas those with type 2 diabetes have several options.

Diabetes and men

Diabetes can affect the sexual activity of men. According to the American Diabetes Association, erection problems occur among 50 to 60 percent of all men over age 50 who are diabetic. Blood vessel disease and nerve disease are the most common causes of problems in men with diabetes. Blood vessel disease blocks the flow of blood to the penis. If the nerves to the penis are damaged, they may not be able to send signals and, thus, may limit blood flow, which can prevent an erection.

If you have diabetes, you should practice good blood-sugar control in order to prevent nerve and circulatory damage and prevent any problems. If you have diabetes and are experiencing erection problems, you should see your doctor to determine the exact cause and receive treatment.

Some people with type 2 diabetes do eventually become insulin dependent, but the majority can control their sugar levels, and some can even reverse the disease process so that insulin is produced and functions normally. But it won't happen without a disciplined regimen of medication, diet, exercise, and weight loss.

Drugs to treat type 2 diabetes include insulin and the oral hypoglycemic medications: alpha-glucosidase inhibitors, metformin, sulfonylureas, and troglitazone.

✔ Examples of alpha-glucosidase inhibitors include acarbose (Precose) and miglitol (Glyset). These drugs work by interfering with enzymes in the intestine responsible for breaking down the carbohydrates found in starchy foods into glucose and other sugars, and they help to lower blood-sugar levels by slowing the absorption of glucose into the bloodstream after eating. Possible side effects include abdominal pain, gas, diarrhea, and liver problems. People with kidney disease, cirrhosis, inflammatory bowel disease, or absorption diseases shouldn't use these drugs.

✔ Metformin (Glucophage), belonging to the biguanides chemical family, is usually used by people with diabetes after other medications have proved unsuccessful. This drug causes the liver to release stored glucose more slowly and appears to lower insulin resistance while lowering blood sugar without increasing insulin production. Possible side effects include diarrhea, nausea, vomiting, loss of appetite, gas and, occasionally, low levels of vitamin B12. Rarely, this drug can cause a metallic taste in the mouth.

✔ Sulfonylureas make up a group of seven drugs. Examples include acetohexamide (Dymelar) and tolazamide (Tolinase). These drugs work by triggering the production and release of insulin from the pancreas. One possible side effect is hypoglycemia, which is character-ized by hunger, shaking, dizziness, confusion, irritability, sweating, and nausea. Other side effects may include weight gain and allergic reac-tions, such as rash, hives, vomiting, and cramping.

✔ Troglitazone (Rezulin) belongs to the thiazolindinediones chemical family. The drug works by reducing the body's resistance to insulin and can be used alone or in combination with other drugs. Initial research suggests that the drug can reduce fasting blood-glucose levels by 30 percent without causing hypoglycemia. In many cases, the drug re-duces or eliminates the need for insulin in those taking it, experts say. Possible side effects include infections, headaches, pain, weakness, dizziness, sore throat, runny nose, and nausea. People with hepatitis or other liver disease should use this drug with caution. The Food and Drug Administration recommends that people taking troglitazone have liver-function tests monthly during the first six months of treatment, bimonthly during the second six months of treatment, and periodically after that.

Preventing diabetes

Type 1 diabetes can't be prevented at present, but scientists are looking for ways to identify the predisposing genetic factors of the disease. However, you can reduce your risk of getting type 2 diabetes by following these suggested tips:

- ✔ Maintain a healthy weight.

- ✔ Eat low-fat foods.

- ✔ Get regular exercise. Exercise can help you lose excess weight that could trigger diabetes. Also, evidence suggests that building muscle mass through exercise triggers your muscle's use of insulin and may help prevent diabetes.

Part IV
Your Sexual Health

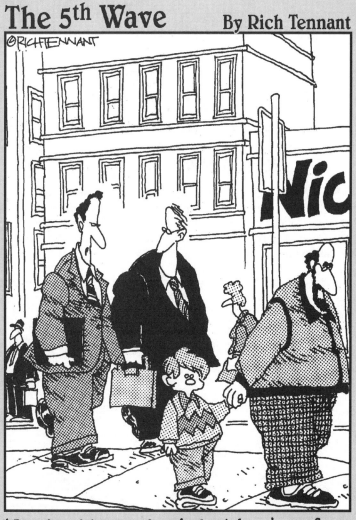

"I got a little confused about how to perform an NPT test*. I thought you could use a postage meter."

*See Chapter 7

In this part . . .

We start out by discussing male sexual development and normal sexual functioning. Then we get into topics like contraception, infertility, sexually transmitted diseases, and sexual dysfunction. Read on. You're bound to learn something.

Chapter 20

Sexual Development

S exual development. It's as plain as the birds and the bees and the flowers and the trees. It's what every healthy child goes through provided that his life isn't cut short. And although gender is defined at the moment a sperm fertilizes an egg, the development of male physical characteristics doesn't happen immediately from the start. For example, the testicles don't form until around the sixth week of pregnancy, and the fetus doesn't take on the appearance of a male until eight weeks later when the testicles start producing hormones. At this point, the penis, scrotum, and prostate begin to form. Then, just before birth, the testicles descend into their proper place in the scrotum. For about 10 years, hormone levels in the male remain constant, and sexual development "hibernates" until puberty begins.

But a man's sexual self also undergoes changes in the latter years of life when levels of testosterone gradually decrease. This process is referred to as male menopause and can affect a man's sexual drive. Regardless of what stage of life you're in, many options exist to help you maintain or regain peak sexual performance. So stick around to find out what happens during puberty, what male menopause is, and how to keep yourself at your sexual best whether you are in the prime of your life or in your latter years.

Puberty

Think of puberty as the transition stage from boyhood to manhood. It usually starts around age 11 and may last until age 17. Puberty is the further development of the genitals, changes in the hair and physique to that typical of adult males, and the regular production of hormones and sperm, which enable full sexual function. And although the change seems to begin below the waist, the process of puberty actually begins above in the brain and is separated into five stages of development called the *Tanner stages* after the British physician who first categorized them. Keep in mind that the timing of changes may vary among boys of the same age (see the upcoming "Rates of development" section).

Tanner stage one (from ages 9 to 10)

During this stage, testosterone production in the testicles is stimulated for the first time. The *hypothalamus* — the area of the brain that controls hormone production — stimulates the pituitary gland (located at the base of the brain) to secrete the hormones FSH (follicle-stimulating hormone) and LH (luteinizing hormone). FSH stimulates sperm production and LH causes the testicles to produce testosterone.

Tanner stage two (from ages 12 to 13)

During this stage, puberty becomes physically obvious. The FSH and LH hormones cause the testicles to enlarge and pubic hair to sprout at the base of the penis. These hormones may also cause an overall growth spurt in the body. But because this sudden growth may occur at different rates for different parts of the body (for example, feet faster than legs), physical awkwardness, so common in early puberty, results. Generally, the body grows taller and heavier, and the shoulders widen, resulting in a stronger upper body. This stage usually lasts 13 months, though it can range from 5 to 24 months.

Tanner stage three (from ages 13 to 14)

During this short stage, lasting about 10 months, the most pronounced physical changes occur. At this stage, the boy's penis begins to lengthen and his pubic hair becomes thicker and coarser. One testicle (usually the left) begins to hang lower than the other. His voice deepens as the larynx enlarges but is also marked by the typical teenage male's "cracking" voice. He continues to grow in height (as much as 5 inches a year), and gains weight and muscle. Hair also begins to form on his upper lip, arms, and legs.

Tanner stage four (from ages 14 to 15)

During this stage, the libido, or sex drive, awakens. Most adolescent males experience their first ejaculation during this stage, almost always as an involuntary nocturnal (during sleep) emission. Ejaculation is a sign that the testicles are starting to produce sperm (the male equivalent of a girl's menstrual periods beginning). Frequent, spontaneous erections may also occur, a normal and common, though frustrating, source of teenage male embarrassment.

Also during this stage, the penis continues to widen and lengthen, and the testicles continue to grow. The skin on the genitals darkens, and the pubic hair spreads across the groin area. Body and facial hair become more apparent. Perspiration gets heavier. The hair and skin become oilier, often leading to dandruff and acne problems. Although this stage may seem to last forever for those experiencing it, the length is 2 to 3 years.

Tanner stage five (from ages 15 to 18)

During this final stage, the adolescent has become a young man and is sexually mature. His genitals have reached their full size, and he has the general physique of a man. He may continue to grow a few inches taller and develop more chest hair until his early 20s.

Masturbation

Although males of any age (even infants) are capable of having an erection, ejaculation can't occur until puberty. *Masturbation,* or the stimulation of one's own genitals, often begins at adolescence because the libido increases as a result of the hormones a boy produces during puberty. Masturbation typically continues well into later life as a way of relieving sexual tension. In males, masturbation often involves sexual fantasy, thus accounting for the sales of many "male-oriented" magazines.

Although many myths and social taboos surround masturbation, medically, this activity is normal and harmless. Despite dire warnings from parents, clergy, and teachers, masturbation doesn't make you go blind, cause genital warts or acne, or make hair grow on your palms! To the contrary, masturbation is good for you (provided it doesn't become a compulsion, which may actually interfere with ability to climax with a partner). It helps to maintain healthy sexual function by sustaining sperm quality, vitality, and quantity. Stored sperm tend to lose their speed and not function well. Regular masturbation helps to promote sperm production and health. And as mentioned in Chapter 16, regular ejaculation is also useful in promoting a healthy prostate by preventing congestive prostatitis, a condition in which prostatic fluid builds up to cause inflammation and congestion.

Masturbation may also be used therapeutically for both men and women suffering from sexual problems. Masturbation with a partner can serve as a substitute for intercourse, particularly for medical or contraceptive reasons.

Gynecomastia

Did you know that breast enlargement, or adolescent gynecomastia, occurs in 50 to 85 percent of teenage males? It's one of the most psychologically troubling manifestations of puberty and is caused by hormone production and imbalance, which may also lead to some pain or small lumps in the breasts. These problems usually disappear on their own in 12 to 16 months. However, boys (especially those engaged in sports activities) should be warned that drugs, such as amphetamines or steroids, can cause breast enlargement at any age.

Rates of development

Although the Tanner stages include average ages for the different developmental stages, the range of ages for normal, healthy males is actually quite wide. Plus, it's not unusual to have boys at various stages of development sharing the same classroom. Some may be shaving heavy facial hair while others have yet to sprout enough "peach fuzz" to justify picking up a razor!

Although this fact may cause anxiety in "late bloomers," these boys could have simply inherited genes for later development from their parents. Maturity will come, just a bit slower. However, if a boy seems to be lagging in physical development far behind others of the same age, a doctor should examine him to rule out glandular problems.

Penis size

With the exception of a few, what man hasn't worried over the size of his penis at one time or another? And no wonder, given society's obsessive notion that big is better (big houses, big cars, and big incomes). From locker room talk to shock jock Howard Stern, most men think their penises are too small and, therefore, unappealing to women. But more women are satisfied sexually through clitoral stimulation than through vaginal intercourse. And more isn't necessarily better because many women fear that large penises may hurt them during intercourse. With that said, here are a few penis facts:

- ✔ **First appearance:** At approximately 14 weeks

- ✔ **Average flaccid size at maturity:** 3.5 inches long x 1.25 inches in diameter

- ✔ **Average erect size at maturity:** 5.1 inches long x 1.6 inches in diameter

- ✔ **Longest medically recorded erection:** 12 inches

- ✔ **Average number of erections per night while sleeping:** 5

- ✔ **Average duration of each nighttime erection:** 20 to 30 minutes

Male Menopause

The subject of *male menopause* — the idea that men undergo a drop in hormone levels as they age, just like women do at menopause — is mired in controversy. Testosterone levels decline as men age, and these lower levels can lead to a lowered libido, erection problems, depression, fatigue, and osteoporosis in some men. Some scientists deny that male menopause exists, chalking up the physical manifestation to a psychological, mid-life crisis. But the good news is that research is evaluating the use of supplemental testosterone to treat *hypogonadism* — a condition in which the body produces insufficient amounts of testosterone and that is often the cause of male menopause. This form of hormone replacement therapy is similar to estrogen therapy, which treats the symptoms of menopause in women.

Experts usually refer to male menopause as *andropause* or *viripause* because it's not the same as female menopause. Menopause marks the end of menstruation and a slowdown in the function of the ovaries. Men, of course, don't have ovaries and don't have to deal with menstruation, and the decline of testosterone is very gradual — about 1 percent a year. The decline begins around the age of 48 but may start anytime between the ages of 40 and 50. (Some studies suggest that a man's testosterone levels may fall as much as 30 to 40 percent between the ages of 40 and 70.) About 15 percent of older men have testosterone levels low enough to be considered hypogonadism.

Recognizing the signs

Most men never feel the effects of male menopause because the decline in testosterone is so slight. However, some men experience the following symptoms:

- Decreased erections
- Increased anxiety and fear
- Insomnia
- Loss of muscle and bone
- Fatigue
- Weight gain

Knowing for sure

Because other physical ailments (such as kidney and liver disease) can cause symptoms of reduced libido and impaired sexual performance, you need to get a thorough physical examination. After your practitioner rules out other factors, a complete blood test of testosterone levels may show lower-than-expected amounts. But because the decline in testosterone may be small and still within the range of what is considered normal, this test cannot itself give a definitive answer. You should have any symptoms of sexual dysfunction checked to determine whether lowered testosterone levels are causing them.

Before your doctor can recommend hormone replacement, you must undergo a screening for prostate cancer. Hormones don't cause prostate cancer, but this cancer can grow faster in their presence (see Chapter 18).

Treating male menopause

If your doctor finds hypogonadism, he may prescribe testosterone replacement therapy (TRT). TRT comes in several different forms. You may be given an injection of testosterone into a muscle; however, with this form of hormone therapy, levels are high immediately after the injection and then drop sharply and remain at low levels until the next injection. Alternatives to injections include placing pelletlike implants of testosterone under the skin of the buttocks or abdomen and wearing skin patches that deliver testosterone through the skin.

Possible side effects of TRT include weight gain, due to muscle growth, and fluid retention. Sleep apnea, a condition in which the airways become momentarily blocked during sleep, may develop or worsen during TRT. In rare cases, liver disorders such as cysts in the liver may occur. Supplemental testosterone can also interfere with fertility. And because even small amounts of testosterone can affect women (such as unwanted hair growth), make sure that during sleep or in the heat of passion, the patch doesn't come off and stick to your partner.

Maintaining Peak Sexual Functioning

Eat right. Get regular exercise. Shed unwanted pounds. Learn to relax. Give up smoking. Lose the booze.

Sound like a lecture from your doctor? Well, it's also the basis of a plan to keep your body performing at its sexual best. Good sexual functioning doesn't exist by itself. The parts of the body are all connected and interact with each other. So to keep your sex life in shape, you need to keep both mind and body in shape as well.

Try these following tips:

- ✔ **Eat a well-balanced diet:** A diet rich in zinc and B vitamins helps to keep up proper testosterone and sperm production.

- ✔ **Get regular exercise:** Feeling good is important for sexual arousal. Besides making you feel better, exercise helps maintain muscle tone and proper weight. By staying in shape, you also help to keep your blood pressure normal, which in turn, helps to avoid sexual problems associated with medications that control hypertension. A good program of regular exercise, particularly aerobic exercise (such as walking, running, and cycling) to strengthen your heart and lungs, is a path to better health (which makes you feel good) and improved sexual functioning.

- ✔ **Maintain a healthy weight:** Being overweight can make you lethargic and less interested in sex (and perhaps less interesting to your partner!). Needless to say, getting prematurely out of breath and physically exhausted before you or your partner is satisfied does nothing positive for a relationship or for your sexual self-esteem. Stick to a low-fat, high-fiber diet.

- ✔ **Avoid drugs that make you drowsy (such as antihistamines and alcohol):** They may make your love life drowsy as well. Although alcohol may make you feel sexier by lowering inhibitions, it also reduces libido, causes erection problems, and impairs the ability to have an orgasm because it's a depressant. Alcohol dilates the blood vessels, making it harder to send blood to reach the penis for an erection. Prolonged alcohol abuse has also been shown to cause irreversible damage to the nerves in the penis and lead to erection problems.

  Too much beer can be especially troublesome because of the naturally occurring plant estrogens found in hops. Over time, plant estrogens counter the effects of testosterone (the hormone important to male sexual functioning) and may cause erection problems. Plant estrogens can also lead to a fat distribution pattern more typical of women.

- ✔ **Avoid smoking:** Although Hollywood would have you believe that smoking is sexy, nicotine can stifle your libido, not to mention the other negative effects on your health (such as lung cancer). Smoking damages the small arteries that feed blood to the penis to create and maintain an erection. Many doctors point to smoking as the major cause of sexual dysfunction in men. Studies have found that the majority of men with erection problems are smokers or former smokers. Smoking can also reduce sperm count and quality.

- ✔ **Learn relaxation techniques:** Stress is one of the leading causes of erection problems. Anxiety and tension rob the mind of its ability to focus on the pleasure of being aroused, sometimes to the point that arousal becomes difficult or impossible. By shutting out distractions and worries of everyday life and learning how to relax (see Chapter 6), you can maintain, restore, or even heighten sexual function.

✔ **Get a massage:** A sensual massage can do wonders to enhance the feeling of intimacy between partners, as well as create an overall sense of relaxation that can aid in achieving sexual arousal. Everyday stresses can melt away under the caressing hands of one's partner, allowing sexual desire to rise to the surface.

✔ **Use lubricants, such as K-Y Jelly:** As men grow older, they often experience a gradual loss of sensitivity in the penis. Lubricants can help men with this problem to gain a freer range of motion. Some lubricants also contain additives that cause a warm sensation for additional stimulation.

✔ **Do Kegel exercises:** These exercises can increase sexual enjoyment. Kegels are a way to strengthen the muscles that connect the base of the penis with the tailbone. These muscles act to control the flow of fluids through the urethra, so by learning to control them, you can delay ejaculation to heighten your orgasm. To learn how these muscles feel, trying stopping the flow of urine when you urinate. Those are the muscles you need to tighten. To do Kegels, squeeze the muscles, hold them for a few seconds, and then relax the muscles. Repeat. Practice the squeeze-hold-release-and-repeat pattern several times a day while standing, sitting, or reclining. By contracting these muscles, you gradually build up their strength.

How often do people have sex?

Locker room talk notwithstanding, no single group in our society has anything more than modest amounts of sex, according to studies on sexual behavior. About a third of all Americans have sex at least twice a week, another third have sex a few times a month, and the rest have sex a few times a year or not at all.

Want to have more sex? Get married or move in together. Studies show that being part of a "partnered couple" increases the likelihood of having frequent sex. So although your unattached single friends may brag, the truth is you're probably having more sex than they are if you're living with someone.

Aphrodisiacs

Few subjects are more controversial than that of aphrodisiacs. Loosely defined, an aphrodisiac is any food, drug, or other substance that increases sexual desire and/or potency. Not everyone believes that they even exist, however. The Food and Drug Administration, for example, not only states that there is no such thing as an aphrodisiac, but in 1990, they also banned any product claiming to enhance sexual performance or libido.

In truth, few studies have been done on the effects of aphrodisiacs, and those that have been done face criticism because of the question of the *placebo effect* — the idea that an inactive substance affects those who believe it has an effect. In other words, you get what you expect. However, some people believe that certain foods or unusual additives can actually enhance the sexual experience (such as tomatoes, oysters, honey, rhinoceros horn, and deer sperm). Few would argue with the proposition that any food or substance that benefits your overall state of health can also improve your sexual functioning.

Good health and physical fitness are the best aphrodisiacs! However, if you're having erection problems or a low libido, talk with your health practitioner. Sexual dysfunction and erection problems are highly treatable (see Chapter 24).

The following is a quick list of some foods and other substances once — or in some cases, still — thought to be associated with sexual performance:

- **Alcohol:** This drug has long been thought to be an aphrodisiac, but as we've already said, it's a depressant. Alcohol can reduce your libido, cause erection problems, and impair your ability to have an orgasm.

- **Oysters and rhinoceros horns:** Just because these items look like male genitalia doesn't mean that they help yours!

- **Chocolate:** The chemical reactions that chocolate produces in your brain have been likened to some of those produced during sex, but there's no evidence that eating chocolate makes you better at sex.

- **Hot chili peppers, curries, and other spicy foods:** Although they can increase your heart rate and make you sweat, that's about all they have in common with making love.

- **Spanish fly:** Not a fly at all, Spanish fly is actually dried beetle remains. (Maybe it got its name from the burning sensation it gives to the urethra — much like urinating hot chili peppers.) Spanish fly is a dangerous poison. Stay away from it.

- **Ginkgo biloba:** This herb is widely recognized for its ability to improve circulation to the extremities, including the genitals! Ginkgo has been found in tests to help those with arterial erectile dysfunction (caused by blockage of arteries to the penis) to regain the ability to achieve and maintain erections. It has also been found to help people suffering from decreased libido due to prescription antidepressants. In one study, 84 percent of men treated with ginkgo extract showed improved sexual function. Because it thins the blood, men regularly taking aspirin or other anticoagulants, or those with clotting disorders, should exercise caution in taking ginkgo. Check with your doctor.

✔ **Zinc:** This mineral is essential for healthy sperm production and the creation of testosterone. A zinc deficiency can lead to problems in arousal and maintaining erection and low sperm count. In children it can lead to delayed sexual development. Fortunately, zinc is found in many common foods such as meat, liver, eggs, nuts, beans, whole-grain products, and wheat germ. Zinc supplements are also readily available.

✔ **Yohimbe:** This substance, derived from the bark of the African yohimbe tree, is thought to be a sexual enhancer by stimulating reflex action in the lower regions of the spinal cord. Reports exist as well of painfully hard erections that last too long for comfort. Talk with your practitioner before trying yohimbe, and start off slow with weaker formulations until you see how you react to it.

Chapter 21

Contraceptives

In This Chapter
▶ Contraception options
▶ Reversible contraception
▶ Permanent contraception

*W*e can't put it any plainer — a contraceptive is a device or method that prevents pregnancy. And unless you want to be a daddy, you'd better think twice (or thrice, or more) about having intercourse because the stats show that of 100 women who together with their partners don't use birth control, 85 percent become pregnant within a year. That's a pretty big percentage. And if that isn't enough to worry about, you put yourself at risk for contracting a sexually transmitted disease (STD) — such as human immunodeficiency virus (HIV), the virus that causes AIDS — if you forgo protective contraceptive such as the condom. But fortunately, this chapter explains what options you and your partner have in contraceptives so that you can prevent pregnancy and STDs.

Options in Contraception

For men, the temporary, reversible options in contraception are limited and include the following:

- ✔ Abstinence and periodic abstinence (not having intercourse or refraining from intercourse during a partner's fertile period)
- ✔ Outercourse (sex play without intercourse)
- ✔ Condom (a sheath worn over the penis to catch the semen)
- ✔ Withdrawal method (removing the penis from the vagina before ejaculation)

A permanent method of birth control for men is the vasectomy, a surgical procedure that blocks sperm from entering the ejaculate.

Both partners' preferences and needs should be taken into account when choosing a method of birth control. For example, religious or medical concerns may dictate a choice in contraception. For these reasons, information about contraceptives used by women is also included in this chapter.

Reversible Contraception

What follows are the common methods of reversible contraception for both men and women, along with advantages and disadvantages. And you should be aware that some forms of contraception can be or should be used in combination to increase protection against pregnancy and STDs.

Abstinence

This method is 100-percent effective in preventing pregnancy and STDs because when practiced without fail, no vaginal intercourse occurs. This method has no side effect.

Outercourse

Outercourse is sex without intercourse (more commonly known as foreplay or sex play), and it's a way to enjoy sex without exchanging body fluids. Examples include masturbation, petting, erotic massage, and sex toys. This method is 100-percent effective in preventing pregnancy and most STDs. However, a woman can become pregnant if semen is spilled on her vulva during sex play.

If you use sex toys, keeping them clean is vital — especially if you share them during sex play — because they can transmit STDs. Cover toys with a condom if they are inserted into the body, and remember to use a fresh condom for each partner and each area of the body.

Norplant

Norplant is a hormonal method in which six soft capsules are implanted in a woman's upper arm. These matchstick-size implants release synthetic hormones that prevent the ovaries from releasing eggs (ovulation) and thicken the cervical mucus at the opening of the uterus to prevent sperm from joining with the egg. It protects against pregnancy for five years. Advantages include an extremely low risk of pregnancy and contraceptive benefits that last for years. However, this method does require minor surgery and has a number of side effects, including headaches, weight gain or loss, dizziness, and nausea. It also doesn't protect against STDs. This method is nearly 100-percent effective against pregnancy.

Depo-Provera

With this method, a woman gets an injection every 12 weeks. It works by preventing ovulation and thickening cervical mucus. Although Depo-Provera doesn't offer protection against STDs and may have side effects for some women (such as fluid retention, weight gain, and skin rashes), it removes the burden of day-to-day contraception and may reduce menstrual cramps. Because Depo-Provera remains in the body after discontinuing use, women may have to wait up to 18 months to become pregnant. This method is nearly 100-percent effective against pregnancy.

The Pill

In addition to the condom, you've most likely heard of this contraceptive. A woman takes the Pill (or oral contraceptive) daily to prevent ovulation and, therefore, pregnancy. The Pill contains estrogen and progestin (combination pills) or progestin only (minipills). Women who use the Pill tend to have regular periods with a lighter menstrual flow. The Pill may also help prevent endometrial cancer, ovarian cancer, noncancerous breast cysts, and ovarian cysts. However, a woman needs to remember to take the Pill at roughly the same time each day. Side effects include high blood pressure, fluid retention, and headaches. Women at risk of heart disease, blood clots, stroke, and liver disease should not take the Pill. In addition, women who are over 35 and smoke should not take the Pill. Plus, the Pill doesn't protect against STDs. Effectiveness against pregnancy is 95 percent with typical use and nearly 100 percent with perfect use.

IUD

An IUD, or intrauterine device, is a plastic device placed surgically within a woman's uterus to prevent fertilization of the egg. It also changes the uterine lining to prevent an egg from implanting. It is a long-term form of contraception (the ParaGard brand lasts for 10 years; the Progestasert must be replaced every year). A big advantage is no daily pill to remember to take. Again, side effects are possible (such as infection and accidental uterine puncture), and the IUD offers no protection against STDs. This method is best used by women who have already had a child because of the risk of infection that can occur with IUD insertion. Rarely, infection may cause sterility. Effectiveness against pregnancy is 99 percent with typical use and nearly 100 percent with perfect use.

Condom

A condom is a sheath of plastic, latex, or animal tissue that's worn over the penis during intercourse to catch semen and prevent pregnancy. Latex condoms provide the best protection against the spread of STDs. Latex condoms provide an effective barrier to even small viruses such as HIV (which causes AIDS) and hepatitis B.

Condoms offer you a wide choice, available in many different styles, colors, and sizes. Condoms may be lubricated or dry, or may have a *spermicide* — a chemical that immobilizes sperm — added for extra protection against pregnancy. You can also add spermicides and lubricants before intercourse. Avoid oil-based lubricants such as petroleum jelly or baby oil, though, which can damage the condom and cause it to break. Instead, use water-based lubricants such as K-Y Jelly. Condoms are available at drugstores, supermarkets, vending machines, and health clinics.

Make sure that condoms have an expiration or manufacture date on the package. Don't use a condom after its expiration date or if it has been damaged in any way. You can use a condom up to five years after its manufacture date.

To get the most out of a condom, use it *consistently* and *correctly.* Consistent use means using a condom from start to finish every time you have intercourse. Follow these instructions from the Food and Drug Administration on using a condom correctly:

1. **Do not unroll the condom before placing it on your penis.**

   Use a new condom for every act of anal, oral (penis-mouth contact), and vaginal intercourse.

   Put the condom on after your penis is erect and before you make any contact between your penis and any part of your partner's body.

2. **If the condom does not have a reservoir top, pinch the tip enough to leave a half-inch space for semen to collect.**

   Always make sure to eliminate any air in the tip to help keep the condom from breaking.

3. **Holding the condom rim (and pinching a half inch space if necessary), place the condom on the top of your penis.**

   Then, continuing to hold it by the rim, unroll it all the way to the base of your penis, as shown in Figure 21-1. If you're also using a water-based lubricant, put more on the outside of the condom to keep it moist.

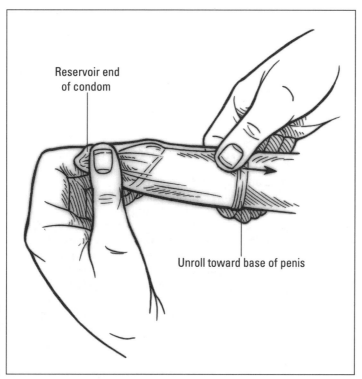

Reservoir end
of condom

Unroll toward base of penis

Figure 21-1:
Putting on a
condom.

4. **Pull out immediately if the condom breaks.**

   Use soap and water to wash away any semen that leaks out. (If semen should accidentally spill onto the woman's vulva, she should contact her health-care practitioner because of the risk of pregnancy.) Put on a new condom before resuming intercourse.

5. **After ejaculation and before your penis gets soft, grip the rim of the condom and carefully withdraw.**

6. **To remove the condom, gently pull it off the penis, being careful that semen doesn't spill out.**

7. **Wrap the condom in a tissue and throw it in the trash where others won't handle it.**

   Don't flush condoms down the toilet because they may cause sewer problems. Wash your hands with soap and hot water.

Advantages of condoms include low cost, no side effects (unless either you or your partner have an allergy to latex), and protection against STDs. But condoms can break if they are used or stored improperly, allowing semen to spill out. In addition, some couples feel that using a condom interrupts intercourse and reduces sensation for the man. Effectiveness against pregnancy is 86 percent with typical use and 97 percent with perfect use. To increase their effectiveness against pregnancy, use condoms in combination with other contraceptives, such as suppositories, jellies, creams, and foams.

Keep condoms properly stored in a cool, dry place. Storing condoms in the glove compartment of your car, your wallet, or your back pocket can damage them.

Diaphragm and cervical cap

The diaphragm is a soft rubber barrier worn over the woman's cervix to prevent sperm from entering the uterus. It is domed-shaped with a flexible rim. The cervical cap is also a soft rubber barrier. It is thimble-shaped. Neither the diaphragm nor the cervical cap has any side effects, though women who use them may be more prone to urinary tract infections. And some women may not be able to use them because of the shape of their cervix (a practitioner must fit each device to the particular woman). A woman must insert a diaphragm or cervical cap before intercourse, and it must remain in place for eight hours after sex. Some partners feel that insertion interrupts intercourse. Effectiveness against pregnancy is 80 percent with typical use and 94 percent with perfect use for either the diaphragm or cervical cap.

Withdrawal

Q: What do you call people who use the withdrawal method?

A: Parents.

Perhaps you've heard this old joke about the withdrawal method, a technique that involves removing the penis from the vagina before ejaculation. But don't laugh: Hypothetically, withdrawal could be an effective method of birth control. However, it's really quite unreliable because of the small amounts of semen that are released prior to ejaculation (which can result in pregnancy). To practice withdrawal effectively, you need a great deal of self-control and experience, and for this reason, withdrawal is especially not recommended for teenagers. Withdrawal is usually used when no other form of birth control is available. Although it has no side effects and is free, the withdrawal method doesn't protect against STDs. Effectiveness against pregnancy is 81 percent with typical use and 96 percent with perfect use.

Female condom

The female condom, also known as the *vaginal pouch,* is a polyurethane sheath that is worn in the vagina. Like the condom, the vaginal pouch collects semen to prevent fertilization from occurring. It also allows a woman to take responsibility for STD prevention. Another advantage is that it can be inserted up to eight hours before intercourse. However, the pouch may slip during intercourse, and it may squeak. In addition, the rings that hold the pouch in place may irritate the penis or vagina. Some people say that sensitivity is reduced. Effectiveness against pregnancy is 79 percent with typical use and 95 percent with perfect use.

Periodic abstinence

This method involves refraining from intercourse during a woman's fertile period, which typically lasts nine to 15 days out of each cycle. The woman can determine this period of time through several methods, including monitoring her morning temperature (basal body temperature method), observing changes in her cervical mucus (cervical mucus method), charting her menstrual cycle on a calendar (calendar or rhythm method), combining these three methods (symptothermal method), or refraining from inter- course until several days after ovulation (postovulation method). Kits are available to help learn these methods. This method of birth control doesn't prevent STDs. Effectiveness against pregnancy is 75 percent with typical use and 99 percent with perfect use.

Contraceptive foam, suppositories, creams, and jellies

These over-the-counter contraceptives work by creating a barrier that blocks the entrance of the uterus and contains a spermicide that immobi- lizes sperm. After inserting the contraceptive into the vagina, a couple needs to wait 10 minutes before intercourse so that the contraceptive becomes effective. Effectiveness lasts up to one hour after insertion. You must insert more of the product each time you repeat intercourse. Side effects include vaginal irritation and messiness because of the liquid in- volved. Effectiveness against pregnancy is 74 percent with typical use and 94 percent with perfect use.

In the future

As you can see from this chapter, few contraceptive options are designed specifically for men, but research is ongoing. One possibility is a contraceptive injection of testosterone that would halt sperm production. A study that investigated this reversible method of contraception found that the injections were effective contraception 98.6 percent of the time. After four to seven months after the injections ended, sperm output was back to normal.

However, a number of men dropped out of the study because of side effects, including decreased testicle size and weight gain, or because they didn't like getting the injections, which were given in a muscle on a weekly basis.

An oral contraceptive for men is also in development. An Italian study gave pills containing testosterone and progestin/antiandrogen cyproterone acetate to four men twice daily. At the beginning of the study, all men had sperm counts between 25 million and 50 million sperm per milliliter. Eight weeks into the study, sperm counts were down to 1, 2, and 5 million/ml in three subjects and had disappeared in the other — enough to prevent conception. Sperm counts returned to normal after the study ended, though it took several months. However, one side effect of the drug was a decreased sex drive.

Permanent Contraception: Vasectomy

Vasectomy is a permanent method of birth control for men. Each year, about half a million American men have vasectomies, and at least 15 million men have already undergone the procedure. It's a minor surgical procedure that requires a local anesthetic, takes about 20 minutes to do, and can be done in the doctor's office.

The vas deferens are small tubes through which sperm travel from your testicles, past your prostate, and into your urethra. In the urethra, the sperm are mixed with seminal fluid from the prostate to form semen.

A vasectomy, also called male sterilization, is a surgical procedure in which the vas deferens are blocked. This obstruction keeps the sperm out of the ejaculate, and instead of being mixed with seminal fluid and sent on their way to cause fertilization, the sperm are absorbed into your body. You won't see any difference in the amount of ejaculate or the ability to have an erection after a vasectomy, and the procedure has no effect on hormone production. The only difference is that a small amount of sperm will be missing from your semen.

Traditional vasectomy

In traditional vasectomy, a urologist (a specialist in male reproduction) injects a local anesthetic into the groin area and makes a half-inch incision on each side of the scrotum to reach the vas deferens. Once he locates the tubes, he removes a small section of each tube. The ends of the cut tubes may be tied off, *cauterized* (cut and sealed with heat), or blocked with surgical clips. Finally, the small incisions in the scrotum are stitched closed. This procedure is shown in Figure 21-2. Though the area may be sore for a few days, side effects are rare, but they can include swelling, pain, infection of the wound, and skin discoloration.

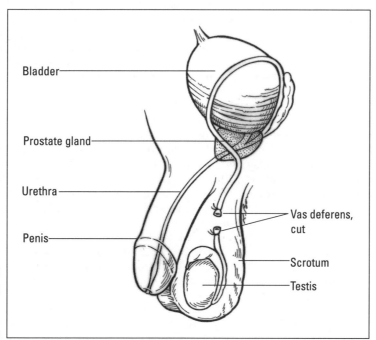

Figure 21-2:
A traditional
vasectomy.

No-scalpel vasectomy

An alternative to traditional vasectomy is the no-scalpel vasectomy (NSV). (The name itself sounds much more inviting, doesn't it?) As you may have guessed by its name, this technique uses no scalpels. However, you need to be sure to find someone who is properly trained in this very delicate procedure.

In NSV, the surgeon punches one tiny hole in the center of the scrotum using a device called a ring clamp and draws the tubes out, instead of making two half-inch cuts in the scrotum to reach the vas deferens. Unlike the traditional vasectomy, the NSV requires no stitches.

Both procedures require a waiting period before engaging in intercourse. Because sperm are stored in the vas deferens beyond the area of the blockage, these procedures are not effective immediately. It takes about 15 ejaculations before the sperm are cleared from the tubes. Another form of birth control should be used after vasectomy until two sperm analyses show the semen to be free of sperm.

Vasectomy reversal

Huh? We just told you that a vasectomy is permanent. Well, technically it is — unless you undergo a vasectomy reversal, or *vasovasotomy,* to surgically reconnect the vas deferens, allowing the sperm back into your semen. The procedure is an option for men who have had a vasectomy and then decide they want to have a child. Most often, studies show, men change their minds because of a change in their situation — they've divorced and remarried, for example, and now want children. Each year, about 6 percent of American men who have had a vasectomy undergo vasectomy reversal.

We won't kid you — a vasectomy reversal is a difficult operation that carries no guarantees. Using microsurgery, the surgeon must reconnect the vas deferens, structures that are only .3 millimeters in diameter. The procedure is done under general or epidural anesthesia (a local anesthetic injected into the spinal column), and it can take up to four hours. The cost of a vasectomy reversal — along with preliminary screening tests (such as to dertermine whether antibodies to sperm have developed) to see whether you're a good candidate for reversal and operating room fees — could cost you a whopping $10,000 or more.

In 90 percent of men, sperm can be returned to the ejaculate with vasectomy reversal. About half of those men can father children. And studies show that the more recently the vasectomy was done, the better the chances of a successful reversal.

With all this in mind, you should think long and hard about having a vasectomy and should consider the procedure permanent for all intents and purposes.

Chapter 22
Sexually Transmitted Diseases

In This Chapter
▶ Recognizing and treating all kinds of STDs
▶ Preventing STDs

exually transmitted diseases (STDs) come in more than 30 different flavors. In this chapter, we focus specifically on the STDs that are more commonly found in men. This chapter also identifies how STDs are passed from person to person, what the symptoms are, and what treatment is available. Finally, we give you information on practicing safer sex as a way of reducing your risk of contracting or passing an STD.

Types of Sexually Transmitted Diseases

You acquire a sexually transmitted disease (also called venereal disease) during anal, oral, or genital contact. (A few STDs can be transmitted through intimate contact such as kissing and touching.) STDs are caused by bacteria, parasites, or viruses that are transmitted through body fluids such as saliva, semen, blood, breast milk, and vaginal secretions.

Chancroid

A chancroid, caused by the *Haemophilus ducreyi* bacterium, produces sores. This STD is particularly dangerous because the sores can increase the risk of contracting HIV. A chancroid is spread during anal, oral, or genital contact and infects more men than women.

Recognizing the signs
The symptoms of a chancroid begin about a week after contraction and appear in stages:

✔ **Stage 1:** A small boil appears on the penis.

✔ **Stage 2:** The boil turns into an open and painful sore that may ooze pus.

✔ **Stage 3:** The lymph nodes in the groin become infected and swollen (if left untreated).

Knowing for sure

Visual diagnosis of a chancroid is difficult because it looks like many other STDs. Therefore, a microscopic examination of the pus is necessary to confirm a diagnosis.

Treating a chancroid

Fortunately, antibiotics (like azithromycin, ceftriaxone, ciprofloxacin, and erythromycin) can cure a chancroid sore. Possible side effects include nausea, vomiting, diarrhea, and stomach cramps. Use a condom to protect yourself from contracting a chancroid during anal, oral, or vaginal intercourse. (To use a condom correctly, see Chapter 21.)

Chlamydia

Caused by the *Chlamydia trachomatis* bacterium, chlamydia is the most common STD in the United States, infecting 4 million people every year. This disease is spread by vaginal or anal intercourse but can also be spread to other parts of the body through touching.

Recognizing the signs

The symptoms of chlamydia take one to three weeks to appear. However, as many as one in four men with a chlamydial infection have no symptoms. Symptoms may include the following:

✔ Urethral discharge

✔ Burning sensation during urination

✔ Heaviness in the affected testicle

✔ Inflamed scrotal skin

✔ Pain and swelling at the bottom of the testicle

Chlamydia may also infect the epididymis, the structure under each testicle where sperm mature, causing heaviness, swelling, and pain of the testicle and redness of the overlying skin.

Facts about sexually transmitted diseases

Throughout their life span, as many as one out of four people catch a sexually transmitted disease (STD). Some studies report that 50 percent of Americans contract an STD by their early 30s. And yearly, close to 12 million people find out they have a STD. What's more, 86 percent of STDs occur in people ages 15 to 29. And a staggering $17 billion annually is spent to treat STDs in the United States.

Knowing for sure

Because chlamydia can easily be confused with gonorrhea, a tissue analysis and urine sample are necessary for diagnosis.

Treating chlamydia

If you suspect you have a chlamydial infection, getting treatment is very important because untreated chlamydia can cause serious damage such as sterility and urinary tract infection.

Fortunately, chlamydia can be cured with antibiotics such as doxycycline, ofloxacin, and azithromycin. Possible side effects include upset stomach, nausea, vomiting, diarrhea, and rash. Stay out of the sun if you're taking doxycycline because it can make you susceptible to sunburn. Wearing a condom during anal, oral, or vaginal intercourse can prevent you from passing chlamydia to your partner or from contracting it yourself.

Cytomegalovirus

Cytomegalovirus (CMV) is a virus that's found in body fluids (such as saliva, semen, blood, vaginal secretions, breast milk, and urine) and is spread during anal, oral, and genital contact, as well as by kissing, receiving blood transfusions, and sharing infected needles, and from mother to developing fetus. Between 40 and 80 percent of people catch CMV through contact (usually through saliva) with other children by the time they reach puberty, according to Planned Parenthood Federation. On the other hand, adults usually get CMV through sexual activity. Once you contract CMV, the virus remains in your body for life.

Recognizing the signs

Typically, you won't experience any symptoms during the first infection with CMV. But the virus can become reactivated through reinfection or through infection with another STD (such as hepatitis B). Common symptoms may include the following:

✔ Swollen glands

✔ Fever

✔ Fatigue and generalized weakness

✔ Nausea and diarrhea

✔ Loss of vision

Knowing for sure

The only way to detect CMV is through a blood test.

Treating CMV

Unfortunately, CMV has no cure. Instead, antiviral drugs, such as foscarnet and ganciclovir, are used to prevent the virus from reproducing and causing symptoms to flare up. Possible side effects include fever, diarrhea, stomach pain, rash, increased sensitivity to the sun, nausea, and vomiting. While taking foscarnet, you need frequent blood tests to monitor blood cell counts, kidney function, calcium levels, and electrolytes. You also should have regular eye exams because foscarnet can cause vision problems. Ganciclovir also requires regular blood tests to monitor blood cell counts. A condom can protect against CMV during anal, oral, or vaginal intercourse. However, the virus can be transmitted through intimate touching and kissing.

Gonorrhea

Gonorrhea, also called "the clap," is caused by the *Neisseria gonorrhoeae* bacterium. The disease is spread during anal, oral, or vaginal intercourse. Each year, more than 1 million cases of gonorrhea are reported in the United States.

Recognizing the signs

Symptoms generally appear anywhere from one to five days after contraction. Ten percent of men experience no symptoms, but the most common include the following:

✔ Cloudy, foul-smelling discharge from the penis

✔ Painful, burning urination

✔ Swollen lymph nodes in the groin

✔ Inflammation of the scrotal skin and swelling of the testicle (if gonorrhea is left untreated)

Knowing for sure

Discharge from the penis is examined under a microscope and implanted in a culture (a jellylike substance in which bacteria grow) to diagnose gonorrhea.

The doctor may also swab the tissues of your throat or rectum to see whether the bacteria are present.

Treating gonorrhea

Left untreated, gonorrhea can cause sterility, arthritis, and problems with the heart, liver, and central nervous system. Treatment includes antibiotics, such as cefixime, ceftriaxone, ciprofloxacin, and ofloxacin, taken along with a single dose of azithromycin or doxycycline for seven days. Possible side effects include diarrhea, gas, increased sensitivity to the sun, itching, rash, nausea, and vomiting. Wear a condom during intercourse to prevent contracting gonorrhea.

If you're being treated for gonorrhea, your doctor may also treat you for chlamydia. Many people with gonorrhea have a chlamydial infection as well.

Hepatitis B virus (HBV)

Hepatitis B, a virus that's found in semen, saliva, blood, and vaginal secretions, is passed during anal, oral, and genital contact. It can also be transmitted through sharing infected needles and kissing. Approximately 1.5 million Americans are infected with hepatitis B virus (HBV) and about 6,000 die annually from health complications associated with the virus (such as cirrhosis of the liver and liver cancer). Ironically, almost 240,000 new cases occur yearly even though a vaccination could have prevented them. Once you are infected, HBV remains in your body for life.

Recognizing the signs

A person with HBV can be highly contagious and yet not have any warning symptoms. Symptoms, if they appear at all, typically show up within four weeks after contraction. Early symptoms include the following:

- ✔ Fatigue
- ✔ Headache
- ✔ Fever
- ✔ Nausea, stomach pain, and vomiting
- ✔ Loss of appetite

Later symptoms include the following:

- ✔ Dark-colored urine
- ✔ Clay-colored stool
- ✔ Jaundice (yellowish color of the skin and whites of the eyes)

Knowing for sure

The only way to know for certain whether you have hepatitis B is through a blood test.

Treating HBV

Because HBV has no cure, prevention is important. The Centers for Disease Control and Prevention recommends vaccination against HBV if you are a sexually active man — whether heterosexual, homosexual, or bisexual — and especially if you have recently had another STD, have multiple sex partners, or use illegal drugs.

Treatment for an acute (severe) HBV infection focuses on controlling its symptoms with bed rest and plenty of fluids. The acute HBV infection may last four to eight weeks. People with chronic (long-term) HBV infection may receive antiviral drugs, such as alpha-2b interferon, or antiretroviral drugs, such as lamivudine, in an attempt to wipe out chronic HBV infection. Possible side effects of alpha-2b interferon include chills, dizziness, fatigue, fever, metallic taste in the mouth, rash, nausea, vomiting, and diarrhea. Possible side effects of lamivudine include headache, sleeplessness, numbness and tingling, nausea, diarrhea, vomiting, stuffy or runny nose, and cough. A condom worn during anal, oral, or vaginal intercourse can reduce your risk of contracting HBV. But remember, HBV can be passed through sharing needles, kissing, and intimate touching.

Herpes

The two most common herpes viruses are herpes simplex virus-1 (HSV-1) and herpes simplex virus-2 (HSV-2). HSV-1, or oral herpes, causes cold sores and fever blisters in the mouth and on the lips and is primarily spread by kissing. HSV-2, or genital herpes, produces sores in the genital area and is spread during anal, oral, or vaginal contact and by intimate touch. However, both viruses can be spread from the mouth to the genitals and vice versa. Moreover, people with genital ulcers from herpes — as well as ulcers or sores from other STDs — have a greater risk of contracting HIV through open skin.

The herpes virus stays in your body for life. Eventually, genital herpes makes a home for itself in the nerves near the bottom of your spine, and oral herpes resides in the nerves behind your neck. These viruses may hibernate forever or they may cause future outbreaks, especially during times of fatigue and stress. As many as 60 percent of people with oral herpes and as many as 90 percent of people with genital herpes experience a recurrence at least once in their lives.

Every year, 500,000 Americans learn they have genital herpes. A study by the Centers for Disease Control and Prevention shows that only 10 percent of people infected with herpes are aware they have the disease. Almost $80 million is spent annually in the United States diagnosing and treating herpes.

Recognizing the signs

Symptoms of oral herpes may include the following:

- ✔ Small, solid bumps (papules) on the lips that blister, crust over, and heal within 10 to 16 days
- ✔ Fever
- ✔ Muscle aches
- ✔ Swollen glands in the neck
- ✔ Flulike symptoms

Symptoms of genital herpes include enlarged lymph nodes in the groin, fever, muscle aches, and headaches. Additional symptoms include papules that may be described in the following stages:

- ✔ **Stage 1:** Painful, red papules appear on the shaft of the penis, anus, or buttocks about 4 to 14 days after exposure to the virus.
- ✔ **Stage 2:** The papules turn into painful blisters filled with highly contagious fluid.
- ✔ **Stage 3:** Blisters rupture, producing painful open sores encircled by a red ring. During this time, you are highly contagious.
- ✔ **Stage 4:** Open sores begin to crust over approximately 10 days after the papules first appeared.

In many people, the classic symptoms of herpes are typically hard to ignore, particularly during what is called a *primary episode,* the period following a first-time infection in which symptoms appear. Recurrent symptoms, however, are usually fewer, less painful, and don't last as long.

In some people, the symptoms of genital herpes may be mild and easily missed. A person is highly contagious while he or she has sores; nevertheless, the person can also transmit the virus while he or she has no sores.

You can contract genital herpes from an infected partner during vaginal intercourse — even if you wear a condom — because vaginal secretions can come in contact with unprotected body parts, such as your scrotum or buttocks. A female condom (a polyurethane sheath with rings at each end that a woman inserts into her vagina) may provide better protection (see Chapter 21).

Knowing for sure

Most likely, your practitioner will diagnose herpes after looking at your sores. Drainage from a blister is sent to a laboratory for examination. Emerging technology in herpes diagnosis is a blood test.

Treating herpes

Currently, herpes has no cure. But antiviral drugs such as acyclovir, famciclovir, and valacyclovir may be used to suppress virus reproduction and recurrent flare-ups and shorten the length of outbreaks. Possible side effects include itching, rash, dizziness, headache, nausea, vomiting, and diarrhea.

Human immunodeficiency virus (HIV)

HIV, the virus responsible for AIDS (acquired immune deficiency syndrome), attacks the immune system so that the infected person's ability to fight other diseases is weakened. Eventually, the HIV-positive person develops AIDS, the last stage of HIV.

In 1997, close to 6 million people became infected with HIV worldwide, with 2.3 million deaths, including 460,000 children. And the facts become more grim given that 90 percent of HIV-infected people live in developing countries with no access to drug therapy. However, the news on AIDS is slowly improving for industrialized nations such as the United States.

How HIV is transmitted

HIV is commonly transmitted through contact with contaminated blood, semen, or vaginal secretions during anal, oral, or vaginal intercourse. (Wearing a condom during intercourse can reduce the risk of transmitting HIV.) HIV is more easily transmitted from man to woman than from woman to man. HIV can also be spread by sharing blood-contaminated needles during intravenous drug use. And children, born and unborn, may contract HIV from their HIV-positive mothers. For example, a mother can pass HIV to her fetus during pregnancy and to her infant during breastfeeding. Casual contact such as hugging, touching, sharing telephones, and eating together does not spread the virus. Also, most scientists believe that saliva, stool, urine, and tears can't transmit the virus.

Recognizing the signs

Once HIV enters a person's body, it progresses through a series of stages. During the first stage, HIV attacks helper CD4 T cells, which are important soldiers of the immune system that fight against HIV. Within three weeks of being infected, a person may develop acute retroviral syndrome as the immune system tries to fight the virus. It produces flulike symptoms (such as fever, night sweats, muscle aches, headaches, fatigue, rash, sore throat, swollen lymph nodes, diarrhea, and poor appetite) that clear up within three weeks. Unfortunately, though the immune system may recover, it cannot destroy HIV.

Most people produce antibodies to HIV — which a blood test can detect — within six months of contracting the virus. These antibodies are part of the body's defense system as it attempts to fight the virus. HIV may lie quietly in the body for up to ten years before symptoms appear. During this time, the person may feel fine but can pass the virus on to others.

During the second stage, HIV attacks and kills T cells. The immune system becomes overwhelmed and can no longer fight other potentially deadly infections (called *opportunistic infections*) that the person may contract. One common opportunistic infection is *Pneumocystis carinii* pneumonia, which is caused by an organism normally found in the lungs of healthy people but which becomes deadly in a person with a weakened immune system. The body is also susceptible to certain cancers when the immune system is weak.

During the third stage, AIDS-related complex (ARC) develops as HIV takes over. Symptoms include fever, weight loss, diarrhea, swollen lymph nodes, night sweats, severe rashes, neurological complications, yeast infections in the mouth, kidney infections, arthritis, pneumonia, forgetfulness, personality changes, and dementia.

During the final stage of AIDS, the immune system is overwhelmed, and the person can no longer fight infection. Diseases and infection overrun the body, and, eventually, death occurs.

Knowing for sure

If you've been exposed to HIV, getting tested is very important as soon as the antibodies are expected to be present. Typically, it takes one to three months but can take up to six months for antibodies to develop after exposure to HIV. The earlier you find out the results, the sooner you can start treatment to fight HIV and ward off opportunistic infections.

Two standard blood tests to detect HIV are the ELISA (enzyme-linked immunosorbent assay) and the Western blot test. The results of these tests can take several days to two weeks to be available, so be certain to call the clinic or your practitioner to learn the results. If you prefer, you can be tested anonymously. For example, some home HIV-testing kits, as well as some clinics, use a code number instead of your name.

Rapid tests are now available that can give you results in ten minutes. But they often give false-positive results — implying that you're HIV positive when you're not. If you get a positive result, be prepared to have a standard test.

What to do if you test positive for HIV

If you test positive for HIV — don't panic! Admittedly, that may be easier said than done. But stop, catch your breath, and contact your practitioner or an AIDS clinic as soon as possible for counseling and treatment to help slow the progression of HIV. A positive HIV test means you have developed antibodies to HIV — it doesn't mean you have AIDS, which can take a decade to develop.

Here are steps to help yourself:

✔ **Stay healthy:** Be sure to schedule regular checkups, which help your practitioner detect and treat any problems as early as possible.

✔ **Keep your immune system strong:** Eat nutritious meals, exercise regularly, and avoid cigarettes, alcohol, and illegal drugs.

✔ **Be informed:** Ask your doctor about HIV and its treatments. Read all you can about it and call the toll-free numbers available in your local telephone book to provide you with information and referrals to treatment centers and support groups in the area.

✔ **Be responsible and practice safe sex to prevent spreading the virus to others:** A recent study, reported in the *Archives of Internal Medicine*, found that 40 percent of people with HIV did not tell their partners of their diagnosis, nor did they protect their partners by wearing a condom.

An oral test called Orasure is also available. In this test, a special pad is placed between the gum and cheek to soak up antibodies. Home testing is also available in which a drop of blood is placed on special paper and mailed to a laboratory. Within a week, results are available by telephone.

Treating HIV

As of yet, HIV has no cure. But many new advances in drug therapy allow people with HIV to live longer, healthier, and more productive lives — rather than merely providing comfort, treating infections, and assisting with a peaceful death, as was the case previously.

Currently, three groups of drugs are available to stop HIV from reproducing: nucleoside reverse transcriptase inhibitors (NRTIs), nonnucleoside reverse transcriptase inhibitors (NNRTIs), and protease inhibitors.

Among the first to be found effective against HIV, NRTIs interfere with the activity of an enzyme (called reverse transcriptase) that HIV needs for reproduction. These drugs block the spread of HIV to new cells but have no effect on cells already infected. NRTIs work at an earlier stage of the HIV life cycle than protease inhibitors and are often prescribed in combination with them. Examples include didanosine, lamivudine, stavudine, zalcitabine, zidovudine, and the combination of lamivudine and zidovudine (Combivir).

Side effects vary from drug to drug and may include headaches, numbness and tingling, diarrhea, nausea, vomiting, rash, flulike symptoms, low-blood cell count, and inflammation of the pancreas and mouth.

NNRTIs work similarly to NRTIs, targeting the reverse transcriptase enzyme, but they also bind directly to the enzyme. Because resistance to these drugs is common, they are often combined with NRTIs. Examples include delavirdine and nevirapine. Possible side effects include nausea, headache, rash, and liver problems.

Protease inhibitors act on the enzyme HIV protease to produce a virus that's no longer infectious. However, these drugs are not a cure. They are often combined with other antiviral drugs. Examples of protease inhibitors include indinavir, nelfinavir, ritonavir, and saquinavir. Side effects vary from drug to drug and include nausea, vomiting, diarrhea, fatigue, loss of appetite, changes in blood sugar, increased lipid levels, blood in urine, and tingling in the hands, feet, and around the mouth.

During drug therapy, the doctor closely monitors viral levels. A person is more likely to avoid developing AIDS or to prolong the time to the development of AIDS if viral levels drop to the point where they are nondetectable.

A major drawback to all these drugs is the difficult regime. For example, an HIV-positive person has to take from 10 to 24 pills daily, at different times of the day, with or without food and drink. Some anti-AIDS drugs can't be taken with other drugs (such as those for pain and nausea). Another drawback is the cost. The drug saquinavir can cost almost $6,000 per year, and when it's combined with zidovudine and lamivudine, the cost can rise to nearly $12,000 per year. Fortunately, two new drugs — Abacavir (an NRTI that is currently under research and awaiting approval by the Food and Drug Administration) and the recently approved Sustiva (an NRTI) — offer an easier drug regimen. Sustiva requires three pills daily, and Abacavir requires two pills daily. Possible side effects include fever, nausea, vomiting, malaise, and rash.

Triple play: Increasing the effectiveness of HIV drug therapy

Currently, the most effective way to combat HIV is through "triple therapy," which usually consists of two NRTIs and a protease inhibitor. So far, scientists have found that this combination of drugs produces striking improvements in health and major drops in HIV levels (called viral load). Some doctors are adding an NNRTI as a fourth drug — making a quadruple "cocktail" — to attack the virus during more phases of its life cycle and to delay the time when the virus becomes resistant to drug therapy. Many combinations of these drugs are used.

Looking to the future

New and exciting research continues. Interleukin-2, a protein that boosts the immune system, is being used to increase helper T-cell levels. Research is also looking at bone marrow transplants to bolster the immune system and gene therapy that would allow HIV-positive people to resist opportunistic infections. Research on alternative therapies also holds hope. (For example, a protein that occurs naturally in the Chinese bitter melon plant has been shown to have anti-HIV activity by affecting the way protein assembles within a HIV-infected cell.) And work on a vaccine continues.

Many HIV-positive people seek alternative therapies, such as acupuncture, herbal medicine, massage, diet, chiropractic therapy, homeopathic treatment, and relaxation exercises, to use along with the drug therapies their doctors prescribe. The purpose of these therapies is to strengthen the immune system, provide relaxation, remove impurities, and provide pain relief.

Human papillomavirus (HPV)

Many different types of human papillomaviruses (HPV) exist, and they cause a variety of warts and other conditions. Some of these are associated with cancers of the penis, cervix, and vulva. A few HPVs cause genital warts, but most genital HPV infections are not visible and have no symptoms, according to Planned Parenthood Federation.

The virus is spread during anal, oral, or vaginal intercourse. The number of people infected with HPV has skyrocketed. It's estimated that 40 million adults have HPV, with an additional 1 million people contracting HPV each year.

Recognizing the signs

Common symptoms of HPV include the following:

- Warts inside or outside of the anus and penis that appear a few weeks after infection
- Pink or red, soft, cauliflower-like warts under the foreskin
- Yellowish, hard warts on the dry areas of the penis

Knowing for sure

Diagnosing HPV requires a microscopic and clinical examination of the warts (the latter during a physical exam). Sometimes, HPV causes very subtle changes on the skin that can't be seen with the naked eye. Your practitioner can find these microscopic warts only with the help of special instruments. To detect warts or other abnormal tissue, the practitioner sometimes puts a solution of acetic acid (like vinegar) on the genitals. Doing so causes abnormal tissue to turn white and makes the tissue easier to see when viewed through a magnifying lens.

Treating HPV

HPV has no cure. However, several options are available for removing warts. One option is topical creams such as podofilox and imiquimod. Possible side effects include pain, burning, itching, and irritation. Other treatments include cryotherapy (freezing the warts and then removing them), surgery, laser surgery (removing the warts with a high-powered beam of light), and injecting interferon into the warts. Without treatment, genital warts can grow big enough to block the opening of the urethra. A condom gives some protection against HPV, although the virus may be shed from areas not covered by the condom.

Nongonococcal urethritis (NGU)

NGU, an infection of the urethra, is caused by the *Ureaplasma urealyticum* and *Chlamydia trachomatis* bacterium (the pest responsible for chlamydia) and the *Trichomonas* parasite. Not all cases of NGU are sexually transmitted. In fact, nearly half of all cases of urethritis are caused by allergic reactions to vaginal fluids, soaps, and spermicides. NGU caused by sexually transmitted organisms is transmitted through anal, oral, or vaginal intercourse.

Recognizing the signs

Symptoms of NGU include the following:

✔ Discharge from the penis

✔ Burning while urinating

✔ Burning or itching around the opening of the penis

Knowing for sure

Because the symptoms of NGU mimic those of gonorrhea, seeing a practitioner is important. A microscopic examination and a culture of the discharge can rule out gonorrhea.

Treating NGU

Untreated, the symptoms of NGU may go away after two or three months. But don't be fooled by lack of symptoms or mild symptoms: When left untreated, the infection can cause permanent damage to the reproductive organs of both men and women, resulting in infertility. Treatment with antibiotics such as doxycycline or azithromycin is necessary to prevent complications, such as arthritis and infections of the prostate gland and epididymis. Wearing a condom can help prevent NGU.

Pubic lice

Pubic lice, also called crabs or cooties, are tiny parasitic insects that infect millions of people yearly. Lice are transmitted through close or sexual contact, as well as through contact with infected clothing, furniture, and bedding. Once lice are in the pubic hair, they hold on with their claws and stick their heads into the skin to feed on blood.

Recognizing the signs

Signs of pubic lice include the following:

- Extreme itchiness in the genital area
- Mild fever
- Irritability
- Tiredness

You may also have visible evidence. If your close vision is good, you may be able to see very tiny, yellowish-gray spots (they look darker when they're swollen with blood) in the pubic hair. You may also notice small white clumps of eggs at the base of the hair.

Knowing for sure

Your practitioner can diagnose pubic lice by examining you and collecting a specimen for microscopic examination.

Treating pubic lice

Over-the-counter drugs such as A-200 pyrinate, Kwell, NIX, and RID kill lice. Possible side effects include itching, irritation, and rash. Apply the drug to the hairy parts of your body (such as pubic region, underarms, chest, head, and eyebrows). Then wash your clothing and linen in very hot water and dry on the hot cycle. Reapply the medication in a week to kill any new lice that may have hatched, and don't forget to wash your clothing and linen again.

Syphilis

The *Treponema pallidum* bacterium (also called a spirochete) causes syphilis. Although the number of reported cases of syphilis is dropping, there are still approximately 101,000 new cases of syphilis yearly. This number is alarming because syphilis is a very serious STD. It can cause irreversible damage to vital organs (such as the heart and brain) and, if left untreated, can result in death. Syphilis is spread by contact with open sores during anal, oral, or genital contact, by kissing, and from mother to fetus.

Recognizing the signs

You can have syphilis and not even know it. Early symptoms may go unnoticed or not show at all. Syphilis symptoms occur in stages if left untreated:

- ✔ **Primary stage:** During this early stage, you may experience a painless, red sore called a *chancre,* which may appear on the genitals, lips, mouth, or anus about three weeks after contraction. A chancre may heal on its own within one to six weeks. Glands may also be swollen during this time.

- ✔ **Secondary stage:** This stage begins about three to six weeks after sores appear and may last as long as two years. During this stage, you may experience rashes on the palms of your hands and soles of your feet, fatigue, sore throat, swollen glands, hair loss, muscle aches, and pain.

- ✔ **Latent stage:** During the latent stage, which may last for years, no symptoms are apparent. A person is no longer contagious after being in this stage for at least a year.

- ✔ **Tertiary stage:** This is the last stage of syphilis. About 33 percent of the people who don't receive treatment for syphilis enter this stage. These people often suffer damage to their nervous system, brain, heart, liver, and other organs. The final symptoms of syphilis can be severe, often resulting in death. However, depending on the damage, treatment is possible even in this late stage.

Knowing for sure

Syphilis is diagnosed by a blood test and by microscopic examination of spinal fluid and chancre fluid.

Treating syphilis

The earlier you begin treatment, the better.

The first two stages of syphilis are treated with a single injection of the antibiotic benzathine penicillin G. Latent and tertiary stages may require an injection once a week for three weeks. Other antibiotics include doxycycline, tetracycline, and erythromycin. Possible side effects include an allergic reaction such as itching, rash, swelling, fever, chills, and breathing difficulty. Contact your practitioner immediately if you experience these reactions. Condoms can protect you from syphilis during sexual intercourse.

Safer Sex: Preventing STDs

You may wonder why we don't use the term safe sex. That's because there is no such thing as safe sex (with the exception of masturbation). Instead, we prefer the term *safer sex* because sex with a partner carries a risk and can't really be called safe (your partner may not even know that he or she has an STD). Safer sex also implies that methods are available to reduce the risk of contracting an STD.

Practicing safer sex protects you from getting an STD from your partner or passing an STD to your partner. As part of practicing safer sex, you must get treatment for STDs. Some STDs that produce sores — such as herpes and syphilis — provide an open doorway for HIV to enter. STDs may also cause inflammation of the genital tract, making it easier to contract HIV during anal, oral, or vaginal intercourse.

You increase your risk of STDs if you engage in the following high-risk behaviors: have multiple sex partners, share contaminated needles, have sex without a condom, or have sex with high-risk partners — such as intravenous (I.V.) drug users, prostitutes, or people with multiple sex partners.

Practicing safer sex is no guarantee against contracting an STD; it only lowers your risk. Therefore, honest and open communication with a partner is important. Ask your partner about his or her past sexual history — for instance, ask about I.V. drug use, previous STDs, multiple sex partners, and sex with prostitutes. Be aware that one-third of people lie when questioned about their sexual histories. Practicing safer sex is your own responsibility and a must if you're sexually active.

Nonoxynol-9: Is it a safe bet?

Opinions are conflicting on whether to recommend spermicides containing nonoxynol-9 (a disinfectant) for the prevention of sexually transmitted diseases, including HIV. Nonoxynol-9, used as a contraceptive, was found to help prevent STDs such as chlamydia, herpes, and gonorrhea in laboratory studies. It was also found to destroy HIV and virus-fighting lymphocytes (white blood cells).

However, when the disinfectant was tested in the body, the results were mixed. Some studies show that nonoxynol-9 is effective against some STDs, including HIV. Others, including a study reported in the *New England Journal of Medicine,* suggests that the disinfectant doesn't reduce the risk of HIV and other STDs.

All studies have shown side effects in women, such as vaginal irritation.

Because of this side effect and nonoxynol-9's ability to kill helpful lymphocytes in laboratory studies, some researchers fear that nonoxynol-9 may actually increase the risk of HIV in women by killing the lymphocytes in the body.

With these conflicting results, you're better off not relying on nonoxynol-9 for protection against STDs. Instead, stick to the more reliable latex condom. ***Note:*** Many condoms have spermicides on them, so you may want to consider using condoms that don't contain nonoxynol-9.

What can you do to protect yourself and your partner against STDs? The general rule is to keep your body fluids out of your partner's body and keep your partner's body fluids out of your body. Here are more specific guidelines to follow:

- **Try outercourse.** Outercourse includes nonintercourse activities such as masturbation and mutual masturbation. Because some infections, such as herpes, can be spread by intimate touch, you need to note whether your partner's genitals have rashes, blisters, warts, chancres, or any discharge. If you detect any signs of infection, express your concerns. Your partner may not be aware of the possibility of an infection.

- **Wear a latex condom each and every time you have anal, oral, or vaginal intercourse!** A condom provides considerable protection against chlamydia, gonorrhea, chancroid, syphilis, and HIV. A condom reduces the risk, though not as effectively, of HPV, herpes, and HBV. Unfortunately, condoms offer no protection against pubic lice. The female condom also provides some protection against STDs.

- **Use a condom or a dental dam (a square of latex) over your partner's genitals to protect yourself against direct skin-to-skin contact or from contact with body fluids during oral sex.**

- **Avoid drinking alcohol during sexual activity.** Not only can alcohol affect your ability to get aroused, but it may also lower your inhibitions enough that you engage in high-risk behaviors — something you may not normally do when sober.

- **Avoid sex with multiple partners.** The more partners you have, the greater your risk of contracting STDs. Likewise, avoid sex with someone who has multiple partners (such as a prostitute).

- **Don't share I.V. drug equipment.**

- **See your doctor regularly for checkups if you are sexually active, even if you have no signs of an STD.**

Chapter 23

Infertility

So you and your mate are having trouble conceiving a child. You're not sure whether the problem is with her, you, or both. Well, chances are 50-50 that trouble with your sperm is causing at least part of the infertility problem. Fear not, however, because medical technology may offer you a solution (as this chapter shows), and before you know it, you'll be changing enough diapers to be a spokesperson for Pampers.

Despite what your parents may have told you, only 20 percent of women get pregnant on the first try (but don't be foolish and tempt fate — always use birth control if pregnancy is undesirable). For a woman to become pregnant, a man must have intercourse with her during her most fertile time of the month, known as *ovulation*. Ovulation typically lasts between 9 and 15 days out of each cycle. Although ovulation is a difficult target to hit, about 60 percent of couples who are trying manage to become pregnant within three months. Couples who are unsuccessful at becoming pregnant after six months of intercourse without birth control should consult a doctor.

Infertility is a frustrating and complex problem. It affects 6.1 million Americans, or about 10 percent of people of reproductive age, according to the American Society for Reproductive Medicine. The World Health Organization did a three-year study and concluded that in 27 percent of infertility cases, the problem lies with the man and woman. Twenty percent of the cases stem from the man alone.

Understanding the Causes of Male Infertility

At the heart of most male infertility is trouble with the number and *motility* (sperm's ability to swim into a woman's fallopian tubes and fertilize an egg) of sperm. Here are several factors that can affect the number and motility of sperm:

- **Infection:** Illnesses (such as flu) and diseases (such as mumps contracted during adulthood) can slow sperm production and lower the number of sperm.

- **Sexually transmitted diseases (STDs):** STDs (see Chapter 22), such as syphilis, may damage the testes. Gonorrhea and chlamydia can block and damage the spermatic ducts.

- **Environmental toxins (such as chemicals, pollutants, and radiation):** These substances can damage the testes and harm sperm.

- **Alcohol and drug use:** These cause a decrease in sperm production and may result in damaged and misshapen sperm.

- **Smoking:** Smoking can lower sperm counts.

- **Varicocele:** Damaged or enlarged veins that surround the spermatic cord (structure that attaches the testicle to the body) can lower sperm counts by increasing heat in the testes.

Keep your privates cool. Sperm are livelier and more numerous when they're kept about 4 degrees below body temperature — the reason your scrotum moves closer to or farther away from your body. Avoid hot tubs, saunas, or any other environment that may "cook" sperm.

- **Congenital problems:** Some disorders present from birth can cause infertility, including cystic fibrosis, sickle cell anemia, underdeveloped testes, and the absence of a spermatic duct.

- **Chromosomal defect:** Klinefelter's syndrome, in which a man has an extra X chromosome, results in small testes and infertility.

- **Hormone insufficiency:** Problems with testosterone production in the testes or diseases that affect the pituitary gland (which controls puberty and other functions) can lower sperm counts.

- **Retrograde ejaculation:** Instead of sperm moving forward and out of the penis, sperm leak into the bladder (due to weak bladder neck) during ejaculation. Diabetes and prostate surgery are two examples of conditions that may cause retrograde ejaculation.

Female infertility

Infertility in a woman is just as complex and difficult (some would say more so) to target as in a man. Here are some causes of female infertility:

✔ **Irregular ovulation:** Age, hormone imbalance, genetics, poor nutrition, below-normal body fat, medical conditions, and stress can affect ovulation.

✔ **Alcohol and drug use and smoking:** These substances can interfere with ovulation and damage egg cells.

✔ **Antibodies in the *cervix* (doorway to the uterus):** Sometimes a woman's immune

system sees sperm as an invader and, as a result, triggers cervical mucus to form a plug to block sperm.

✔ **Sexually transmitted diseases (STDs):** STDs, such as chlamydia, can severely damage the fallopian tubes.

✔ **Endometriosis:** This condition occurs when uterine tissue grows elsewhere in the pelvic cavity.

✔ **Uterine defects:** If the uterus is misshapen or contains extraneous tissue, a fertilized egg may not be able to implant and grow.

Diagnosing Infertility

Because infertility is a complex condition, your practitioner may refer you to a *urologist,* a doctor who specializes in treating male reproductive and urinary problems.

After the doctor performs a physical examination and asks you about your medical history to rule out any secondary causes of infertility (such as STDs), your sperm are tested for number count and motility. Here are some possible tests:

✔ **Semen (fluid that contains sperm) analysis:** You provide a sample of your sperm by ejaculating (via masturbation) into a specimen cup in the privacy of a small room in the clinic or in your own home. The ejaculate is examined and checked for semen volume, consistency (such as thickness), pH level, sperm counts, percentage of moving sperm, and sperm shape. The sample is also analyzed for sugar content (to check for diabetes) and to determine whether antibodies and infection are present. A normal sample has more than 20 million sperm per milliliter. More than 50 percent of the sperm should be moving forward (to show they can reach the fallopian tube to reach the egg), and more than 30 percent should have normal shape. Expect to provide two samples taken on separate days. Avoid ejaculation for two to three days prior to the test.

✔ **Postcoital test:** This test checks the compatibility of the man's sperm with the woman's cervical mucus. The couple has sex near the time when the woman is fertile, and that same day, the doctor checks a sample of the woman's cervical mucus under a microscope. If the doctor finds five or more active sperm under the microscope, it's a good indication that the man is fertile. However, a negative result isn't conclusive because of possible infertility problems with the woman.

✔ **Blood tests:** These tests check for hormone imbalances.

✔ **X rays:** These look for damage to and blockages of the vas deferens (the long tube in which sperm travel during ejaculation), epididymis (a tubelike structure where sperm mature and are stored), and testes.

Less common, yet more thorough tests include chromosome analysis (to count the number of chromosomes), vital staining (to check how many sperm are alive or dead), hypno-osmotic swelling test (to check the sperm's structure), biochemical analysis (to check for chemical signs of blocked sperm ducts), human zona pellucida binding (to check the sperm's ability to bind to the outer covering on an egg), and testicular biopsy (to check for testicular cancer).

If all these tests prove inconclusive, your doctor may suggest the hamster assay. This test may sound strange, but it helps to check your sperm's ability to penetrate and fertilize a human egg. A sample of your sperm is mixed with hamster egg cells. If less than 10 percent of the eggs are penetrated, the diagnosis is infertility.

Treating Infertility

Doctor-prescribed infertility treatment depends on the results of your tests. If damage to the vas deferens or a blockage is the problem, microsurgery can repair the damage (however, it doesn't guarantee fertility). In microsurgery, the doctor makes a tiny incision with the aid of a microscope. A varicocele can also be corrected through microsurgery.

If infertility is caused by low sperm counts, injections of *menotropins* (a hormone preparation that stimulates the testes) can sometimes be used to enhance sperm production. Hormone insufficiency can be treated with regular injections of hormones such as testosterone and other hormones that regulate sperm production. Decongestants and antidepressants can help treat retrograde ejaculation because the drugs stimulate the nerves that control the bladder neck. Of course, whatever abnormalities may be affecting your partner must also be resolved.

Increasing your chances of becoming a daddy

No matter what the tests show, you can boost your sperm production by trying the following tips. Keep in mind that you may try all these things and still have no success. That's when you and your partner should seek testing. If the woman is over age 30 or has had previous miscarriages, talk to your doctor sooner rather than later.

✔ **Avoid stress.** Stress is linked to lower sperm counts, though the experts aren't sure what the connection is. (See Chapter 6 for stress-busting techniques.)

✔ **Don't smoke or use alcohol or illicit drugs.** These no-no's can have a toxic effect on your sperm, lowering sperm counts and possibly contributing to birth defects. One study showed that smoking was linked to a 15 percent drop in sperm counts.

✔ **Check your medicine cabinet.** Some drugs can interfere with erection and decrease testosterone levels. Examples include beta blockers, MAO inhibitors, anabolic steroids, and tricyclic antidepressants. Talk with your doctor.

✔ **Stock up on antioxidants.** Antioxidants — vitamins C and E, the mineral selenium and beta-carotene — neutralize harmful molecules known as free radicals. Free radicals are known to adversely affect sperm production. Eat plenty of fruits and vegetables, brewer's yeast, and whole grains daily to get an adequate supply of antioxidants.

✔ **Get enough zinc.** Zinc has been linked to good prostate health as well as to healthy sperm. Beef, crabmeat, pumpkin seeds, and oysters are good sources of zinc. Just be sure not to exceed the recommended dietary allowance (RDA) of 15 mg daily without a health practitioner's advice.

✔ **Avoid environmental toxins.** Some metals (such as lead), pesticides, and glue and paint chemicals can lower sperm counts. Use safety precautions if you work in an environment that exposes you to dangerous substances.

✔ **Have more intercourse.** Although this is perhaps the toughest advice to follow (wink, wink), you increase the chance of fertilization if you and your partner have intercourse at least every other day during your partner's ovulation. An ovulation kit, designed to record the woman's fertile period of time, can help to determine the opportune moment. Ask your practitioner or pharmacist about the kit.

In the end, you may have to consider fertility treatment by assisted reproductive technology (ART). About 10 percent of infertile couples try to get pregnant via artificial insemination, in vitro fertilization (IVF), and a new procedure called intracytoplasmic sperm injection. We won't kid you — the odds of pregnancy aren't exceptional. Only half of the couples who seek ART conceive. Here are some examples of ART procedures:

✔ **Artificial insemination:** In artificial insemination, sperm are placed into the woman's vagina or cervix or within her uterus during her fertile time. Sperm are usually collected by masturbation. If ejaculation is impossible — because of an obstruction, retrograde ejaculation, or erection problem — sperm are collected through surgery. Artificial insemination may be repeated until pregnancy occurs. According to the American Society for Reproductive Medicine, artificial insemination has an average pregnancy rate of 10 percent per cycle. Most women who get pregnant through this method do so in the first three to five cycles.

✔ **Sperm enhancement:** Sperm are placed in a test tube and the strongest ones that swim to the top are collected for insemination. The sperm may also be cleansed to remove anything that may hinder fertilization (such as blood cells, dead sperm, chemicals, and other contaminants).

✔ **Intracytoplasmic sperm injection (ICSI):** This technique involves injecting a single sperm directly into an egg that was removed from the woman. The fertilized egg is then placed into the woman's fallopian tube. This process is particularly useful when the man's sperm are not strong enough to penetrate the egg for fertilization, or too few sperm are present to attempt IVF. Because ICSI is still new, studies about its effect on children continue. Some concern has been expressed about slightly higher sex chromosome abnormalities in ICSI children. Another study suggests that ICSI children may have delayed mental development compared with children conceived normally or through IVF.

✔ **Epididymal aspiration:** This surgical procedure, called for in the case of a congenital absence of the vas deferens, removes sperm from the epididymis. This procedure is done along with IVF and ICSI.

✔ **Percutaneous epididymal sperm aspiration (PESA):** This procedure is used for men with an irreparable obstruction, congenital absence of the vas deferens, or failed vasovasostomy (see Chapter 21). PESA involves a small needle that draws out sperm from the epididymis and takes about 20 minutes to complete. It is done along with IVF and ICSI.

✔ **In vitro fertilization (IVF):** This is the famous "test tube baby" procedure in which fertilization takes place outside of a woman's body. In IVF, a woman — with obstructed fallopian tubes but healthy ovaries — uses fertility drugs to stimulate the eggs to mature. Mature eggs are then removed with a laparoscope before they are released in ovulation. The collected eggs are mixed with her mate's or donor's sperm in a laboratory glass dish. After a few days, several fertilized eggs are placed in the woman's uterus. With a little luck, at least one egg will implant itself and develop into a fetus. Multiple births can occur when several eggs are successfully transplanted.

Variations of IVF include zygote intrafallopian transfer (ZIFT) and gamete intrafallopian transfer (GIFT). In ZIFT, eggs are fertilized in a laboratory dish and are placed in the woman's fallopian tube, rather than her uterus. The eggs gradually travel through the tube and into her uterus for implantation. Unused fertilized eggs are often frozen for later use if the initial procedure does not produce a child. In GIFT, eggs are retrieved by using a needle guided by transvaginal ultrasound or through laparoscopy. The eggs and sperm are mixed together in a special catheter and are threaded through the fallopian tube.

Chapter 24

Sexual Difficulties, or "I Swear This Never Happened to Me Before!"

• •

In This Chapter

▶ Premature ejaculation

▶ Sexual desire disorders

▶ Male orgasmic disorder

▶ Dyspareunia

▶ Erectile dysfunction

• •

*S*exual difficulties — they probably worry men more than any other aspect of their physical being. Why shouldn't they? A man's masculinity is under scrutiny from the time he is born. Our society and especially the media promote the unrealistic idea that any man worth his salt should be an excellent provider, a wonderful father, a considerate husband, a star athlete, a soccer coach, a mathematical whiz, a handyman, a problem-solver, a strong shoulder to lean on, and, after all this, a magnificent, caring, well-endowed lover. With all the expectations and responsibility placed on him, it's no wonder that he may fall short (no pun intended) in some areas.

This chapter looks at the common *sexual dysfunctions* you may experience. Sexual dysfunction is a term that describes a group of disorders that prevent men and women from enjoying sex. Most men are affected by some form of sexual dysfunction in their lifetimes. Stress, illness, medication, psychological issues, and social taboos are only a few of the things that can cause sexual dysfunction.

Common male sexual dysfunctions include premature ejaculation, male orgasmic disorder, sexual desire disorder, dyspareunia, and erectile dysfunction (ED). All these sound pretty grim, but many problems can be overcome with the help of an understanding partner. If sexual problems persist, discuss them with your doctor to rule out underlying physiological problems.

Premature Ejaculation

Any ejaculation that happens before you want it to is considered premature. Here's an interesting little nugget: The average time an American couple spends making love is between five and ten minutes. Premature ejaculation can happen during sex play or during penetration or just after penetration — but know this: There are no hard, fast rules about length of time — just what you perceive it should be. If you and your mate don't mind the speed of the intercourse, you *don't* have a problem. Remember the old adage: If it ain't broke, don't fix it!

Just in case you don't know the physiological process involved in ejaculation (be it premature or not), we provide Figure 24-1.

Premature ejaculation is the most common male sexual problem and is usually due to over eagerness and performance anxiety. Premature ejaculation is more prevalent among younger men.

If you don't want to be Speedy Gonzales, try the following tips to help you last longer:

- ✔ **Wear a condom:** A condom decreases sensitivity, and it reduces the risk of unwanted pregnancy and sexually transmitted diseases (STDs are covered in Chapter 22).

- ✔ **Masturbate before intercourse:** Masturbate to orgasm before engaging in intercourse because a second erection lasts longer.

- ✔ **Change positions:** Have your mate move into a position that you find less stimulating to delay ejaculation.

- ✔ **Talk to each other:** Sometimes you need to slow down or stop movement altogether to decrease stimulation. Your partner may not know this fact, so tell him or her. No need to "uncouple" — just take a breather for a moment or two, caressing and cuddling.

- ✔ **Use the stop/start technique:** When you're on the brink of orgasm, stop and relax until the ejaculatory feeling subsides. Repeat this exercise several times. Doing so helps you recognize the sensation of ejaculation, allowing more self-control.

- ✔ **Use the squeeze technique:** When you're about to have an orgasm, gently squeeze (or ask your partner to squeeze) the tip of your penis and hold for several seconds. Some experts say to squeeze the base of the penis. Either way, both approaches help to soften the penis slightly. Repeat the process several times.

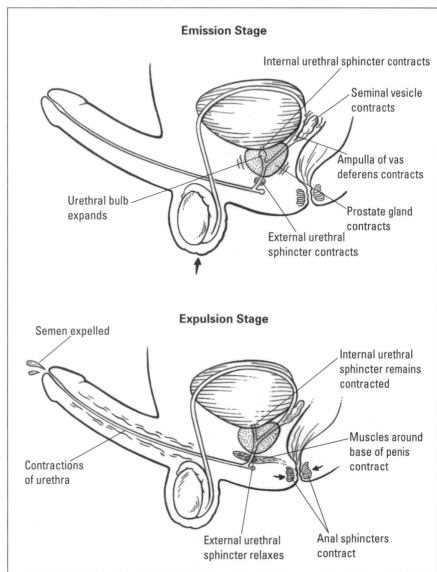

Emission Stage

Internal urethral sphincter contracts

Seminal vesicle contracts

Ampulla of vas deferens contracts

Prostate gland contracts

External urethral sphincter contracts

Urethral bulb expands

Expulsion Stage

Semen expelled

Internal urethral sphincter remains contracted

Muscles around base of penis contract

Contractions of urethra

External urethral sphincter relaxes

Anal sphincters contract

Figure 24-1: What happens before and during ejaculation.

Male Orgasmic Disorder

Sometimes referred to as retarded ejaculation, male orgasmic disorder is the inability to have an orgasm when you want to. The condition results in delayed ejaculation or no ejaculation at all, which can end in frustration, physical discomfort, and loss of sexual desire. Most men who cannot ejaculate during intercourse can achieve orgasm through masturbation or manual or oral stimulation with their partners, therefore the condition may be psychologically based. Although you may want to boast about a prolonged erection, if you can't achieve an orgasm when you want to, you should visit your doctor.

Sexual Desire Disorders

Sexual desire, or libido, is your interest in having sexual activity. A loss or lack of libido can occur for several reasons — decreased levels of testosterone (male hormone responsible for libido and other functions), fatigue, stress, illness, medication, relationship problems, sexual abuse, and the birth of a child, for example. Following are several types of sexual desire disorders:

- **Hypoactive sexual desire disorder (HSD):** HSD is a generalized, nonspecific disorder that expresses itself through tense or anxious feelings about sex. You may or may not respond when sexually stimulated. HSD usually happens at a specific time in your life. It can occur because you have been the victim of an abusive relationship or because of unresolved relationship issues. HSD can also occur if you are homosexual and have not fully accepted your sexual orientation.

- **Sexual aversion disorder (SAD):** This condition is not only a lack of sexual interest but a combination of feelings that range from discomfort and repulsion to fear, anxiety, and panic about sex. You may express these feelings through physical reactions, including sweating, nausea, dizziness, increased heart rate, trembling, and diarrhea. SAD is usually the result of sexual abuse or trauma during childhood.

- **Male sexual arousal disorder:** This disorder may be caused by the same factors associated with HSD but also includes performance anxiety. For example, if you've experienced a previous erection problem, the fear of it repeating may actually contribute to erection problems.

Usually, a decreased libido passes with time, especially if you and your partner have positive, open communication. *Sensate focus* — simple exercises in which you and your partner touch each other without the goal of sex in mind — may help to boost libido and reduce stress. However, if you think that you have a problem with libido, visit your practitioner to rule out any medical conditions such as diabetes or circulatory problems. If your libido doesn't improve within three months, you may want to visit a counselor or a practitioner who specializes in sex therapy.

Treat your loss of libido seriously. If left untreated, it can worsen and lead to depression.

Dyspareunia

Dyspareunia is a big word that simply means "painful intercourse." We can't put it any plainer — intercourse should *never* hurt. If it does, see your practitioner or a urologist, a doctor who specializes in male reproductive and male and female urinary problems.

For men who are uncircumcised, some possible reasons for painful intercourse include tight foreskin, the build up of smegma (cheesy glandular secretions and cells), or infection under the foreskin. Other possible causes of painful intercourse include Peyronie's disease (the growth of fibrous tissue and calcium deposits inside the penis, leading to pain and bending of the erect penis); some STDs such as herpes and gonorrhea; infections of the prostate gland, testes, seminal vesicles, bladder, and urethra; allergic reaction to spermicides, condoms, lubricating gels, and contraceptive foams and creams; physical disabilities, arthritis, and lower-back pain.

Erectile Dysfunction (ED)

Commonly called "impotence," erection problems, or *erectile dysfunction* (ED) — the persistent lack of a rigid erection needed for penetrative intercourse — affect approximately 10 to 20 million American men annually. Most men who experience ED are 65 years or older. If you have chronic high blood pressure, diabetes, arteriosclerosis, or heart disease, you're four times more likely to suffer ED than men without these conditions. And if you smoke, you increase the risk of problems.

How your body builds an erection

You know how an erection feels, but do you know the mechanics of an erection? Technically speaking, an erection must complete two tasks. Blood must flow like a river into three spongy cavernlike areas of your penis, which suck up the blood to expand. And while this occurs, the soft tissues and veins of your penis must constrict slightly to prevent the blood from spilling outside of the spongy areas.

Physiological ED

If you went to your doctor because of ED about 20 years ago, he would have probably said it was all "in your head." But today, fortunately, doctors know better. Although ED may actually have a psychological cause, between 75 and 80 percent of ED cases have a physiological cause. The good news is that a physiological cause is highly treatable. The bad news is that a physiological cause could be something more serious such as diabetes. But on a positive note, treating the ailment may also relieve ED. Other causes include the following:

- **Circulatory problems:** Heart disease and cholesterol-blocked arteries may make blood circulation difficult, resulting in fewer and less effective erections.

- **Medications:** Both nonprescription and prescription medications, especially antidepressants and blood pressure drugs, may cause ED. If you think that a medication may be causing problems, talk with your practitioner before discontinuing use.

- **Nerve disorders:** Brain or spinal cord problems can cause ED in rare cases. Alcoholism, drug abuse, diabetes, and surgery to the bladder, prostate, or rectum can also damage nerves that affect sexual performance.

- **Pelvic trauma:** Don't be fooled into thinking that only a major accident, such as a car wreck, can stress your pelvis. Seemingly mild factors, such as a fall during a sports activity or a long ride on an uncomfortable bike seat, can stress your pelvis enough to cause ED.

Mind over matter: The psychological factor

Although most cases of ED stem from physiological causes, a strong psychological component is often present as well. Day-to-day living can be stressful, and that stress takes a hard toll on the body. For example, stress and pressure, although psychological, can promote circulatory problems such as hypertension and heart disease, which can interfere with erection.

Sixty-four percent of men with erectile dysfunction wait a year before seeing their physicians for the problem, according to one study.

Knowing for sure

If ED plagues you only occasionally, the problem probably is due to fatigue and stress (see Chapter 6 for relaxation and stress-reducing tips); however, if you have a chronic problem (five weeks or longer) achieving an erection, you need to see your family doctor or urologist.

Expect a complete physical examination and a medical history review to rule out physiological factors. Your doctor is likely to ask very personal questions about your sex life, such as whether you have more than one sex partner. Don't flinch at this question — it's a very important one. For example, if you do have more than one sex partner and experience ED with only one, the problem is very likely psychological. For your benefit, be completely open and honest with your doctor.

Erectile dysfunction that occurs suddenly is probably psychologically based, whereas problems that slowly build are usually physiologically based.

Possible tests include the following:

- **Blood flow:** This test evaluates the blood flow to your penis by measuring the blood pressure in your penis.

- **The stamp test (or nocturnal penile tumescence — NPT — test):** A strip of perforated stamps is glued to your penis before sleep. If the perforations are broken the next morning, you know you had an erection during your sleep (which tells the doctor that your ED is probably psychological).

- **Ultrasound:** Sound waves create an image of your penis's tissues to check for abnormalities.

- **Erection-producing drug:** An injection of an erection-producing drug (such as papaverine) can show whether your problem is physiological or psychological. If a high dose is necessary to produce an erection, your problem has a physiological cause.

Treating physiological ED

Several treatment options are available to deal with physiological ED. Here are some examples:

- **Hormone replacement therapy:** Low-testosterone levels can be increased through monthly injections or a skin patch. Do not use hormone replacement therapy if you're at risk for prostate cancer (see Chapter 18).

- **Injection therapy:** This therapy requires that you inject the base of your penis with an erection-producing drug 5 to 15 minutes before intercourse. Erection lasts one to four hours. Possible side effects include pain in the penis, prolonged erection, scarring, and hematoma (pooled blood). You should not use injection therapy if you have heart or liver disease or are on blood-thinning medication.

✔ **Vacuum device:** In this therapy, you place your flaccid penis inside a hard plastic tube that's attached to a small, sealed vacuum pump. When you turn the pump on, your penis becomes hard from blood drawn within the penis due to the vacuum inside the tube. Then you slip a rubber band around the base of your erect penis before intercourse.

✔ **Penile implant:** This surgical procedure inserts rods or inflatable tubes into the penis. With a rod implant, your penis is always rigid (and sometimes noticeably so). When you want to have intercourse, you simply bend your penis into an upright position. Possible side effects include infection, scar tissue, and migration — the shifting or movement of the implant. With inflatable tubes, the doctor surgically places a pump into your scrotum and inflatable tubes within your penis. Squeezing the pump releases gel into the inflatable tubes, creating an erection. Squeezing the release valve drains the gel back into the pump, making your penis flaccid. Possible side effects include mechanical failure, infection, scar tissue, migration, and penile deformity. Implant surgery has fallen out of favor with the development of effective, cheaper, nonsurgical treatment.

✔ **Bypass surgery:** When blood flow to your penis is blocked, your doctor may do surgery to reroute the vessels in your pelvic area around the blockage.

✔ **Transurethral delivery:** Alprostadil — an erection-producing drug — in pellet form is delivered through the opening of your urethra with a tubelike applicator. You simply insert the stem of the applicator into the opening of your urethra, and then squeeze the applicator button to release the drug 7 to 25 minutes before intercourse. This method is more comfortable than injecting erection-producing drugs at the base of your penis. Erection lasts one to two hours. Possible side effects include penile pain and dizziness.

Seeking professional sex therapy

Whether your ED is caused by physiological or psychological factors, your doctor may also advise you to seek counseling or sex therapy. Sex therapists offer emotional support and specific problem-solving techniques. Be prepared to reveal intimate details of your sex life. Sometimes it takes a while to develop enough trust with your therapist to disclose what is troubling you, but being open and honest only works to your advantage.

Several forms of sex therapy exist and most use the PLISSIT (permission, limited information, specific suggestion, and intensive therapy) model. Here is PLISSIT broken down by level:

Invigorating Viagra

Perhaps no other drug than sildenafil citrate, commonly known as Viagra, has received more attention today. Touted as a wonder drug, Viagra is the first oral medication for erectile dysfunction (ED). Whether or not Viagra is a wonder drug, it's very popular. In its first three months on the market, nearly 3 million prescriptions were filled, and an estimated $1 billion worth of sales were predicted by March 1999. That should come as no surprise given that Viagra is easy to use and has a reasonable success rate of about 70 percent.

Viagra does not cause erections; rather, the drug manipulates enzymes in the penis that control the flow of blood. Viagra is usually prescribed to men whose ED has a physiological cause such as diabetes, arteriosclerosis, or chronic high blood pressure. About 80 percent of Viagra prescriptions are dispensed to men ages 50 and older.

According to manufacturer's directions, a man should take a pill about one hour before sexual activity; however, he may need to experiment until he calculates the best timing. The effect lasts four to six hours, or until orgasm. 50 milligrams is the usual starting dose, but the dosage may be modified up to 100 mg or down to 25 mg, depending on its effectiveness. Typically, only one pill is taken daily.

Viagra is relatively safe to use. However, possible side effects include headaches, nausea, low blood pressure, visual disturbances (such as tinted-vision and light sensitivity), and flushed skin.

Deaths — 69 in the first four months the drug was on the market — have been reported, but analysis of these cases has yet to show that the drug was at fault. The major caveat — from both the Food and Drug Administration (FDA) and the drug's manufacturer — is that Viagra is potentially dangerous to men taking nitroglycerin and long-acting nitrates used for heart conditions. So it goes without saying that if you take nitrates in any form, don't use Viagra.

✔ **Permission:** This level reassures you that your feelings and emotions about sex are valid.

✔ **Limited information:** This level provides information about your specific sexual problem. Knowing the facts — average penis size, average intercourse duration, and the like — can alleviate tension and performance anxiety.

✔ **Specific suggestion:** This level offers specific instructions and exercises that you can practice at home alone or with your partner. For example, the "stop/start" technique (which we describe earlier in this chapter).

✔ **Intensive therapy:** If your sexual problems stem from emotional difficulties, you may require more extensive treatment than the first three levels can provide. Types of intensive therapy include *psychosexual therapy,* which delves into unconscious feelings and emotions that are negatively affecting your sexual activity; *systems therapy,* which views that sexual problems serve a purpose in unresolved relationship issues; and *Eye Movement Desensitization and Reprocessing (EMDR),* which treats severe cases of sexual abuse, compulsions, and other mental health disorders. In EMDR, the therapist moves her fingers back and forth across your eyes while you think about your problems. The eye movement is believed to help stimulate the brain to unearth past emotional trauma.

Part V
The Part of Tens

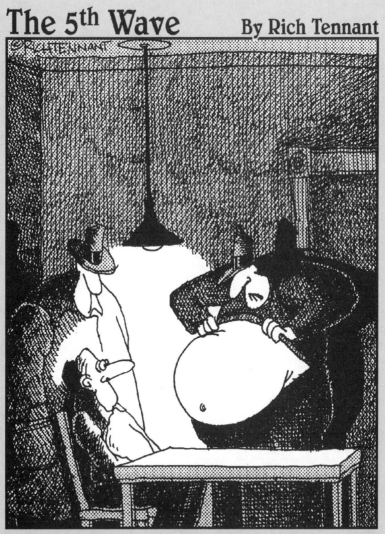

The 5th Wave   By Rich Tennant

"Look—just tell us what we want to know.
Don't make me use this on you!"

In this part . . .

Every *...For Dummies* book ends with top-ten lists, and this one is no exception. We offer ten health resources on the Internet, and we explain ten common surgeries and procedures.

Chapter 25

Ten Health Resources
Worth Surfing For

· ·

Surf's up, Dude! No, we're not talking about riding some Pacific waves. We're talking about surfing the Internet (also called "cyberspace") or World Wide Web. As well put together as this book is, you're nevertheless bound to have a few more questions about men's health. And even if you don't have any questions at the moment, the ten Web sites in this chapter are definitely worth taking a look at.

A Man's Life (`www.manslife.com`)

A Man's Life is an online magazine that includes health and fitness articles and news, plus an interactive section that lets you send questions to a medical doctor. And if health isn't your only interest, this site also contains articles about the great outdoors, sports, machinery, food, relationship problems, and more.

American Holistic Health Association (`www.healthy.net/ahha`)

If you want to know more about alternative/complementary medicine, then the American Holistic Health Association Web site is a good place to start. This site contains information about alternative/complementary medicine, educational booklets, resources on how to find a practitioner in your area, and links to other holistic-related sites.

House Call (`www.housecall.com`)

The House Call Web site offers information on health care topics and forums, newsgroups, home care, and specific health concerns. The site also has links to the National Health Council and the American Academy of Family Physicians home pages.

National Institutes of Health (`www.nih.gov`)

The National Institutes of Health (NIH) Web site is put together by the United States government. Talk about loaded! This site offers health information from A to Z, the latest health news, research, free health pamphlets, scientific resources, contact groups, and more. The NIH site is very large and can link you to its many individual organizations that collectively make up the NIH.

New York Times Syndicate — Your Daily Health (www.nytsyn.com)

The New York Times Syndicate Web site offers the latest health and medicine news, additional health topics, and a special section devoted to men's health. The site also includes links to other health Web sites, a wide array of news, features, book excerpts, and columns.

PharmInfoNet (pharminfo.com)

Have questions about that pill you just swallowed? Then surf to the PharmInfoNet Web site. This site offers information about medications, medications for certain diseases and health conditions, discussion groups, featured articles, full-text articles from clinical publications, economic data, links to other pharmaceutical sites, and an A-Z glossary on drug classes, drug research, diseases, health conditions, and medical tests.

American Botanical Council (www.herbalgram.org)

If you want to know more about herbal medicine and herbs, then the American Botanical Council Web site is an excellent choice. This site offers the latest information on herbal medicine, press releases, and books, as well as links to many other sites.

Hairloss Information On-line (www.hairloss.com)

All you ever wanted (or needed) to know about hair loss can be found in the Hairloss Information On-line Web site. This site focuses on the consumer, giving the scoop and the poop on baldness drugs and hair transplants, lists additional Web sites, offers free items, and more. The Web site also includes an interactive feature that can answer your questions by e-mail.

Prostate Cancer Infolink (www.comed.com/prostate)

The Prostate Cancer Infolink Web site — part of CoMed Communications Internet Health Forum — offers you the latest information on prostate cancer. You can find current clinical reviews and information to help you get medical help. This site includes an interactive forum called "Ask Arthur," which allows you to ask questions and share experiences.

Yahoo Health (dir.yahoo.com/Health)

It's easy to surf through the Yahoo Health Web site, which is chock-full of general health topics as well as men's health topics. From circumcision and erectile dysfunction to male contraceptives and testicular cancer, this Web site offers the latest information.

Chapter 26

Ten Common Surgeries and Procedures

● ●

*A*t some point in your life, you may need surgery or have to undergo a
diagnostic procedure. And chances are good that the surgery or
procedure will be one of the ones listed in this chapter. So as a savvy health
consumer, it's in your best interest to know what's what about the following
procedures and surgeries.

Before you agree to any surgery or procedure, ask your health-care practitioner a few questions:

- ✔ Why do I need this surgery/procedure?

- ✔ Why this particular type of surgery/procedure? In the case of a procedure, does it provide general or specific information? If it provides
general information, ask what the next step will be.

- ✔ How reliable is the surgery/procedure?

- ✔ Is the procedure invasive or noninvasive? If it is invasive, what are
the risks involved? Can a noninvasive procedure provide similar
information?

- ✔ What possible risks does the surgery/procedure have?

- ✔ Does the surgery/procedure require any special preparation?

- ✔ How much does it cost?

- ✔ Are any alternatives available if I refuse this surgery/procedure?

All surgeries and procedures carry possible risks such as infection, human
error, and anesthesia mishaps. Be sure to discuss the risks with your doctor
before submitting to any surgery or procedure.

Arteriography

Arteriography is a diagnostic procedure that uses contrast dye and X rays to evaluate the condition of the arteries in your abdomen, chest, arms, or legs. Special arteriographic procedures for the arteries in the brain (cerebral arteriography), lungs (pulmonary arteriography), and heart (coronary arteriography) are also done. Arteriography can determine abnormalities of blood flow, including blood clots, aneurysms, and ruptured blood vessels.

The procedure, done under local anesthesia, is performed in the X-ray suite of a hospital. A radiologist inserts a special needle— called an arterial needle — in an artery. He or she then inserts a catheter (a fine tube) through the special needle and threads the catheter to the section of your body to be examined. The contrast dye is then injected and X rays are taken. Rare but possible complications include allergic reaction to the contrast material, infection, damage to an artery, or loosening of a piece of clotted blood.

Cardiac catheterization

This diagnostic procedure determines the location and condition of blocked arteries that supply the heart, defects of the heart, severity of damage to heart function, and how well your heart pumps blood through your body. The principal problem that cardiac catheterization helps to diagnose is the narrowing of the coronary arteries caused by *plaque* (a complex mass of cells, cholesterol, and other organic matter).

Cardiac catheterization is performed under local anesthesia. A cardiac surgeon, radiologist, or cardiologist injects a special needle into an artery or vein of your arm or groin and then passes a catheter through the needle into the vessel. Next, he or she threads the catheter to an artery or heart chamber. When the catheter is in the right position, a contrast dye is injected and X rays are taken. During the procedure, the doctor may give you a nitroglycerin tablet to help dilate the blood vessels, or you may be given an injection to help constrict the coronary arteries. After all imaging is done, the doctor withdraws the catheter. Rare but possible complications include allergic reaction to the dye, renal failure, blood clot, and circulatory collapse (cessation of effective blood flow).

Aortocoronary bypass

Aortocoronary bypass, commonly known as coronary artery bypass graft (CABG), is surgery in which blocked coronary arteries are replaced with transplanted veins or arteries from your leg. CABG — performed in the hospital and under general anesthesia — takes between two and fours hours to complete.

While your heart is stopped, circulation is taken over by a heart-lung machine, which ensures adequate blood flow. Rare but possible complications include infection, stroke, failure of the breastbone to heal, and death.

Appendectomy

Appendectomy is surgery in which a surgeon removes an inflamed appendix from your body. Before the surgery, your doctor will prescribe antibiotics for you to help reduce the infection and limit tissue damage in your abdomen. The surgery is usually performed in the hospital under general or spinal anesthesia. The surgeon makes an incision in your lower right abdomen and then cuts the appendix away from your body. Possible complications include infection and reaction to anesthetic drugs.

Bronchoscopy

Bronchoscopy, also known as endoscopic lung biopsy, is a diagnostic procedure generally performed under general anesthesia in which a small piece of lung tissue is removed for microscopic examination using a bronchoscope (a tubelike fiber-optic viewing scope). In this procedure — done in a hospital, outpatient surgery clinic, or well-equipped doctor's office — a surgeon or pulmonologist inserts the bronchoscope in your mouth, past the trachea, and into your bronchi (large airways). If the surgeon sees a suspicious area (such as a tumor), he or she will remove a piece of tissue using the cutting instrument in the bronchoscope. Rare but possible complications include bleeding, air in the chest cavity, and the breakage of brushes that are used for obtaining surface tissue samples.

Computerized axial tomography

Also known as CAT scan, computerized axial tomography is a diagnostic procedure used to determine a variety of conditions. For example, a CAT scan of the kidneys can confirm tumors, stones, infection, obstruction, and other diseases and conditions of the kidneys. In a CAT scan, a technician takes a series of cross-sectional X rays and then uses a computer to construct highly detailed images of the inside of your body.

Diagnostic ultrasound

Ultrasound imaging, a diagnostic procedure, uses sound waves to show images of your internal organs, such as the liver, spleen, or pancreas. An ultrasound technician applies a lubricant gel to your skin over the area that needs to be examined and passes a transducer — a device that records the sound waves — over the lubricated area. An image of the area is captured on a monitor.

Endoscopy of the large bowel

This diagnostic procedure — done under light or heavy sedation and on an inpatient or outpatient basis in a hospital or outpatient surgery clinic — uses a colonscope (a tubelike fiber-optic viewing scope) to check for benign or malignant tumors of the colon, bowel obstruction, inflammatory bowel disease, colitis, and foreign objects. A colon-rectal surgeon or gastroenterologist inserts the colonoscope through your rectum and snakes the device through your colon, looking for polyps and other lesions. Suspicious tissue is taken for microscopic examination. Rare but possible complications include bleeding, infection, and perforation of the colon wall.

Transurethral resection of the prostate

Transurethral resection of the prostate (TURP) is surgery in which a urologist removes a portion of your prostate gland that is partially or completely blocking the urethra. In TURP — done in a hospital under general anesthesia — the urologist inserts a cystoscope (a tubelike fiber-optic viewing scope) into your penis to examine the inside of your bladder for tumors and signs of infection. Once the urologist locates the portion of the prostrate gland that is blocking your urethra, he or she cuts the diseased or malignant tissue with a cutting device called an electrosurgical loop. The urologist may put an irrigation catheter (which has tubes for inserting and draining irrigation solution) into your bladder for a day or so until the irrigation fluid is clear of blood clots and tissue fragments. Possible complications include infection and a puncture of the bladder by the cystoscope. After the surgery, possible side effects include erection problems, retrograde ejaculation (see Chapter 24), and sterility.

Respiratory therapy

Respiratory therapy is any procedure that improves or maintains your respiratory system. One example of respiratory therapy is mechanical ventilation. Respiratory therapy can be done at the hospital, at the clinic, or in the privacy of your home.

Mechanical ventilation uses a ventilator (mechanical breathing machine) and is used when you cannot breathe on your own or when your breaths are not strong enough to deliver air to your lungs. Possible conditions that can make it difficult for you to breathe on your own include blood clots in the lung, infections, or diseases such as adult respiratory distress syndrome.

Possible complications of mechanical ventilation include irregular heartbeat, collapsed lung, infection, and decreased cardiac output.

Index

• C •

Notes

Notes

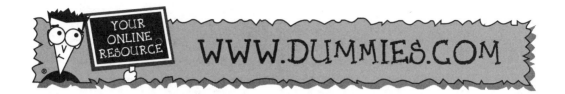
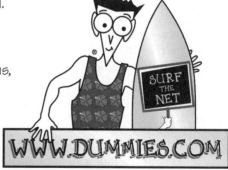

IDG BOOKS WORLDWIDE BOOK REGISTRATION

We want to hear from you!

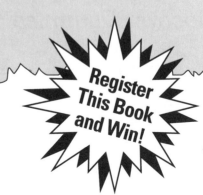

Register This Book and Win!

Visit **http://my2cents.dummies.com** to register this book and tell us how you liked it!

- ✔ Get entered in our monthly prize giveaway.

- ✔ Give us feedback about this book — tell us what you like best, what you like least, or maybe what you'd like to ask the author and us to change!

- ✔ Let us know any other ...*For Dummies*® topics that interest you.

Your feedback helps us determine what books to publish, tells us what coverage to add as we revise our books, and lets us know whether we're meeting your needs as a ...*For Dummies* reader. You're our most valuable resource, and what you have to say is important to us!

Not on the Web yet? It's easy to get started with *Dummies 101*®: *The Internet For Windows*® *98* or *The Internet For Dummies*®, 5th Edition, at local retailers everywhere.

Or let us know what you think by sending us a letter at the following address:

...*For Dummies* Book Registration
Dummies Press
7260 Shadeland Station, Suite 100
Indianapolis, IN 46256-3945
Fax 317-596-5498

™

FOR DUMMIES

BESTSELLING
BOOK SERIES